Chlamydia

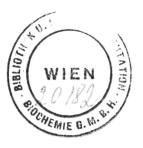

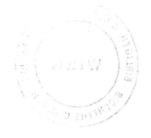

Chlamydia

Per-Anders Mårdh, M.D., D.M.S.

Institute of Clinical Bacteriology
University of Uppsala
Uppsala, Sweden

Jorma Paavonen, M.D., D.M.S.

Helsinki University Central Hospital
Helsinki, Finland

and

Mirja Puolakkainen, M.D., D.M.S.

Institute of Virology
University of Helsinki
Helsinki, Finland

PLENUM MEDICAL BOOK COMPANY
NEW YORK AND LONDON

Library of Congress Cataloging in Publication Data

Mårdh, Per-Anders.
  Chlamydia / Per-Anders Mårdh, Jorma Paavonen, and Mirja Puolakkainen.
     p.   cm.
  Bibliography: p.
  Includes index.
  ISBN 0-306-42965-9
  1. Chlamydia infections. 2. Chlamydia. I. Paavonen, Jorma. II. Puolakkainen,
Mirja. III. Title.
  [DNLM: 1. Chlamydia. 2. Chlamydia infections. WC 600 M322c]
RC124.5.M37   1989
616.9′2 — dc19
DNLM/DLC   88-38170
for Library of Congress   CIP

© 1989 Plenum Publishing Corporation
233 Spring Street, New York, N.Y. 10013

Plenum Medical Book Company is an imprint of Plenum Publishing Corporation

Printed in the United States of America

Preface

During recent decades, it has been firmly documented that chlamydiae are common and important pathogens in humans and animals. In humans, chlamydiae are known to cause trachoma (which is still one of the major blinding diseases in the world) and are also one of the most common etiological agents of sexually transmitted diseases and the sequelae thereof, such as infertility. In the last few years, it has also become evident that chlamydiae, i.e., the so-called TWAR agents, are common respiratory tract pathogens.

Chlamydiae are also important pathogens in birds and lower mammals, in whom they cause a variety of infectious conditions, a spectrum which has increased every year. Some of these infections occur as zoonoses, e.g., psittacosis/ornithosis and, as recently discovered, abortion.

Knowledge of the molecular biology and immunobiology of chlamydiae has expanded rapidly during recent years. Insight into the pathophysiology of chlamydial infections has also increased, and new methods for the diagnosis of chlamydial infections have been introduced.

The importance of establishing control and preventive programs for chlamydial infections has become obvious in order to combat the present chlamydial epidemic.

We hope that this book can usefully serve those who want to increase their general knowledge of *Chlamydia* and that it can act as a handbook and reference source for those involved in chlamydial research as well as for those working with chlamydial infections in medical and veterinary clinical disciplines, including clinical laboratories.

Attempts have been made not only to include the most recent data within the field but also to outline briefly some of the landmarks in chlamydiology that have been achieved during this century. A great number of selected references have been cited, a feature that we believe is an essential part of a publication of this nature.

Per-Anders Mårdh
Jorma Paavonen
Mirja Puolakkainen

Uppsala and Helsinki

Contents

IV. Antibiosis and Vaccines

V. *Chlamydia trachomatis* Infections

V. *Chlamydia psittaci* Infections

Color Plates

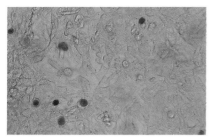

FIGURE 27. McCoy cells stained with Lugol's solution (iodine), demonstrating dark brown intracytoplasmic inclusions of *C. trachomatis* (×400).

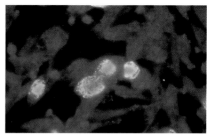

FIGURE 28. McCoy cells stained with fluorescein-labeled monoclonal antibodies showing yellow–green chlamydial inclusions (×400).

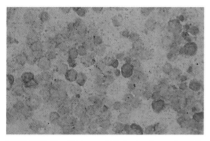

FIGURE 29. Chlamydial inclusions in McCoy cells stained with immunoperoxidase (×400).

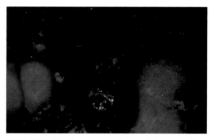

FIGURE 30. Smears of genital secretion stained with fluorescein-labeled monoclonal antibodies showing apple green elementary bodies (EBs) (×1000).

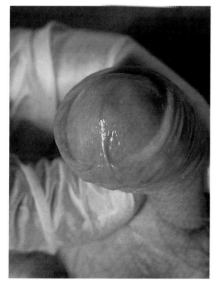

FIGURE 42. Urethral watery discharge in the urethral meatus of a man with chlamydial urethritis. (Courtesy of Dr. D. Oriel.)

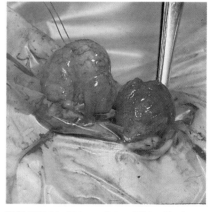

FIGURE 44. Chlamydial epididymitis in an experimentally infected grivet monkey showing the inflamed epididymis to the right and the noninfected organ to the left. (Courtesy of Dr. B. Møller.)

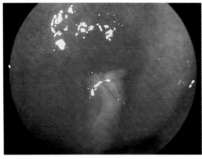

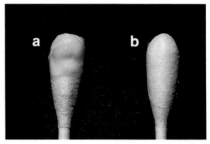

FIGURE 49. The cervical os of a woman with chlamydial cervicitis showing yellow endocervical mucopus.

FIGURE 50. Swab test in a case of mucopurulent cervicitis (a) and control (b).

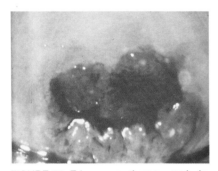

FIGURE 51. Edema, erythema, and induced bleeding in a patient with chlamydial cervicitis.

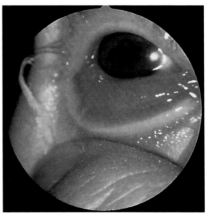

FIGURE 64. The conjunctiva of a newborn child with mild chlamydial ophthalmia neonatorum. (Courtesy of Dr. L. Salminen.)

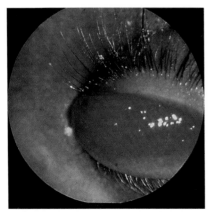

FIGURE 68. Chlamydial conjunctivitis in an adult patient with edematous congested mucosa that bleeds easily. (Courtesy of Dr. L. Salminen.)

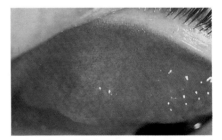

FIGURE 69. Follicles on the upper tarsal conjunctiva in a case of chlamydial conjunctivitis (paratrachoma). (Courtesy of Dr. J. Treharne.)

Chlamydia

Introduction

1

A Historical Outline

CLINICAL SPECTRUM OF CHLAMYDIAL DISEASES

Since the discovery of the life cycle of *Chlamydia* (formerly *Bedsonia*) by Bedson and others more than 50 years ago, it has become evident that the species of *Chlamydia* they studied (*Chlamydia psittaci*) is widespread among animals, including mammals and birds. The agent is now known to cause a variety of diseases in animals, such as spontaneous abortion, eye infection, pneumonia, peritonitis, and various neurological conditions, to mention a few (cf. Macfarlane and Macrae, 1983).

Humans can also be affected by *C. psittaci* and subsequently develop pneumonia, i.e., psittacosis or ornithosis (Fig. 1) (Bedson et al., 1930; cf. Macfarlane and Macrae, 1983). In addition, several other clinical manifestations can be seen in patients with chlamydial pneumonia (see below). In recent years, placentitis in humans has been attributed to infections with ovine *C. psittaci* strains (Wong et al., 1985), and spontaneous abortion has been described in women who have had contact with infected sheep or lambs (Johnson et al., 1985; Helm et al., 1987).

Pneumonia caused in humans by *C. psittaci* organisms, i.e., the so-called TWAR agents or TWAR chlamydiae, has recently been described (Saikku et al., 1985; Grayston et al., 1986b). "TW" in TWAR stands for Taiwan, where the first TWAR agent was isolated in 1965 from a child with conjunctivitis, and "AR" stands for acute respiratory disease, which was diagnosed in a person from whom one of the first TWAR strains was isolated. In 1967, IOL-207 was isolated from the eye of a child with trachoma. This latter strain is very similar to the TWAR agents.

The clinical picture of TWAR pneumonia is similar to that of pneumonia caused by *Mycoplasma pneumoniae*, and the TWAR etiology seems to outnumber other causes of primary atypical pneumonia. Upper respiratory tract

DEUTSCHE MEDIZINISCHE WOCHENSCHRIFT 1907:

Zur Aetiologie des Trachoms.

Von Dr. Halberstaedter in Berlin und Dr. Prowazek
in Hamburg.

BERLINER KLINISCHE WOCHENSCHRIFT 1909:

Ueber Chlamydozoenbefunde bei Blennorrhoea neonatorum non gonorrhoica.

Von

L. Halberstaedter-Berlin und S. v. Prowazek-Hamburg.

WIENER KLINISCHE WOCHENSCHRIFT 1910:

Aus der zweiten Augenklinik in Wien. (Vorstand:
Hofr. Prof. E. Fuchs.)

Zur Aetiologie der gonokokkenfreien Urethritis.

Von Dr. K. Lindner, Sekundararzt.

THE LANCET 1930:

Clinical and Laboratory Notes.

OBSERVATIONS ON
THE ÆTIOLOGY OF PSITTACOSIS.

BY S. P. BEDSON, M.D., M.Sc. DURH.,
SENIOR FREEDOM RESEARCH FELLOW, LONDON HOSPITAL;

G. T. WESTERN, M.D. CAMB.,
PHYSICIAN IN CHARGE OF THE INOCULATION DEPT. OF THE
HOSPITAL;

AND

S. LEVY SIMPSON, M.D. CAMB., M.R.C.P. LOND.,
MEDICAL FIRST ASSISTANT AT THE HOSPITAL.

FIGURE 1. Titles of some studies of interest in the history of chlamydial research, i.e., by Halberstaedter and von Prowazek from 1907 and 1909, by Lindner from 1910, and by Bedson and co-workers on psittacosis from 1930.

infections also tend to occur in persons infected by TWAR chlamydiae (Grayston et al., 1986a).

The IOL-207 strain was used in experiments on monkeys, in whom it produced conjunctivitis and urethritis (Darougar et al., 1977a). During the following years it was shown seroepidemiologically that antibodies to IOL-207 are common in the general population of the United Kingdom (Forsey et al., 1986).

Trachoma is the earliest known human disease entity caused by chlamydiae (Fig. 2). The term *trachoma* was coined around 60 AD by a Sicilian physician

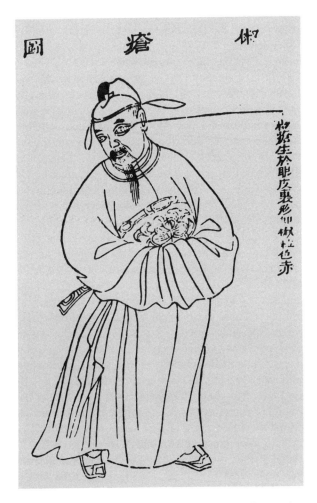

FIGURE 2. Trachoma was a recognized disease in China several thousand years ago. It still affects hundreds of millions of people.

named Pedanius Diascarides. That the disease runs through different stages was also described at about the same time. However, the Egyptians and the Chinese already knew about the disease, i.e., they knew about the application of copper salts around the eyes which also served as a cosmetic (compare our use of mascara today). In that relation, the inhibitory effect of metal ions, i.e., copper ions on the ability of *Chlamydia trachomatis* to form inclusions in tissue cell cultures (Mårdh et al., 1980a) is of interest. Trachoma is known to have been spread among the Romans, and there is reason to believe that some of the well-known Romans (e.g., Cicero) suffered from the disease. The Crusaders spread the disease from the Near East to Europe. Napoleon's soldiers once again "boostered" Europe with the infection. In fact, in certain areas of Europe the disease remains endemic.

In his etiological studies of trachoma, Robert Koch isolated, among other things, *Haemophilus aegypticus* from the eyes of patients with so-called Egyptian ophthalmia. In 1907, further observations were made—also by Germans—that in the light of existing knowledge revealed the real cause of trachoma, i.e., a parasite causing formation of intracytoplasmic inclusions (Halberstaedter and Prowazek, 1907). The authors described such inclusions in experimentally infected orangutans. In the years between 1909 and 1911 these and other German investigators (Halberstaedter and Prowazek, 1909; Staargardt, 1909; Lindner, 1910) reported the occurrence of similar inclusions in conjunctival cells of babies with nongonococcal ophthalmia and in urethral secretions of men with nongonococcal urethritis (Fig. 1).

Trachoma is caused by *C. trachomatis,* mainly serotypes (see below) A, B, B_a, and C, although recent reports suggest that the "genital" serotypes (i.e., D–K) can also cause trachoma in locations previously identified as trachoma areas (Harrison et al., 1985).

A link between eye and genital infections was established when genitally infected mothers were found to be transferring the disease to their offspring. It was also shown that the same type of intracytoplasmic inclusions seen in experimentally infected monkeys could be found in secretions from the eyes of babies with conjunctivitis, in urethral secretions of men with urethritis, and in cervical secretions from mothers of infected newborns (Fritsch et al., 1910).

During the 1930s, Thygeson and Stone (1942) made further observations on the pathology and transmission of genital chlamydial infections, but it was not until the 1950s and the introduction of new diagnostic methods (see below) that the modern era of genital chlamydial research began. In 1957, T'ang and co-workers successfully recovered *C. trachomatis* from an embryonated hen's egg. Two years later, Jones and co-workers (1959) became the first to recover *C. trachomatis* from the cervix of a mother and from the eyes of her offspring, who had signs of conjunctivitis. Observations made at the beginning of the century could now be confirmed by culture studies. Thus *C. trachomatis* could be isolated from the eyes of newborns and adults with conjunctivitis and from females with nongonococcal genital infections (Jones, 1964; Dunlop et al., 1964; Holt et al., 1967). Transmission of infections between the sexes, from mothers to offspring, and from genital tract to the eyes of adults was also demonstrated. However, it was not until the 1970s that the important role of *C. trachomatis* in the etiology of nongonococcal urethritis (NGU) in the male (Holmes et al., 1975) and cervicitis in the female (Hilton et al., 1974; Swanson et al., 1975; Oriel et al., 1978) was firmly established and accepted as a clinical reality.

Early in the history of chlamydiology it was established that lymphogranuloma venereum (LGV) is an infection caused by *C. trachomatis* serotypes L_1–L_3 (Miyagawa et al., 1935; Rake et al., 1941) (see further below).

In the 1970s, it was established that a number of complications of genital infections, such as salpingitis (Mårdh et al., 1977a) and epididymitis (Harnisch et al., 1977), are caused by *C. trachomatis*. In this decade it was also established that *C. trachomatis* spread to the offspring from a genitally infected mother can result in neonatal complications, e.g., pneumonia (Beem and Saxon, 1977). Recent studies also indicate that neonatal chlamydial pneumonia can cause late sequelae, e.g., asthma (Harrison et al., 1982).

A number of other novel manifestations of chlamydial infections were detected in the years that followed, e.g., peritonitis and perihepatitis in non-salpingitis cases (Müller-Schoop et al., 1978), endometritis (Mårdh et al., 1981a), perihepatitis (Wølner-Hansen et al., 1980), and pneumonia in adults (Komaroff et al., 1981). Still more recent descriptions of manifestations of chlamydial infections include cases of severe peritonitis with chronic ascites without signs of perihepatitis (Marbet et al., 1986) and cases with exudative ascites as the predominant clinical features (Haight and Ockher, 1988). Perisplenitis and perinephritis in cases of Fitz-Hugh–Curtis syndrome have also been described (Gatt and Jantet, 1987). The diseases and sequelae of chlamydial infections in humans are listed in Table 1.

In most countries *C. trachomatis* is one of the most common STD agents. In many countries it outnumbers *Neisseria gonorrhoeae* as a causative agent, although gonorrhea is still more prevalent in some areas (cf. Holmes and Mårdh, 1983; Meheus et al., 1986; Frost et al., 1987). Gonococcal and chlamydial infections in the female may result in complications, e.g., endometritis and salpingitis, about equally often or in approximately 5–10% of cases. There is also reason to believe that infection by *C. trachomatis* in most industrialized countries today has become the most common cause of such genital infection sequelae as infertility and ectopic pregnancy (Bowie and Jones, 1981; Paperny et al., 1981; Paavonen et al., 1982a; Kristensen et al., 1985; Mårdh, 1986; Persson, 1986). This has recently been established in developing countries as well, e.g., in central Africa (Frost et al., 1987). The role of genital chlamydial infections in male infertility has not yet been established.

TABLE 1. Diseases and Sequelae Believed to Be Associated with
Chlamydial Infection

Agent(s)	Affected	Disease(s) and symptom(s)[a]	Sequelae
TWAR agents (TW-183, AR-69, IOL-207)	Children and adults of both sexes	Pharyngitis, bronchitis, long-standing cough, sore throat, mild to severe pneumonia, conjunctivitis, laboratory infection and naturally acquired infection	Myocardial complications??
C. psittaci	Children and adults of both sexes	Ornithosis/psittacosis (e.g., pneumonia and in some cases arthritis, endocarditis, perihepatitis, severe headache, and rash)	
	Adult females	Abortion	
C. trachomatis			
Serotypes A, B, B$_a$, C	Children and adults of both sexes	Conjunctivitis, keratitis, trachoma	Impaired vision, blindness
Serotypes B, D–K	Neonates	Conjunctivitis, pharyngitis, pneumonia, otitis media?, gastroenteritis??, vaginitis	Impaired vision?, tarsal scarring?, chronic respiratory dysfunction (?)
	Children	Conjunctivitis, pneumonia?, vaginitis/urethritis (e.g., in child abuse)	Asthma, chronic respiratory dysfunction
	Adult males	Nongonococcal urethritis, vaseitis?, epididymitis, proctitis	Subfertility?, infertility??
	Adult females	Vaginitis (in hysterectomized women), cervicitis, endometritis, late postpartum endometritis, periappendicitis, perihepatitis, perisplenitis, pericolitis (?), proctitis, premature rupture of membranes (PROM), chorionamnionitis, fetal infection (?)	Impaired fertility, infertility, chronic abdominal pain, tubal (ectopic) pregnancy, cellular dysplasia?, carcinoma of the cervix?? Prematurity?, stillbirth?
Serotypes D–K	Adults of both sexes	Conjunctivitis, keratitis, pharyngitis??, pneumonia in immuno- and	Joint dysfunction

TABLE 1. (*Continued*)

Agent(s)	Affected	Disease(s) and symptom(s)[a]	Sequelae
Serotypes L₁–L₃	Mainly adult males, but affects adults of both sexes	nonimmunocompromised persons, Reiter's syndrome (?) (e.g., uveitis, urethritis, and arthritis) Proctitis, lymphogranuloma venereum (e.g., genital ulcers, urethritis, inguinal lymphadenitis, bubo, and proctitis)	Strictures and/or severe structural changes of the urinary, genital, and distal gastrointestinal tracts, lymphoedema (elephantiasis)

[a](?), Etiological association very likely, but more data to support statement would be preferred; ?, etiological relationship likely, but so far data from comparatively few groups are available; ??, etiological relationship, if any, still to be considered hypothetical.

DIAGNOSIS OF CHLAMYDIAL INFECTIONS

The development of new methods for diagnosing chlamydial infections has formed the backbone of our understanding of the epidemiology of chlamydial infections. *Chlamydia trachomatis* was first isolated in embryonated hen's eggs by T'ang in 1956. This method involved many limitations and a high risk of transmission of the agent between eggs, resulting in false-positive test results.

The technique introduced by Gordon and Quan (1965) utilizing irradiated McCoy cells was a breakthrough in the diagnosis of chlamydial infections. In 1974, a method utilizing McCoy cells treated with 5-iodo-2-deoxyuridine (IUdR) was described by Wenthworth and Alexander. In 1977, Ripa and Mårdh introduced cycloheximide for the treatment of McCoy cells for clinical laboratory use. Today this latter method is used by most laboratories performing chlamydial cultures. The treatment can be made in conjunction with infection of the cells by chlamydiae whereas irradiation and IUdR treatment must take place some days before the cells are ready for use. Introduction of the cycloheximide treatment further facilitated the diagnostic procedure, permitting routine, large-scale diagnosis of chlamydial infections for the first time. Diethylaminoethyldextrane (DEAE-dextran) treatment of HeLa 229 (Seattle) cells is another method that has been successfully used by some laboratories to isolate *C. trachomatis* (Kuo et al., 1972) and, more recently, to recover TWAR chlamydiae as well (Kuo et al., 1986b).

Recently, labeled, species-specific monoclonal antibodies (Tam et al., 1984) have replaced iodine as a stain for intracytoplasmic inclusions in chlamydial cultures, which has meant an increase in diagnostic sensitivity and rapidity. Such antibodies have also been used for the direct detection of chlamydiae in clinical samples (Tam et al., 1984; Bell et al., 1984). Yet the overall value of labeled monoclonal antichlamydial antibodies in the routine diagnosis of chlamydial infections partly remains to be established, particularly in tests of extragenital samples.

Other direct-specimen antigen detection tests (ELISA techniques) have recently come into wide use for the diagnosis of chlamydial infections (Jones et al., 1984). The recent introduction of new amplified signal systems that increase the sensitivity of the test system have rendered the ELISA tests more useful in clinical practice (cf. Mabey et al., 1987). ELISA office tests have now become commercially available. ELISA techniques have not only been introduced for the diagnosis of *C. trachomatis* but also for the diagnosis of *C. psittaci* infections in animals.

In 1970, Wang and Grayston developed the so-called microimmunofluorescence (micro-IF) test on the basis of which they were able to subdivide *C. trachomatis* into 15 serotypes (see below). This method has contributed greatly to our understanding of the epidemiology of *C. trachomatis* infections. In addition, the method allows determination of serotype-specific antichlamydial antibodies, and the possibility of identifying new isolates. In recent years, cross-reactivity with TWAR antigen in micro-IF tests has been highlighted (Schachter, 1986d), which means that a considerable portion of the earlier published seroepidemiological data must be reevaluated.

MOLECULAR BIOLOGY OF CHLAMYDIAE

Molecular biological studies of *C. trachomatis* began in the 1970s with, for example, studies of the cell wall lipopolysaccharides (LPS) (Dhir et al., 1972) and the major outer membrane proteins (MOMP) (Caldwell et al., 1975a). In addition, chromosomal DNA was examined and the number of kilobase pairs determined (Becker, 1978). During the 1980s more genetic work on chlamydiae was performed, including restriction enzyme analyses of chlamydial chromosomal DNA (Peterson and de la Maza, 1983) and studies of chlamydial plasmid DNA (Lovett et al., 1980). In 1982, Wenman and Lovett successfully cloned genes of a *C. trachomatis* antigen in *Escherichia coli*.

LANDMARKS IN CHLAMYDIOLOGY

Some of the landmarks in chlamydiology are listed in Table 2. Since 1962 there have been six international chlamydial meetings; 5 years passed between

TABLE 2. Landmarks in Chlamydiology

Year(s)	Landmark(s)
1907	Detection of intracytoplasmic inclusions in conjunctival scrapings from trachoma patients.
1909–1910	Demonstration of intracytoplasmic inclusions in neonatal conjunctivitis, and in urethritis and cervicitis in parents of such children.
Early 1930s	Description of the life cycle of *Bedsonia* (*Chlamydia psittaci*). Isolation of lymphogranuloma venereum (LGV) agent in mice; similarities noted in life cycle between LGV and *C. psittaci*.
1957	First isolation of *C. trachomatis* in embryonated hen's eggs.
1965	Isolation of *C. trachomatis* in cell cultures (irradiated McCoy cells).
1970	Development of microimmunofluorescence (micro-IF) technique, allowing subdivision of *C. trachomatis* into serotypes and chlamydial serological studies.
Early 1970s	Establishment of role of chlamydiae in uncomplicated genital infections.
1972–1977	Simplification of cell culture techniques (using treatment of cells with DEAE-dextran, IDU, or cycloheximide).
1977	Reports on *C. trachomatis* as a cause of complicated genital chlamydial infections, i.e., acute salpingitis and acute epididymitis and perinatal infections, e.g., to pneumonitis.
1978–1987	Demonstration of *C. trachomatis* as a cause of intra-abdominal infections, e.g., periappendicitis, peritonitis, perihepatitis, pericolitis, and perisplenitis.
Early 1980s	Biochemical, antigenic, and genetic characterization of the chlamydial cell ("molecular cell biology era").
1982–1983	Direct-specimen antigen ELISA tests and antigen test of chlamydiae in clinical samples (monoclonal species-specific antibodies for immunofluorescence microscopy).
1984–1987	Clarification of the etiological role of TWAR chlamydiae in human respiratory tract infections.
1984–1988	Identification of genital chlamydial infection as a major health problem. Direct antigen tests for *C. trachomatis* for office use.

each, except for the last two, which were held in 1982 and 1986. The first three meetings were almost entirely devoted to eye infections, i.e., mainly to trachoma. At the fourth meeting (in 1977), eye and genital infections were more or less equally represented on the agenda. At the fifth meeting, genital chlamydial infections dominated, whereas at the meeting in the summer of 1986 molecular biology and new diagnostic methods were the highlighted topics. Of the clinical topics at the last meeting, there was little new information regarding male genital infections, although there was much new information on female genital infections. Old information on TWAR agents was reevaluated and it was made clear that these organisms are common etiological agents of human respiratory tract infections. The next (the seventh) international chlamydial meeting is planned for 1990.

Since the international chlamydial meeting in 1986, there has been a continuing increase in our knowledge of the molecular biology and immunopathology of chlamydial infections.

THE FUTURE

We are now in the dawn of a more general understanding that not only trachoma but also genital chlamydial infection constitutes a major health problem. Hopefully the near future will herald the formation of more national surveillance programs as well as preventive and control programs on a state- and nationwide basis. In some countries, such activities have just begun or are about to start. In a few countries, there are ongoing discussions regarding the establishment of genital chlamydial infection as a venereal disease in the legal sense.

The importance of combatting any type of genital infection, including *Chlamydia,* has become increasingly obvious, since such measures might also mean a decreased risk of transmission of human immunodeficiency virus (HIV). Reducing the pool of genitally infected subjects is probably one of the most important measures we can undertake as we await a vaccine or an effective therapy for AIDS.

Microbiology, Immunopathology, and Animal Models

The Chlamydiae

CLASSIFICATION

Chlamydiae are small, gram-negative eubacteria (Weisburg et al., 1986) that grow intracellularly only. Due to their unique developmental cycle, chlamydiae are recognized in their own order, i.e., Chlamydiales. This order consists of one family, Chlamydiaceae, and of one genus, *Chlamydia,* with two characterized species, *C. psittaci* and *C. trachomatis.* The organisms now included in the genus *Chlamydia* were earlier called *Miyagawanella* and *Bedsonia* (Page, 1974; Moulder et al., 1984). For some decades TRIC (trachoma inclusion conjunctivitis) was used as a designation for the non-LGV *C. trachomatis* organisms. The so-called TWAR chlamydiae may form a new, third species (with the tentative name *C. pneumoniae*) (Fig. 3). The two established species can be differentiated on the basis of inclusion type and sensitivity to sulfonamides. (*C. trachomatis* inclusions contain glycogen whereas *C. psittaci* inclusions do not; *C. trachomatis* is more susceptible to sulfonamides than *C. psittaci.*)

Genetically, *C. trachomatis* and *C. psittaci* are not very closely related. The guanine + cytosine (G + C) DNA content is 44% for *C. trachomatis* and 41% for *C. psittaci* (Schachter and Caldwell, 1980). The two species show only 10% DNA sequence homology (Kingsbury and Weiss, 1968). However, they resemble each other in many biological and biochemical properties. In addition, comparative analysis of their 16S RNA sequences—a method used for determination of phylogenetic relationships between organisms—shows over 95% homology (Weisburg et al., 1986).

The species *C. trachomatis* is further divided into three biovars: the trachoma biovar consisting of serotypes A, B, B_a, C–K (Wang and Grayston, 1970), the lymphogranuloma venereum (LGV) biovar with serotypes L_1–L_3 (Schachter and Meyer, 1969), and the mouse pneumonitis biovar (Higashi et al., 1959; Manire and Galasso, 1959; Moulder, 1982). The classification of *C.*

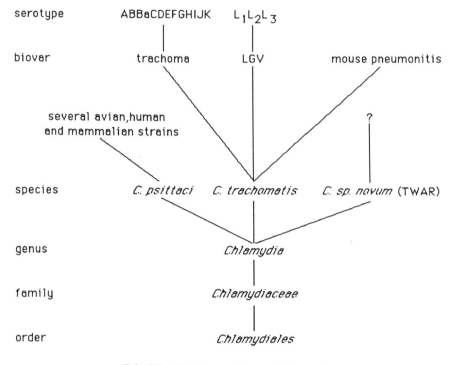

FIGURE 3. The taxonomic tree of *Chlamydia*.

trachomatis strains into serotypes was originally performed with the mouse toxicity prevention test (MTPT), employing active immunization and toxic challenge of mice with live *C. trachomatis* strains (Wang and Grayston, 1963). Later, Wang and Grayston (1970) introduced a simpler method for immunotyping *C. trachomatis* organisms (microimmunofluorescence, or micro-IF). The micro-IF test shows complete agreement with the MTPT; moreover, as an in vitro system, it is easier to perform than the laborious MTPT in vivo test. Even simpler and more precise immunological classification of *C. trachomatis* organisms can now be achieved with the aid of micro-IF tests involving monoclonal antibodies that are species- or subspecies-specific (Wang et al., 1985; Newhall et al., 1986). These tests also allow differentiation among closely related serotypes (Fig. 4). It is possible that additional serotypes and even subgroups will be recognized as an improved selection of monoclonal antibodies becomes available.

A homogeneity of only 30% to 60% between the murine and the human biovar DNA genome has been reported (Weiss et al., 1970). This is a greater homogeneity than that between *C. trachomatis* and *C. psittaci* strains. The latter consists of several mammalian and avian strains (Storz, 1971; Perez-Martinez and Storz, 1985; Eb et al., 1986) that lack closer classification.

Strains of *C. psittaci* have been compared by restriction endonuclease and DNA probe analysis which might be used for a more precise subgrouping of this species (Timms et al., 1988). Also monoclonal antibody typing has been made of *C. psittaci* strains (Fukushi et al., 1987). An immunochemical diversity of the major outer membrane protein between avian and mammalian *C. psittaci* has been demonstrated (Fukushi and Hirai, 1988).

The TWAR chlamydiae are human strains that relate more closely to *C. psittaci* than *C. trachomatis* (Grayston et al., 1986b). These organisms include TW-183 and AR-39 (Kuo et al., 1986b) as well as IOL-207 (Darougar et al., 1977a). At present there are ongoing discussions regarding the taxonomic status of TWAR chlamydiae. Some workers favor the formation of a new species to be called *C. pneumoniae*.

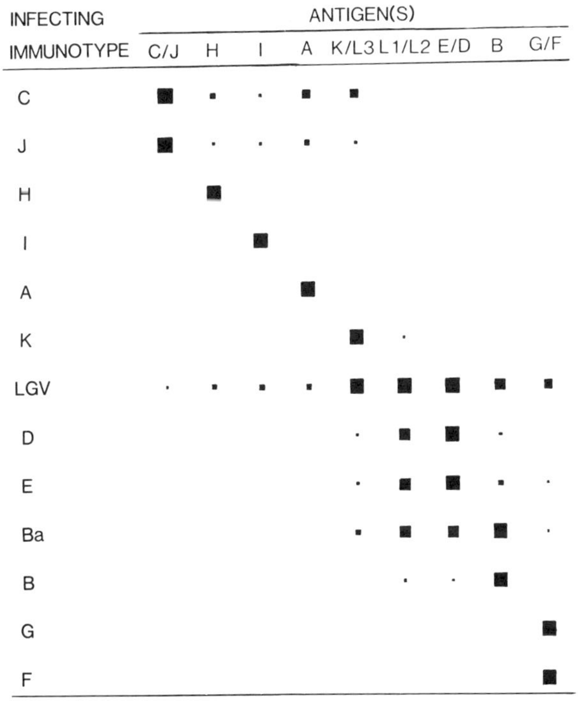

INFECTING IMMUNOTYPE	C/J	H	I	A	K/L3	L1/L2	E/D	B	G/F
C	■	·	·	▪	▪				
J	■	·	·	▪	·				
H		■							
I			■						
A				■					
K					■	·			
LGV	·	▪	▪	▪	■	■	■	■	▪
D					·	▪	■	·	
E					·	▪	■	·	·
Ba					▪	■	▪	■	·
B						·	·	■	
G									■
F									■

FIGURE 4. Cross-reaction between different serotypes of *C. trachomatis* in microimmunofluorescent (micro-IF) tests, according to Dr. S. P. Wang and associates (1971). The extent of the cross-reaction is indicated by the size of the squares; the larger ones mean a homologous reaction.

MORPHOLOGY AND REPLICATION

Chlamydiae are difficult to grow in large quantities and purify from host cell material, which has hampered their production and purification for research. Their developmental cycle involves alternation between two cell types: the infectious elementary body (EB) and the metabolically active reticulate body (RB). The EBs (ϕ = 300–400 nm) are adapted to extracellular survival, whereas the larger RBs (ϕ = 800–1000 nm) are labile, noninfectious forms that exist only intracellularly (Fig. 5).

At both stages of development the chlamydial cell is surrounded by an envelope similar to that of gram-negative bacteria. The envelope consists of two trilaminar membranes, an outer membrane (OM) and an inner, cytoplasmic membrane (CM) (Caldwell et al., 1981). However, the cell does not contain

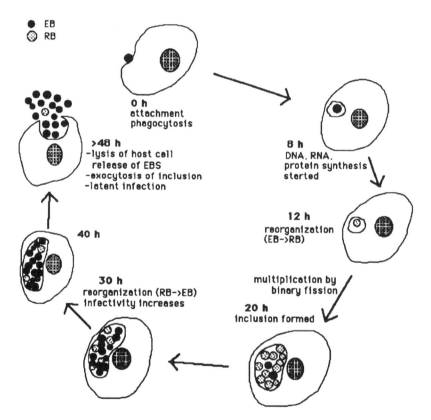

FIGURE 5. Sketch of the developmental cycle of *Chlamydia* (EB = elementary body; RB = reticulate body).

TABLE 3. Biological Characteristics of Chlamydial Species

| Characteristic | C. trachomatis | | C. psittaci | TWAR |
	Non-LGV strains	LGV strains		
Developmental cycle (EB, RB)	+	+	+	+
LPS (genus-specific ag)	+	+	+	+
Extrachromosomal DNA (plasmid)	+	+	+[a]	−
Elementary bodies				
Periplasmic space	Narrow	Narrow	Narrow	Large
Shape	Round	Round	Round	Pear-shaped
Inclusions				
Morphology	Vacuolar	Vacuolar	Oval, dense	Oval, dense
Glycogen	+	+	−	−
Mouse virulence	+	+ + +	+ + +[a]	±
Growth in eggs	+ +	+ + +	+ + +	+
Growth in cell culture enhanced by	+ +	+ + +	+ + +[a]	+
Centrifugation	+ + +	+ +	+ +	+ + +
Cycloheximide	+ +	+	+	+ +
DEAE-dextran	+ + +	±	+[b]	+

[a]Most strains.
[b]Some strains.

peptidoglycan in the periplasmic space (Garrett et al., 1974), a factor that contributes to the integrity of other gram-negative bacterial cells.

Chlamydial cells are composed of protein (35%) and lipid (40–50%) (Manire and Tamura, 1967), and contain both DNA and RNA. More RNA is present in the metabolically active RBs than in EBs (Moulder, 1966). The chlamydial genome, a double-stranded DNA of mol. wt. 660×10^6 Da (Sarov and Becker, 1969), is one of the smallest prokaryotic genomes. In addition to the chromosomal DNA, a plasmid (mol. wt. 4.4×10^6 Da) has been identified in all C. trachomatis strains (Lovett et al., 1980). The plasmid in C. psittaci is shown to differ from that in C. trachomatis (Joseph et al., 1986). Plasmids in C. trachomatis serotypes are closely related (Lovett et al., 1980). So far no plasmid has been identified in TWAR chlamydiae (Campbell et al., 1987a) (Table 3).

The function of plasmids is not yet known, except that they are potential recipients of transposable drug resistance genes. The analysis of plasmids can be applied to the classification of chlamydiae.

The outer membrane of both species of Chlamydia contains a major outer membrane protein (MOMP) with a mol. wt. of 40×10^3 Da. It is analogous to porin protein found in gram-negative bacteria. The MOMP comprises approximately 50% of all proteins in the OM (Caldwell et al., 1981). Through exten-

sive disulfide bridging in the EB phase, the MOMP, and other protein components in the surface structures, the integrity of the EB is maintained (Bavoil et
al., 1984); the OM of RBs has been shown to lack cysteine-rich proteins.
Disulfide unbridging has also been associated with pore formation in the OM of
C. trachomatis (Bavoil et al., 1984). A transport function of these pores has been
suggested.

Electron microscopy has shown two kinds of surface projections in chlamydial OM (Matsumoto, 1979; Gregory et al., 1979; Nichols et al., 1985). The
hemispheric projections have been detected on EBs. The spikelike rods occur
mainly on intermediate developmental forms (transition forms between EBs and
RBs) (Matsumoto, 1979; Gregory et al., 1979; Nichols et al., 1985). The function of these projections is unknown, but a role in the attachment process or in
the transport of molecules has been suggested.

Chi and co-workers (1987) recently studied the ultrastructure of the TWAR
chlamydiae. The morphology of the EBs of TWAR chlamydiae differs distinctly
from that of other chlamydial EBs. TWAR organism EBs are pear-shaped and
pleomorphic in contrast to those of other chlamydial strains that are round. The
periplasmic space in the TWAR EBs is large and contains miniature bodies,
whereas other chlamydial strains contain a narrow, if any, periplasmic space
(Chi et al., 1987) (Table 3). TWAR RBs are circular and closely resemble other
chlamydial RBs. The maturation of RBs to EBs takes longer than for other
chlamydial strains. In tissue cell cultures, the number of EBs increases for 4 days
(Chi et al., 1987). Apart from ultrastructural studies, differentiation of the
TWAR agents from *C. trachomatis* and other *C. psittaci* strains can be made by
serological and restriction endonuclease analyses. Also, DNA hybridization tests
can differentiate TWAR from other chlamydiae. In fact, such hybridization tests
indicate that the TWAR organisms are unique among the chlamydiae (Campbell
et al., 1987a).

The TWAR chlamydiae produce inclusions that morphologically resemble
those of *C. psittaci*. With Giemsa staining, both TWAR and *C. psittaci* inclusions are dense and oval, whereas *C. trachomatis* inclusions are vacuolar (Kuo et
al., 1986a) (Table 3). TWAR inclusions do not contain glycogen, the lack of
which results in a negative iodine stain. When immunological staining is used,
TWAR inclusions can be detected with chlamydial genus-specific or TWAR-
specific labeled monoclonal antibodies, whereas staining with *C. trachomatis*
MOMP-specific monoclonal antibodies gives a negative result (Kuo et al.,
1986b). Immunological studies also suggest that the TWAR strains are unique
among chlamydial strains.

The chlamydial growth cycle is initiated by the adherence of EBs to susceptible cells. *C. trachomatis,* serotypes A–K, prefer columnar epithelial cells,
whereas LGV serotypes and *C. psittaci* strains have a wider range of host cells;

they are capable of replicating in macrophages, for example (Kuo, 1978; Wyrick and Brownbridge, 1978). The attachment process is influenced by surface structures of both the host cell and the EB (Hatch et al., 1981), but specific receptor sites have not yet been established. Recently, chlamydial cell wall proteins that may act as adhesins were detected on EBs but not on RBs (Wenman and Meuser, 1986). In addition, antibodies against these proteins were shown to have a neutralizing capability (i.e., they inhibit infectivity in tissue cell cultures), and thus might serve a protective role (Wenman and Meuser, 1986). The attachment rate is temperature-dependent. Pretreatment of cells with diethylaminoethyldextran, iodeoxyuridine, or irradiation enhances attachment, whereas pretreatment with heparin decreases it (Kuo et al., 1973). The exact nature of the attachment reaction is not yet fully understood. Current knowledge of parasite (chlamydiae)–host interactions was recently reviewed by Ward (1986).

After attachment, the EB particle enters the host cell through a vesicle, a phagosome. The phagocytosis process is induced by live chlamydiae (Byrne and Moulder, 1978); however, fusion of phagosome with lysosomes—as usually occurs—is delayed in chlamydial infection until late stages of the developmental cycle (Friis, 1972). The induced phagocytosis and prevention of phagolysosomal fusion are important factors for chlamydial virulence.

Once inside the vesicle, the EBs reorganize into RBs for 12 hr (Figs. 5 and 6). The reorganization is accompanied by changes in particle size and in the cysteine content of the OM proteins followed by decreased stability (Hatch et al., 1981). The lability and suggested pore formation associated with the absence of extensive disulfide bridging of MOMP might assist in providing chlamydiae with nutrients and energy from the host cell. Chlamydiae cannot synthesize high-energy compounds, but they use host cell ATP and have therefore been called "energy parasites" (Moulder, 1966). The RBs divide by binary fission inside the vesicles. Synthesis of chlamydial DNA, RNA, proteins, lipids, and polysaccharides follows, while metabolic activity in the host cell is reduced. Approximately 18 to 24 hr after attachment, the RBs start to undergo reorganization to EBs, and gradually the EB/RB ratio increases. After 24–30 hr, host cell death is imminent, phagolysosomal fusion occurs, and the infectious EBs are released (Fig. 7), possibly infecting new host cells.

Inclusions can also be exocytosed (Todd and Caldwell, 1985). Thus, under some conditions, a persistent infection can take place instead of the above-described productive infection that results in cell death (Hanna et al., 1968; Storz, 1971). Nutritional depletion, pH and temperature modification, penicillin treatment, and host defense mechanisms might contribute to persistence. Sublethal doses of penicillin can inhibit binary fission and prevent synthesis of essential components of EBs in L cells (Matsumoto and Manire, 1970; see Chapter 10.)

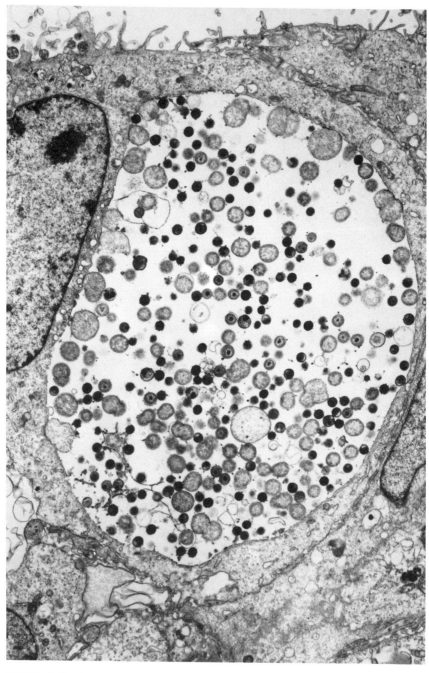

FIGURE 6. Electron micrograph showing a cell inclusion with *C. trachomatis*, serotype C (×3500). (Courtesy of Dr. M. Ward.)

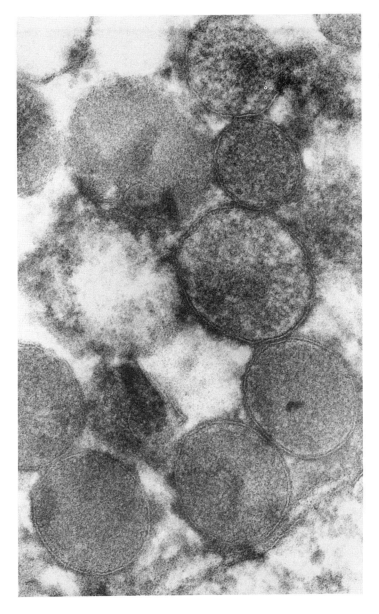

FIGURE 7. Elementary bodies of C. trachomatis in genital secretion. (Courtesy of Drs. Martinov and Popov.)

ANTIGENIC COMPOSITION

Antigens present on the surface of chlamydiae can be classified as genus-, species-, subspecies-, and serotype-specific (cf. Allan, 1986) (Table 4). A genus-specific antigen is shared by *C. psittaci* and *C. trachomatis*. It is a lipopolysaccharide (LPS) (Nurminen et al., 1983) that consists of a heat-stabile, periodate-sensitive carbohydrate part (Barwell, 1952; Kuo et al., 1971) and lipid A in a cryptic form (Brade et al., 1985). The chlamydial genus-specific antigen is located on the outer membrane of the organism (on both EBs and RBs) (Dhir and Boatman, 1972) and is present for the entire developmental cycle (Reeve and Taverne, 1962). In immunofluorescence studies, the genus-specific antigen can be demonstrated in intracytoplasmic inclusions. The antigen also occurs in association with cell cytoplasm in infected cell cultures (Richmond, 1980).

The serologically active part of the carbohydrate is its acidic component, a 2-keto-3-deoxyoctanoic acid (KDO) (Dhir et al., 1972), which is a typical constituent of the LPS core of gram-negative bacteria. Studies with polyclonal and monoclonal antisera have shown that the chlamydial genus-specific antigen resembles the deep-core (Re) part of the enterobacterial LPS (Nurminen et al., 1983; Caldwell and Hitchcock, 1984).

At least three antigenic domains are present in chlamydial LPS. Two of them (lipid A and KDO) seem to be shared by other gram-negative organisms, whereas one is present exclusively in chlamydial LPS (Caldwell and Hitchcock, 1984; Nurminen et al., 1985). Lipopolysaccharide from rough mutants of gram-negative enteric bacteria and from *Acinetobacter* has been reported to cross-react with chlamydial LPS (KDO and lipid A parts) (Volkert and Matthiesen, 1956; Brade and Brunner, 1979). Recently, the genes coding for the enzyme(s) produc-

TABLE 4. *C. trachomatis* Antigens

Antigen	Chemical nature	Comments
Genus-specific (common to *C. trachomatis, C. psittaci* and TWAR chlamydiae)	Lipopolysaccharide	Three distinct antigenic domains
Species-specific (differentiate *C. trachomatis, C. psittaci,* and TWAR chlamydiae)	Proteins	>18 distinct components, 155 kDa in *C. trachomatis,* epitopes in a 40-kDa protein, (MOMP), 60- to 62-kDa protein
Serotype-specific (differentiate between different serovars of *C. trachomatis*)	Proteins	Epitopes in a 40-kDa protein (MOMP), 30-kDa protein in serotypes A and B

ing the genus-specific antigen were cloned and expressed in *E. coli* (Nano and Caldwell, 1985). Carlson and associates (1986) recently characterized the glycoproteins of chlamydial organisms.

Chlamydial LPS has been found to agglutinate mouse and rabbit erythrocytes but not human, guinea pig, or pronghorn antelope erythrocytes. The hemagglutination was not specific for *Chlamydia* spp. as LPS of bacteria, like *E. coli*, also agglutinated such erythrocytes (Watkins et al., 1977).

The species-specific antigens that differentiate *C. trachomatis* and *C. psittaci* from one another are heat-labile proteins. At least 18 species-specific antigenic components have been resolved (Caldwell et al., 1975a), which are predominantly proteins associated with the chlamydial membrane.

A 155-kDa protein common to *C. trachomatis* serotypes was described by Caldwell et al. (1975b). Later, Salari and Ward (1981) discovered three polypeptides with molecular weights of 155, 40, and 29 kDa that are shared by most *C. trachomatis* serotypes. The 155-kDa polypeptide seems common to all *C. trachomatis strains*. It elicits antibody production during experimental infection by *C. trachomatis* (Caldwell et al., 1975b; Caldwell and Kuo, 1977). Because it is a heat-labile protein, it is not detectable in immunoblotting studies involving electrophoresed proteins from preheated chlamydial particles (Newhall et al., 1982).

Recently, a common MOMP determinant of all *C. trachomatis* biovars was demonstrated with the aid of a monoclonal antibody against this determinant (Stephens and Kuo, 1984). The biological significance of this structure is not clear since in the mouse pneumonitis biovar the determinant is masked and cannot be exposed without chemical manipulation.

The approximately 40-kDa MOMP of *C. trachomatis* is the predominant serotyping antigen. Major outer membrane proteins of *C. trachomatis* are different from those of *C. psittaci* (Caldwell and Schachter 1982; Stephens et al., 1982a). In immunoblotting tests, a strong antibody response is often found in the 40-kDa region corresponding to the MOMP (Jones et al., 1982a; Cevenini et al., 1986a, 1986b; Ward et al., 1986). However, Newhall and co-workers (1982) reported weak but consistent reactions with MOMP, even with sera from humans, without evidence of chlamydial infection. In still other studies, antibody-negative control sera remained negative in immunoblotting tests (Cevenini et al., 1986a; Ward et al., 1986). A positive correlation between acute chlamydial urethritis and serum immunoblotting reactivity with purified MOMP has been noted by Cevenini et al. (1986a). Immunoblots of serum from patients with different chlamydial infections are shown in Fig. 8.

Sixty- and 62-kDa proteins can also evoke an antibody response in human chlamydial disease (Jones et al., 1982a; Newhall et al., 1982; Cevenini et al., 1986a, 1986b). These proteins might present with species-specific determinants, since immunoblot-positive sera reacted with 60- and 62-kDa proteins from all *C. trachomatis* serotypes (Newhall et al., 1982). Antibodies against the 60- and 62-

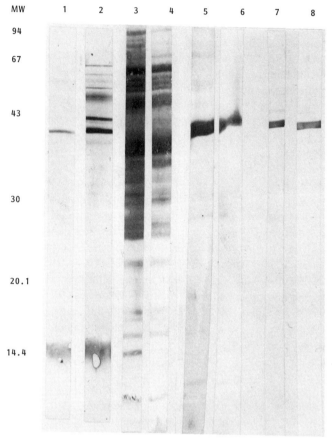

FIGURE 8. Immunoblots from paired sera of patients with chlamydial urethritis (lanes 1–2, IgG response), perihepatitis (lanes 3–4, IgG response), and infant pneumonia (lanes 5–6, IgG and lanes 7–8, IgM response).

kDa proteins could be detected in sera of almost all patients with positive chlamydial culture, but were detected very seldomly in the sera of low-risk patients with negative culture (Newhall et al., 1982).

Several other chlamydial proteins have been identified as immunogenic in humans, inducing chlamydial IgG antibody production (Newhall et al., 1982; Ward et al., 1986). IgA and IgM antibodies seem to show a more restricted reaction pattern (Cevenini et al., 1986b).

In studies with the mouse toxicity prevention test (MTPT), the micro-IF test, and, more recently, tests with labeled monoclonal antibodies, antigens have been grouped as species-, subspecies-, and serotype-specific. These specificities have been demonstrated in association with the MOMP of *C. trachomatis* (Stephens et al., 1982, 1986; Caldwell and Schachter, 1982). According to sub-species-specific antigenic determinants in the MOMP, the *C. trachomatis* serotypes can be classified into two groups: the B and the C complexes (the B complex includes serotypes B, B_a, E, D, K, L_1, L_2, and L_3, and the C complex serotypes C, J, H, I, A, G, and F) (Wang and Grayston, 1982). Studies using monoclonal antibodies with varying specificities confirm the results of micro-IF tests.

The MOMP of *C. psittaci* is immunologically different from that of *C. trachomatis* (Caldwell and Judd, 1982). It seems antigenically heterogeneous. However, further characterization of *C. psittaci* MOMP (e.g., studies of sub-species-specific determinants) is needed.

Type-specific determinants that differentiate between the 15 *C. trachomatis* serotypes either are located evenly on the outer membrane surface of the orga-nism or are distributed heterogeneously (Clark et al., 1982). They are present in both EBs and RBs (Clark et al., 1982). Both polyclonal and monoclonal antisera against the MOMP have been shown to neutralize infectivity in vitro, but the neutralization seems to be type-specific (Caldwell and Perry, 1982; Peeling et al., 1984). In MTPT, toxicity reactions are also type-specific (Wang and Grayston, 1963; Alexander et al., 1967). A type-specific antigen of serotypes A and B with a molecular weight of approximately 30 kDa has been described (Sacks et al., 1978; Sacks and MacDonald, 1979).

GENETICS

Chlamydial chromosomal DNA consists of approximately 600–850 kilo-base pairs (Becker, 1978). In cesium chloride gradient density centrifugation, chromosomal DNA of *C. trachomatis,* serotype L_2, was found to be less dense (2 mg/ml) than that of *E. coli* (Hyypiä et al., 1984). This correlates well with the reported guanosine/cytosine contents of the DNA of *C. trachomatis* (Szybalski, 1968; Schachter and Caldwell, 1980). Comparison of the DNA restriction endo-nuclease patterns have shown marked differences between *C. trachomatis* and *C. psittaci*. Different *C. trachomatis* serotypes were closely related but differed slightly when various restriction enzymes were used (Peterson and de la Maza, 1983). Restriction enzyme analyses of chlamydial plasmid DNA revealed it to be highly conserved in *C. trachomatis* strains (Lovett et al., 1980). Hyypiä and co-workers (1984) found all the known 15 serotypes of *C. trachomatis* to contain DNA sequences homologous with the serotype L_2 plasmid that had been cloned into *E. coli*.

Wenman and Lovett (1982) were the first to report a successful cloning of *C. trachomatis* antigen in *E. coli*. Later, several attempts were made to clone the DNA sequence-encoding MOMP, the principal cell wall component and major immunoreacting antigen of *C. trachomatis*. Expression of this latter protein, or at least immunoreactive parts of it, was achieved in different vector systems (Allan et al., 1984; Stephens et al., 1985; Nano et al., 1985). Allan and co-workers (1984) reported identical *Staphylococcus aureus* V8 protease fragments from both cloned polypeptides and MOMP extracted from EBs. Stephens and associates (1985) cloned the approximately 15-kDa carboxy terminal peptide of MOMP, which was shown to have epitopes of species, subspecies, and type specificity.

　　Polypeptides of *C. psittaci* were also cloned into *E. coli* (Kihlström et al., 1986). Of the expressed polypeptides, one has been found to be immunogenic in human *C. psittaci* infection. Polypeptides expressed from cloned *C. trachomatis* plasmid DNA have been found not to be seroreactive in human infections (Joseph et al., 1986).

　　Preliminary data from DNA hybridization analyses and the restriction endonuclease pattern of TWAR DNA show that it differs distinctly from the DNAs of *C. trachomatis* and *C. psittaci* (Campbell et al., 1987a); this observation favors the separation of the TWAR chlamydiae (from *C. psittaci*) into a new species of the genus *Chlamydia*.

3

Pathology of Chlamydial Infections

CYTOLOGY

Cytology offers a diagnostic aid for *ocular diseases* caused by *C. trachomatis* (e.g., in trachoma and ophthalmia neonatorum) (Sezer, 1951).

The cytological characteristics of trachoma have been described in detail (Sezer, 1951; Hardy, 1966). The most typical finding noted in epithelial scrapings from the conjunctiva is intracellular inclusion bodies, so called Halberstaedter–Prowazek inclusions (1907) (Fig. 9). They can be detected mainly in the early stages of the disease, whereas inclusions are rarely found during the chronic phases, except during acute exacerbations (Sezer, 1951).

Other cytological features characteristic of acute episodes of trachoma are numerous polymorphonuclear (PMN) leukocytes present in eye exudate as well as degenerative changes in epithelial and plasma cells present in epithelial scrapings. Pathognomonic cytological features of trachoma are mitoses and autolytic degeneration in cells from germinal centers (transformed lymphocytes), and an abundance of large macrophages (Sezer, 1951; Hardy, 1966). These findings are suggestive of trachoma even in the absence of intracytoplasmic inclusion bodies (Hardy et al., 1967).

In chlamydial ophthalmia neonatorum and adult inclusion conjunctivitis due to *C. trachomatis* (serotypes D–K), intracellular inclusion bodies are frequently demonstrated (cf. Schachter, 1978). Naib (1970) reported clusters of intracytoplasmic inclusions and numerous neutrophils, histiocytes, and an abundance of thick mucus in conjunctival smears of babies with chlamydial ophthalmia neonatorum. In 387 adult patients with the clinical diagnosis of chlamydial conjunctivitis, the diagnostic value of ocular cytological examination was evaluated with Giemsa-stained smears. Intracytoplasmic inclusions were found in 30

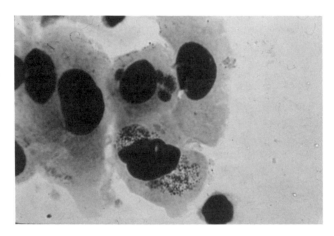

FIGURE 9. Intracytoplasmic inclusion in Giemsa-stained conjunctival cells of a patient with trachoma. (Courtesy of J. Schachter.)

(8%) patients. Both PMN leukocytes and lymphocytes were detected in the smears. Predominant cell type was *not* relevant to the differentiation of chlamydial from adenovirus infection (Wilhelmus et al., 1986).

Before the introduction of cell culture techniques for the diagnosis of chlamydial infection, microscopy of urethral smears formed the cornerstone of the diagnosis of *nongonococcal urethritis* (NGU). In Gram-stained smears, numerous PMN leukocytes were noted but gram-negative intracellular diplococci were absent. In 1910 Lindner noted similarities between the cytology of conjunctival smears from trachoma patients and of urethral smears from NGU cases (i.e., intracellular inclusions of similar appearance were present in both types of smears). Later the occurrence of inclusions in genital samples from chlamydia-infected persons was shown to be a rather infrequent event (Schachter and Dawson, 1978). In addition, the mere absence of gram-negative intracellular diplococci (gonococci) does not necessarily imply a chlamydial infection, although up to 60% of NGU cases have been shown to be culture-positive for *C. trachomatis* (Terho, 1978).

Cytological screening tests are commonly used to detect cellular changes in cervical smears by Papanicolaou-stained (Pap) smears. However, until recently, the value placed on the cytological Pap smear in the diagnosis of genital infections has been highly contradictory (Spence et al., 1986b; Roongpisuthipong et al., 1987). The low diagnostic accuracy of Pap smears for this purpose is now generally accepted.

There is growing interest in the use of cervical cytology for the diagnosis of cervical and vaginal infections with sexually transmitted pathogens, such as *C.*

trachomatis, herpes simplex virus (HSV), and human papilloma virus (HPV). Naib (1970) and Gupta and associates (1979) described cytoplasmic inclusions thought to be consistent with chlamydial infection in cervical Pap smears. Subsequently, there has been a growing tendency of cytopathologists to report inclusions or cytological changes suggestive of *C. trachomatis* in cervical Pap smears (Fig. 10). At least three later studies demonstrated cytoplasmic changes suggestive of *C. trachomatis* infection. These changes occurred more often in women with proven chlamydial infection (31–42%) than in women without chlamydial infection (6–24%) (Forster et al., 1983; Dorman et al., 1983; Geer-

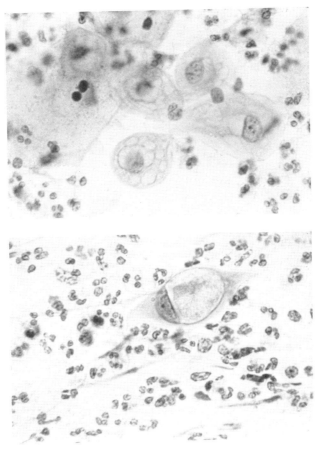

FIGURE 10. Pap-stained vaginal/cervical smears showing inclusion-containing vacuoles with (upper) large and (lower) small intracytoplasmic inclusions in metaplastic cells. (Courtesy of Dr. N. Kiviat.)

ling et al., 1985). However, the vast majority of cytological studies have demonstrated a very poor diagnostic efficacy of Pap smears for detecting *C. trachomatis* infection. For instance, Kiviat and associates (1984) analyzed the potential use of cytology as a screening test for chlamydial infection in a high-risk STD clinic population with 21–25% prevalence of *C. trachomatis*. The presence of vacuoles and inclusions in epithelial cells from randomly selected STD clinic patients and patients referred for cervicitis with or without *C. trachomatis* is shown in Table 5. Logistic regression analysis, adjusted for covariables (age, parity, birth control pill use, number of lifetime sex partners, and time in menstrual cycle), indicated that large, distinct, inclusion-containing vacuoles were associated with the isolation of *C. trachomatis* only in the randomly selected patient ($p = 0.007$). The detection of large, distinct, inclusion-containing vacuoles, however, had a sensitivity of only 12%, a specificity of 94%, and a positive predictive value of only 45%. Overall, distinct vacuoles were seen by Pap smear in only 22% of *C. trachomatis* infections.

It is of interest that some of the cytological abnormalities discussed in association with *C. trachomatis* infection also correlate statistically with the occurrence of *Mycoplasma hominis* (Mårdh et al., 1971).

In the absence of inclusions, a characteristic inflammatory pattern consisting of PMN leukocytes, lymphocytes, plasma cells, and germinal center cells predicts *C. trachomatis* infection (Kiviat et al., 1985a). Several studies have demonstrated an association between *C. trachomatis* and an inflammatory pat-

TABLE 5. Correlation of Vacuoles and Inclusions in Metaplastic or Endocervical Cells with Isolation of *C. trachomatis* in an STD Clinic Population[a]

	Number (%) of patients			
	Large vacuoles		Small vacuoles without inclusions	Vacuoles not present
Population	With inclusions	Without inclusions		
Randomly selected patients				
Chlamydia-positive (*n* = 23)	5 (22)	6 (26)	9 (39)	3 (13)
Chlamydia-negative (*n* = 82)	4 (5)	11 (13)	26 (32)	41 (50)
Patients referred for suspected cervicitis				
Chlamydia-positive (*n* = 54)	4 (7)	13 (24)	15 (28)	22 (41)
Chlamydia-negative (*n* = 101)	7 (7)	15 (15)	27 (27)	52 (51)

[a]From Kiviat et al. (1985a).

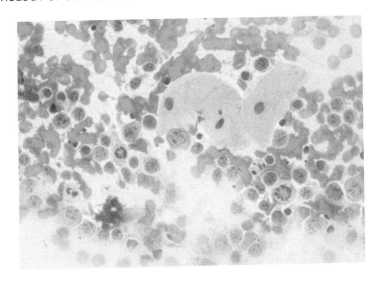

FIGURE 11. Transformed lymphocytes in a Pap smear from a woman with chlamydial cervicitis (×1200). (Courtesy of Dr. R. Aine.)

tern seen in Pap smear (Simmons and Vosmik, 1974; Burns et al., 1975; Oriel et al., 1978; Paavonen and Purola, 1980; Saltz et al., 1981; Purola and Paavonen, 1982; Dorath et al., 1985; Geerling et al., 1985; Lindner et al., 1985; Shafer et al., 1985), although a few studies failed to demonstrate such an association. In the above-mentioned study, Kiviat and co-workers (1985a) used multiple logistic regression, adjusting for demographic and physiological variables and coinfections, to determine more definitely which epithelial and inflammatory cellular changes were independently associated with *C. trachomatis* among STD clinic patients. *C. trachomatis* was associated with transformed lymphocytes (Fig. 11), plasma cells, histiocytes (>30/×400 field), and >3+ PMN leukocytes, and with lymphocytes (>5/×400 field) (Table 6). The most specific criterion for screening for *C. trachomatis* infection among randomly selected STD clinic women was the presence of transformed lymphocytes; this criterion had a sensitivity of 84%, a specificity of 83%, and a positive predictive value of 57% in comparison with isolation of *C. trachomatis*. The most sensitive criterion was the presence of either increased PMN leukocytes or a combination of transformed lymphocytes, plasma cells, and increased histiocytes; this criterion had a sensitivity of 100%, a specificity of 64%, and a positive predictive value of 42%

TABLE 6. Significant Associations of Pathogens and Clinical Diagnoses with Inflammatory Cytological Patterns in an STD Clinic Population[a,b]

Population	Lymphocytes ≥ 5/x400 field	Transformed lymphocytes	Plasma cells	Histiocytes ≥ 30/x400 field	3 + polymorphonuclear leukocytes
Randomly selected patients (n = 63)[c,d]	N. gonorrhoeae (p ≥ 0.001)	C. trachomatis (p = <0.001)[d]	C. trachomatis (p = 0.034)	C. trachomatis (p = 0.002); T. vaginalis (p = 0.007); bacterial vaginosis (p = 0.03, negative correlation)	C. trachomatis (p = 0.002)[d]; endocervical mucopus (p = 0.008); herpes simplex virus (p = 0.048)
Patients referred for suspected cervitis (n = 85)	C. trachomatis (p = 0.017); T. vaginalis (p = 0.046)	Cytomegalovirus (p = 0.004); C. trachomatis (p < 0.001)[d]	C. trachomatis (p = 0.02)	—	T. vaginalis (p = 0.014); endocervical mucopus (p = 0.007)

[a]From Kiviat et al. (1985a).
[b]Logistic regression analysis after adjusting for five covariables: age, parity, birth control pill use, number of lifetime sexual partners, and time in menstrual cycle. The analysis includes those for whom all microbiology, clinical examination, and cytological studies of inflammatory pattern were completed.
[c]p values are unadjusted for multiple comparison.
[d]p < 0.05 after adjusting for multiple comparisons using Bonferroni's inequality.

in comparison with isolation of *C. trachomatis*. The presence of >30 histiocytes (in at least three fields) or the presence of transformed lymphocytes proved to be the optimum criterion for screening of patients at high risk for *C. trachomatis*, with a sensitivity of 95%, a specificity of 75%, and a positive predictive value of 50% (Kiviat et al., 1984). Kiviat et al. (1984) also demonstrated a relatively high interobserver reproducibility for the cytological evaluation of inflammatory pattern.

Several studies have analyzed the epithelial cellular atypias associated with cervical *C. trachomatis* infection (Naib, 1970; Simmons and Vosmik, 1974; Burns et al., 1975; Mourad et al., 1976; Carr et al., 1979; Gupta et al., 1979; Paavonen et al., 1979; Paavonen and Purola, 1980; Kiviat et al., 1985a; Lindner et al., 1985). However, the interpretation of many of these reports is greatly hindered by the lack of uniform criteria used to describe the epithelial cellular abnormalities. There is also confusion regarding the cytological nomenclature used in these studies. The terms inflammatory atypia, Pap class 2 or 3 atypia, metaplastic atypia, and reactive endocervical cell atypia all fall into a loose group of benign cytological atypias not sufficient to be considered consistent with dysplasia. The significance of such benign atypias has not yet been elucidated in large prospective studies, but they may represent an early part of a continuum of cervical intraepithelial neoplasia (CIN). Some of the *C. trachomatis*-associated cervical cytological atypias may represent epithelial changes derived from an active reparative process (cellular repair) either during the course of the infection or during healing after elimination of the infection. In the above-mentioned study by Kiviat and co-workers (1985a), the associations of reactive endocervical cells (Fig. 12) and atypical metaplastic cells (Fig. 13) with *C. trachomatis* were of particular interest (Table 7). Paavonen and Purola (1980) found that not only benign atypia (metaplastic and regenerative atypia) but also CIN was associated with *C. trachomatis* infection (Table 8). It is generally believed that most dysplasias (with the exception of keratinizing dysplasias) arise in areas of squamous metaplasia (Patton, 1978). Atypical squamous metaplasia has often been associated with metaplastic dysplasia (Patton, 1978; Koss, 1979). Thus, it would be important to determine the natural history of benign metaplastic atypia seen with endocervical chlamydial infection adjusting for coinfections, such as HSV-2, *T. vaginalis*, *N. gonorrhoeae*, and HPV.

At least three seroepidemiological studies have shown an association between the presence of serum antichlamydial antibodies and CIN (Schachter et al., 1975a, 1982a; Paavonen et al., 1979). Three studies have demonstrated cytological atypia consistent with CIN more often in women with *C. trachomatis* isolated from the cervix or with local antichlamydial antibodies in cervical mucus than in controls lacking evidence of *C. trachomatis* infection (Carr et al., 1979; Paavonen and Purola, 1980; Cevenini et al., 1981).

Quinn and associates (1987) compared tissue culture with Pap smears, endocervical cytological smears stained with monoclonal antibody to *C. tra-*

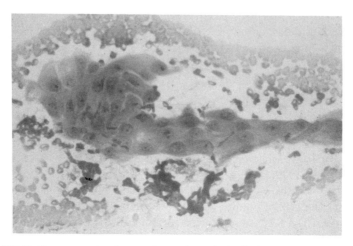

FIGURE 12. Pap smear showing reactive endocervical cells, leukocytes, and atypical meta-plastic cells. (Courtesy of Dr. E. Purola.)

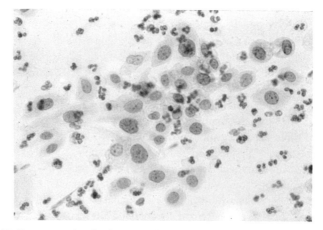

FIGURE 13. Pap smear showing large number of polymorphonuclear leukocytes. (Courtesy of Dr. N. Kiviat.)

TABLE 7. Significant Associations of Pathogens and Clinical Diagnoses with Epithelial Cellular Changes in an STD Clinic Population[a,b]

| | Squamous cells | | | | |
	Minimal nuclear and cytoplasmic changes	Moderate nuclear changes and dyskeratosis	Koilocytic changes	Metaplastic cells: reactive and/or atypical changes	Endocervical cells: reactive changes and leukocytes
Randomly selected patients ($n = 76$)[c]	Yeast ($p = <0.001$)[d,e]; endocervical mucopus ($p = 0.012$)	Condylomata on colposcopy ($p = 0.002$)[e]	Condylomata on colposcopy ($p = <0.001$)[e]; G. vaginalis ($p = 0.027$); endocervical mucopus ($p = 0.003$,[e] negative correlation)	C. trachomatis ($p = 0.017$); G. vaginalis ($p = 0.026$); herpes simplex virus ($p = 0.02$, negative correlation)	C. trachomatis ($p = 0.015$)
Patients referred for suspected cervicitis ($n = 106$)	Bacterial vaginosis ($p = 0.006$)	Herpes simplex virus ($p = 0.012$)	—	C. trachomatis ($p = 0.004$)[e]; T. vaginalis ($p = 0.016$); herpes simplex virus ($p = 0.02$, negative correlation)	C. trachomatis ($p = 0.019$); group B streptococci ($p = 0.045$)

[a]From Kiviat et al. (1985a)

[b]Logistic regression analysis after adjusting for five covariables: age, parity, birth control pill use, number of lifetime sexual partners, and time in menstrual cycle.

[c]Analysis of all those for whom all microbiologic studies, clinical examination, and cytological studies of epithelial cellular changes were completed.

[d]p values are unadjusted for multiple comparisons.

[e]$p < 0.05$ after adjusting for multiple comparison using Bonferroni's inequality.

TABLE 8. Association of *C. trachomatis*
with Cervical Cytological Atypia among NGU Contacts[a]

	Number with atypia (%)	
Cytological finding	Isolated ($N = 93$)	Not isolated ($N = 147$)
Benign atypia	25 (27)	22 (15)[b]
Mild to moderate dysplasia	10 (11)	4 (3)[c]
Total with atypia	35 (38)	26 (18)[c]

[a]From Paavonen and Purola (1980).
[b]$p < 0.02$.
[c]$p < 0.01$.

chomatis, and a direct immunofluorescent stain of cervical specimens for detection of *C. trachomatis* in cervical specimens from mostly (85%) pregnant STD clinic women admitted for induced abortion. Twenty-one percent of the women had positive cultures for *C. trachomatis.* With the criteria of intracytoplasmic coccoid inclusion bodies within metaplastic cells, 34% of 130 Pap smears were read as suggestive of *C. trachomatis.* Seventeen of the 45 positive Pap smears were positive by culture and 28 were negative, giving a sensitivity of 54% and a specificity of 71%. In contrast, immunofluorescent-stained cytological smears had a sensitivity of 92–94% and a specificity of 98–99%. Thus these workers convincingly demonstrated that immunofluorescent staining of cervical specimens or cytological smears is a more sensitive and specific test than routine Pap smear for detection of *C. trachomatis* infection in a high-prevalence (pregnant) population. By adopting the cytological criteria of Kiviat and co-workers (1985b), Quinn and associates found a much lower sensitivity (31%) and a positive predictive value (35%) for Pap smear diagnosis. Only the presence of increased PMN leukocytes correlated with the isolation of *C. trachomatis.* Certainly, differences in study populations might in part explain the different findings, since Kiviat and associates (1985b) did not include pregnant women but had more women with mucopurulent cervicitis.

In summary, cervical cytology showing certain inflammatory and epithelial cellular changes on Pap-stained smears is significantly associated with *C. trachomatis* infection. Thus cytology offers good promise for improved control of genital chlamydial infection.

The possible value of cytology in human *C. psittaci* infections (e.g., in TWAR infections) has not been established.

HISTOPATHOLOGY

This section covers some main histological features of chlamydial infections. Additional data are given in the discussions of specific diseases.

The histopathological features of *trachoma* were described in detail by Sir Stewart Duke-Elder (1965). The most characteristic features are papillary hypertrophy of the epithelium, a lymphoid infiltration of the subepithelial tissues with the formation of typical lymphoid follicles, and the subsequent proliferation of connective tissue resulting in cicatrization.

In the early stage the tarsal conjunctiva shows flattening of the surface epithelium, crypt formation with collections of PMNs, and subepithelial infiltration with lymphocytes and plasma cells. These epithelial changes become more marked. Papillae and pseudocysts are formed. In the submucosa, general hyperplasia is seen. A capillary dilatation occurs with infiltration of lymphocytes and plasma cells. Gradually, follicles begin to appear. Follicles, though not invariably seen, are the most characteristic and striking histopathological feature of trachoma. Initially, follicles appear as scattered aggregates of lymphocytes, plasma cells, and histiocytes with surrounding inflammatory infiltration. The central part of the maturing follicle consists of a mass of mononuclear cells. The cortical area is made up of a zone of proliferating active lymphocytes. There is no true capsule. As the follicle ages, the central area seems to degenerate and undergo autolysis, giving signs of necrosis. Follicles may disappear with resolution of the inflammatory process. Sometimes they rupture, resulting in a wound that heals by subepithelial cicatrization. Some degree of scarring is always present in trachoma. It arises from the diffuse hypertrophy of the connective tissue, and occurs over the whole submucosa. Finally, fibroblasts occupy the main bulk of the tissue. The epithelium over the scar tissue becomes stretched and atrophied, contraction occurs, and deformities are produced. The tarsal conjunctiva usually shows more changes of the trachomatous process than the bulbar conjunctiva. The cornea exhibits some of the earliest and most typical changes of trachoma in the appearance of a superficial keratitis and the eventual formation of pannus. Some degree of pannus is present in every case of trachoma. The initial changes lead to the development of avascular punctate epithelial and subepithelial keratitis. Following the diffuse epithelial opacification, changes occur in the terminal capillary zone of the limbic system of vessels, leading to the development of trachomatous pannus. Secondary to the neovascularization, an infiltration of lymphocytes and plasma cells produces a cloudy opacity. The parallel, non-anastomizing, newly formed vessels act as endothelial rods with endothelial walls and remain between Bowman's membrane and the epithelium, indicating that the neovascularization is the result of infection. In the pannus, typical follicles are found, especially near the limbus. Histologically they are identical to those seen in the conjunctiva and are surrounded by a vascular network. As the process advances, the entire cornea may become neovascularized as the pannus advances from all around the limbus, while the cornea becomes hazy. In extreme cases the cornea is covered with granulation tissue and vision is gravely impaired.

Even though *C. trachomatis* is the major cause of *cervicitis* in women, the histopathological manifestations of cervical chlamydial infection have not been extensively studied in relation to other cervical infections. Several previous studies mentioned the presence of severe inflammation and germinal centers in the stroma of cervical tissue from which *C. trachomatis* was isolated (Hare et al., 1981; Braley, 1938; Paavonen et al., 1982b; Kunimoto and Brunham, 1985). In a study by Kiviat and co-workers (1986a), the effects of other coinfections were controlled by comparing women with *C. trachomatis* to those with no infection or with other infection (*Trichomonas vaginalis,* herpes simplex virus, *N. gonorrhoeae*). The isolation of *C. trachomatis* from the cervix was associated with several epithelial and stromal inflammatory changes, including the presence of intraepithelial and intraluminal inflammatory cells, immature metaplasia, focal loss of surface glandular epithelium, reactive endocervical cells, dense stromal inflammation, and well-formed germinal centers comprising transformed lymphocytes (Fig. 14). These histopathological findings are consistent with cytological changes associated with cervical chlamydial infection. Equal amounts of IgG- and IgA-producing plasma cells were seen in biopsies from women with *C. trachomatis* cervicitis (Kunimoto and Brunham, 1985).

The histopathological diagnosis of *endometritis* is based on the presence of plasma cells in the endometrial stroma (Rotterdam, 1978; Czernobilsky, 1978; Greenwood and Moran, 1981) (Fig. 15). There is a good correlation of plasma cell infiltration of the endometrium with laparoscopic evidence of salpingitis (Paavonen et al, 1985b; Kiviat et al., 1987a). Patients with acute salpingitis usually have a high concentration of plasma cells. The significance of a low

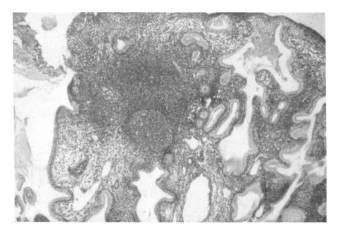

FIGURE 14. Germinal centers in cervical glandular epithelium comprising transformed lymphocytes (×1200). (Courtesy of Prof. E. Saksela.)

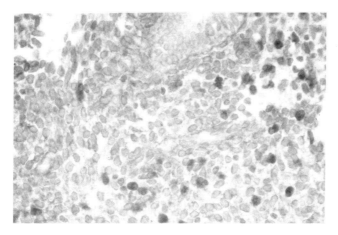

FIGURE 15. Endometrial biopsy specimen showing plasma cells (×400). (Courtesy of Dr. R. Aine.)

concentration of plasma cells requires further study. Isolation of *C. trachomatis* from the endometrium is associated with dense stromal and intraepithelial in-flammation and occurrence of intraluminal inflammatory cells (Fig. 16) of the endometrium (Wølner-Hanssen et al., 1982b; Winkler et al., 1984). Patients with chlamydial endometritis have a higher concentration of plasma cells in endometrial stroma than patients with gonococcal endometritis. The presence of germinal centers comprising transformed lymphocytes in the endometrial stroma

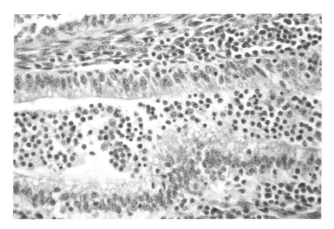

FIGURE 16. Chlamydial endometritis. Monocytic cell infiltration in the endometrium and in-traluminal inflammatory cells (eosin-hematoxylin, ×1000). (Courtesy of Dr. B. Møller.)

(Fig. 17) is associated with the isolation of *C. trachomatis* from the endometrium (Paavonen et al., 1985a; Paavonen et al., 1987). Thus quantitative analysis of several histopathological manifestations of endometritis makes it possible to discriminate between chlamydial, gonococcal, and nonchlamydial nongonococcal endometritis. Endometrial biopsy is useful for confirming by immunocytochemistry the presence of chlamydial infection of the endometrium. In a recent study, elementary bodies or intracellular inclusions of *C. trachomatis* were identified by direct immunofluorescence in 12 of 15 endometrial biopsies from patients who had upper genital tract infection with *C. trachomatis* (Kiviat et al., 1986). Lehtinen and co-workers (1986) studied the B-cell response in chlamydial endometritis. All patients had plasma cell endometritis and *C. trachomatis* isolated from the endometrial aspirates. IgG- and IgA-producing plasma cells were seen in all cases. Lymphoid follicles and IgM-producing plasma cells were also present.

In chlamydial *salpingitis,* the tubal mucosa is usually partly destroyed and the tubal lumen filled by an inflammatory exudate. All layers of the tubal wall can be infiltrated by inflammatory cells. For the most part, monocytic cells, but also polymorphonuclear leukocyte cells, can be seen in the exudate (Møller et all, 1979; cf. Mårdh and Svensson, 1982) (Fig. 18).

In a recent study from the University of Washington (Kiviat et al., unpublished), fimbrial biopsies were systematically obtained from patients with laparoscopically proven salpingitis. Fimbrial biopsies showed inflammation in 9 of 12 patients with laparoscopic evidence of salpingitis and upper genital tract infection with *N. gonorrhoeae* or *C. trachomatis* as compared with 1 of 10 with

FIGURE 17. Germinal centers in the endometrial stroma comprising transformed lymphocytes (×1200). (Courtesy of Dr. R. Aine.)

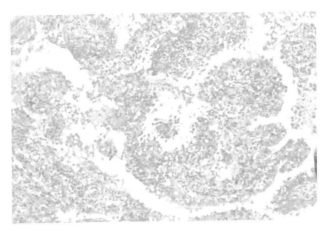

FIGURE 18. Chlamydial salpingitis. Section of a fallopian tube with destroyed cilial epithelium and heavy inflammatory cell infiltration in the tubal wall (×1000).

no laparoscopic evidence of salpingitis (all of whom also lacked upper genital tract chlamydial infection; $p < 0.003$).

The clinical course in *lymphogranuloma venereum* (LGV) can be divided into three stages (Perine and Osoba, 1984). The primary stage includes the initial genital lesions, which are nontender and are often ignored. The ulcer is often herpetiform in character. The secondary stage includes the involvement of regional lymph nodes (bubo), which may rupture spontaneously. The tertiary stage includes chronic or late manifestations such as perirectal abscesses, ischiorectal and rectovaginal fistulas, anal fistulas, and rectal strictures or stenosis. This is also called the chronic anogenitorectal syndrome (Perine and Osoba, 1984). A smaller proportion of the female LGV patients presents with the inguinal syndrome. Deep pelvic and lumbar lymph nodes are often involved, and may be mistaken for appendicitis or a tubo-ovarian abscess.

In lymphogranuloma venereum, then, the chlamydial infection is more invasive than infections caused by other serotypes of *C. trachomatis*. Lymphogranuloma venereum is primarily a disease of lymphatic tissue. It involves thrombolymphangitis and perilymphangitis. The infection spreads from infected lymph nodes to the surrounding tissue. In lymphangitis there is a marked proliferation of endothelial cells lining the lymph vessels and nodes. In the primary infection, the lymph node draining the area of infection may show necrosis (Smith and Custer, 1950). Triangular or quadrangular "stellate" abscesses are found. There is also periadenitis. Later the minute abscesses coalesce, the lymph node ruptures, and fistulas develop that can lead to severe tissue damage.

The subacute histopathological manifestations of the anogenitorectal syndrome are proctocolitis and hyperplasia of intestinal and perirectal lymphatic tissue. A chronic inflammatory process invades the intestinal wall, and noncaseous granulomas and crypt abscesses form. If left untreated, the granulomatous process progressively involves all layers of the bowel wall, and the muscular layers are replaced by fibrous tissue. Contraction of the granulation tissue causes strictures. The mucous membrane below the stricture shows ulcerative and granulomatous proctitis (Smith and Custer, 1950; Schachter and Osoba 1983; Perine and Osoba, 1984).

As mentioned, healing is accompanied by fibrosis, which eventually destroys the normal tissue structure leading to obstruction of lymph vessels. This results in chronic edema and sclerosing fibrosis with induration and enlargement of the affected parts. As a consequence of the fibrosis, the blood supply is affected, resulting in necrosis and ulcerations. In males, penoscrotal elephantiasis can appear in the early years following acute infection (1–20 years).

The Greek term *esthiomene* ("eating away") has been used to describe a progressive lymphangitis, chronic edema, fibrosis, induration, and enlargement of tissues seen in women. There may be chronic ulcerations on the external surface of the labia majora, on the genitocrural folds, and on the lateral regions of the perineum. The edema may extend to the rectum and anus and to the urethra, interfering with normal functions of voiding and defecation. Numerous adhesions may fix the pelvic organs together ("frozen pelvis").

Histopathological characteristics of LGV include severe inflammation with giant cells, lymphocytes, and plasma cells. The histological picture may resemble that of inflammatory bowel disease (e.g., Crohn's disease) (Quinn et al., 1981a,b). LGV may resemble carcinoma clinically and biopsies may be necessary to rule out malignancy. Rectal strictures in LGV are often mistaken for rectal cancer.

The histopathology of *C. psittaci* pneumonia (i.e., in *psittacosis* and *ornithosis*) has long been described in pathology textbooks (cf. Macfarlane and Macrae, 1983). The histopathological features of human psittacosis/ornithosis resemble those of interstitial pneumonia, with myocarditis, encephalitis, aseptic meningitis, and hepatitis as possible complications.

Enzootic abortion of ewes is a well-recognized mammalian infection. The histopathological features of *placentitis* in sheep have been described in detail by Storz (1971). In a recently discovered human manifestation of *C. psittaci* infection (i.e., placentitis), there is tissue destruction and intense acute inflammation (Wong et al., 1985, 1986).

The histopathological features suggest placentitis rather than chorioamnionitis. Initially, deciduitis and acute inflammation of intervillous spaces are seen. Focal microinfarcts are present due to patchy, intense, acute inflammatory cell infiltrates in the intervillous spaces with focal fibrin deposits. The presence of *C. psittaci* was confirmed by immunohistochemistry and electron microscopic studies (Wong et al., 1985). *Chlamydia psittaci* has a predilection for the trophoblast, where the organism multiplies and induces an intense inflammation.

The histopathology of TWAR infections (e.g., *TWAR* pneumonia) remains sparsely documented. The infection is often localized to the lower lobes of the lungs. Often only one lobe is affected. However, upper respiratory tract infections can also be caused by TWAR chlamydiae.

4

Immune Response

INTRODUCTION

Limited information is available regarding the mechanisms involved in recovery from chlamydial infection and resistance to reinfection. According to animal studies, both humoral and cell-mediated immunity are important. Cyclophosphamide-treated guinea pigs (i.e., with impaired humoral immune response) have been reported to suffer from prolonged chlamydial infection, which did not resolve until the appearance of antichlamydial serum antibodies (Rank et al., 1979).

At a cellular level, human polymorphonuclear leukocytes can kill *C. trachomatis* (Yong et al., 1982). Also human monocytes can bind and ingest chlamydiae (cf. Levitt and Barol, 1987). In human polymorphonuclear leukocytes, lysosomes fuse with *C. trachomatis*-containing phagosomes, followed by progressive degradation of chlamydiae (Young et al., 1986). In macrophages, on the other hand, ingested chlamydiae escape phagolysosomal fusion, which may result in proliferation (Wyrick et al., 1978; Rothermel et al., 1983b) and subsequent release of infectious chlamydial particles (elementary bodies).

If macrophages are activated with γ-interferon (γ-IFN) (a lymphokine), replication of both *C. trachomatis* and *C. psittaci* is inhibited (Rothermel et al., 1983a,b; Shemer and Sarov, 1985). γ-IFN increases oxygen-dependent microbicidal and tumoricidal activity of macrophages (Schultz and Kleinschmidt, 1983). This γ-IFN-mediated inhibition can be reversed by tryptophan, but not by other essential amino acids (Byrne et al., 1987). In a recent review, Levitt and Barol (1987) suggested that lymphokines might contribute to prolonged chlamydial infection by allowing the organisms to exist within macrophages without the cells being destroyed by the infection.

Gonadal steroids may influence the course of chlamydial infections (see Chapter 5). The possible link between sex steroids and the immune system (Grossman, 1985) stimulates much interest.

47

HUMORAL AND LOCAL IMMUNE RESPONSE

The kinetics of the humoral antibody response in naturally acquired chlamydial infections is still not very well known. The humoral antibody response in *C. trachomatis* infections is characterized by a conventional IgM or IgG switch. The kinetics of the humoral antibody response has been studied in experimentally infected animals (Ripa et al., 1979) (Fig. 19). In grivet monkeys, antichlamydial IgM antibodies occurred after approximately one week, although IgG antibodies were still found after another week.

In TWAR infections, IgM antibodies usually seem to appear later than in other chlamydial infections (after 2 weeks). IgG antibodies to the TWAR agent generally do not appear for 6–8 weeks (Wang and Grayston, 1986).

In isolation-proven, first-episode chlamydial urethritis, about 67% present with a specific IgM response and 77% present with an IgG antibody response within 3 weeks of onset of the infection, as demonstrated by micro-immunofluorescence tests (Bowie et al., 1977a).

A proportion of the general population has serum IgG antibodies to *C. trachomatis* (Grayston et al., 1984). Such antibodies are more frequently detectable in sera from patients with venereal diseases than in the general population. IgG antibodies to *C. trachomatis* occur more often in females than in males, as indicated by micro-IF tests (Wang and Grayston, 1986). On the other hand, IgG antibodies directed against *C. psittaci* are a rarity (Forsey et al., 1986).

Serum IgG antibody to TWAR chlamydiae is frequently found in the general population (Fig. 20). In contrast to *C. trachomatis* antibodies, TWAR antibodies are more often found in males than in females (Table 9).

Serum IgG antibodies to *C. trachomatis* may persist for years in some persons, whereas in others the titer of such antibodies falls off to nondetectable levels within a couple of years, as was the case in persons with chlamydial pelvic inflammatory disease (PID) (Puolakkainen et al., 1986). The reasons for this interindividual variation is not known. Furthermore, a significant change in the titer of IgG antichlamydial antibodies often cannot be demonstrated during the follow-up period of many patients. This restricts the value of serology for the diagnosis of current chlamydial infections.

IgM antibodies to *C. trachomatis* are less often demonstrated in sera from female patients with uncomplicated genital chlamydial infections than from infected males. This is probably attributable to the fact that chlamydial infections in women are often mild, causing many female patients to consult their doctors weeks after the onset of symptoms, if ever. The current chlamydial infection often represents a reinfection by the same serotype of *C. trachomatis* from a nontreated partner. In such cases with reinfection, IgM antibodies are not likely to be detected. Double infections with different serotypes do, however, occur.

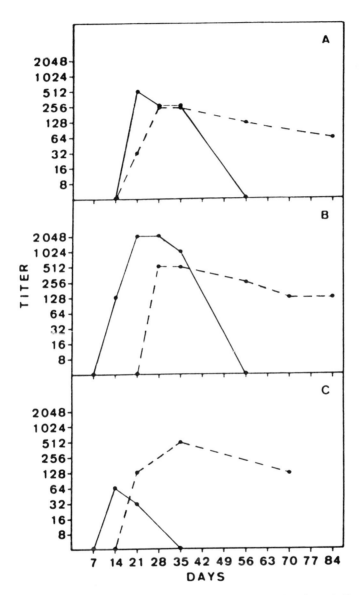

FIGURE 19. Humoral antibody response in three grivet monkeys (monkeys A, B, and C) infected by *C. trachomatis*. Solid line, IgM; dashed line, IgG. (From Ripa et al., 1979.)

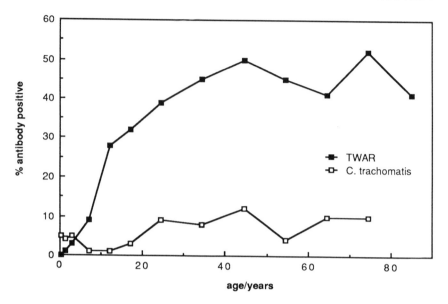

FIGURE 20. Prevalence of TWAR and *C. trachomatis* antibodies in a Danish population studied by microimmunofluorescence technique. (Adapted from Grayston et al., 1984.)

In a Seattle study, IgM antibody to *C. trachomatis* in titers ≥ 8 was approximately four times more prevalent (23% versus 7%) in patients with *C. trachomatis*-positive PID than in *C. trachomatis*-positive controls without PID seen in the same clinical setting. The difference was even more striking for patients with PID versus controls who were *C. trachomatis* culture-negative (17% versus 3%) (Wølner-Hanssen et al., 1987).

Although immune responsiveness in infancy is depressed, infants suffering from chlamydial pneumonitis generally develop high antichlamydial antibody titers, especially of IgM antibodies, and hyperimmunoglobulinemia (elevated total IgG) (Levitt et al., 1983). The demonstration of high (≥ 64) titers of IgM antibodies to *C. trachomatis* in infants has been considered pathognomonic for chlamydial pneumonia (Schachter et al., 1982b).

Recently, the occurrence of spurious IgM antibodies to *C. trachomatis* has been demonstrated not only in children with mononucleosis but also in those with signs of lower respiratory tract infection (Persson and Bröms, 1986). The reactivity pattern of spurious IgM antibodies suggested that they are monoclonal. However, the titers of such IgM antibodies were usually only moderately elevated (i.e., the titer often did not exceed 64). In cases with spurious antichlamydial IgM antibodies, antichlamydial IgG antibodies are not detected (Persson and Bröms, 1987), whereas in infants suffering from pneumonitis, high or moderate levels of such IgG antibodies are frequently seen (Schachter et al., 1982b; Puolakkainen et al., 1984).

The significance of IgA antibodies in chlamydial infection remains unclear. Short-lived serum IgA antibodies might suggest an active *C. trachomatis* infection (Cevenini et al., 1984). Serum IgA antibodies were found in up to half of all patients with IgG antibodies in the series of women with salpingitis studied by Osser and Persson (1984). Local antibodies might offer some protection against mucosal *C. trachomatis* infection. The existence of IgA antibody to *C. trachomatis* in cervical secretion generally correlates with the presence of serum antibody and appears to reflect present or past chlamydial infection (Treharne et al., 1978a; McComb et al., 1979; Puolakkainen et al., 1986). The presence of local IgA antibodies in secretion has also been considered a sign of an active ongoing infection (McComb et al., 1979). Treharne and co-workers (1978a) showed that the presence of cervical IgA antibodies correlated with the isolation of *C. trachomatis* from the cervix. However, the correlation between local and

TABLE 9. Antichlamydial IgG Antibody Prevalences
in Different Study Populations

Study group	Test/titer	Positive (%)	Reference
Children			
0–9 yr	TWAR-micro-IF[a]/≥32	4	Wang and Grayston, 1986
10–19 yr		28	
Adults		46	
Adults	IOL-207-micro-IF[b]/≥16	19	Forsey et al., 1986
Children, 1–17 yr	*C.t.*-micro-IF[c]/≥32	4	Grayston et al., 1986a
Adults			Grayston et al., 1982
Males		8	
Females		15	
Female VD clinic patients	*C.t.*-micro-IF/≥8	90	Schachter et al., 1979
Acute salpingitis patients	*C.t.*-micro-IF/≥64	62	Treharne et al., 1979
Infertile women	*C.t.*-micro-IF/≥32	>70	Moore et al., 1982
Prostatitis patients	*C.t.*-micro-IF/≥64	12	Mårdh et al., 1978
Blood donors	I-IFAT[d]/≥8	40	Saikku and Paavonen, 1978
VD clinic patients	I-IFAT/≥8	60	Richmond and Caul, 1975
Blood donors	CF[e]/≥16	14	Jansson, 1960
Sera sent for viral screening	CF/≥8	12	Puolakkainen et al., 1987a

[a]Microimmunofluorescence (micro-IF) test with TWAR chlamydiae as antigen.
[b]Microimmunofluorescence (micro-IF) test with IOL-207 agent as antigen.
[c]Microimmunofluorescence (micro-IF) test with pools of *C. trachomatis* serotypes as antigen.
[d]Indirect immunofluorescence antibody test (I-IFAT) with cell grown inclusions of *C. trachomatis* as antigen.
[e]Complement fixation test (CF).

serum antichlamydial antibodies has been shown to be much stronger than the correlation of local antibodies with a positive culture for *C. trachomatis* from the cervix (Richmond et al., 1980).

According to Brunham and associates (1983), the existence of secretory IgA (s-IgA) antibodies in cervical secretion correlates inversely with the quantitative recovery of *C. trachomatis* from the cervix, suggesting an inhibitory effect of s-IgA antibodies on the isolation of *C. trachomatis*. Puolakkainen and co-workers (1986) found cervical IgA antibodies in 45% of women with high IgA antibodies in serum, but in only 7% of women with low IgA titers or with no antichlamydial serum IgG antibodies ($p < 0.001$). Cervical IgA antibodies were found only in women with a history of proven genital chlamydial infection.

Persistence of s-IgA antibodies in genital secretion for several years after an acute chlamydial infection has been demonstrated (Terho and Meurman, 1981). The high "background noise" of local antibodies in many patient groups certainly decreases the diagnostic value of the detection of such antibodies as an indicator of acute infection (Schachter et al., 1979a; Puolakkainen et al., 1986).

In the guinea pig animal model, chlamydial s-IgA antibodies have been shown to play an important role in resistance to reinfection (Murray et al., 1973). The physiological meaning of *persisting* secretory antibodies in humans is not known. It is possible that cervical s-IgA antibodies provide some protection against tubal damage (Puolakkainen et al., 1986), although, according to Bienenstock and Befus (1983), the concentration of secretory antibodies falls rapidly in the absence of continuous antigenic stimulation. Salpingitis patients with persisting cervical antichlamydial IgA antibodies were treated and became chlamydial culture-negative from the cervix (Puolakkainen et al., 1986). Whether *C. trachomatis* remains in the upper genital tract is not known.

It is possible that early chlamydial genital infection produces short-lived immunity in humans. This is suggested by the observed lower isolation rate of *C. trachomatis* in patients with early exposure to sexually transmitted diseases (probably to *C. trachomatis*) than in those without such exposure (Alani et al., 1977; Jones and Batteiger, 1986). According to Schachter and associates (1983), men with gonococcal urethritis had high prevalence of micro-IF antibodies against *C. trachomatis* (94% had IgG and 36% IgM antichlamydial antibodies), suggesting repeated earlier exposure to *C. trachomatis*. The organism was not isolated from these men, although 20% of their female partners harbored chlamydiae in the cervix. In clinical practice, reinfection from untreated sexual partners is still a frequent cause of treatment failure. Evidence of a partial resistance to reinfection has thus been noted.

In vitro, antibodies can neutralize the infectivity of *C. trachomatis* and subsequently prevent infection (Caldwell and Perry, 1982). However, serum antibodies do not seem to protect individuals from mucosal infections, since antichlamydial antibody prevalence is high among patients with genital chlamydial infection (Schachter et al., 1979a). The occurrence of antichlamydial IgG antibodies was equal in infants who did and did not develop chlamydial eye infection (Persson et al., 1986). Nevertheless, the IgG antichlamydial antibodies might play a role in hindering the spread of the infection. Osser and Persson (1984) showed that females harboring *C. trachomatis* in the cervix, and with no detectable antichlamydial antibodies or very low titers of such antibodies, developed salpingitis after abortion more often than females with high antichlamydial antibody titers. Moreover, neonates exposed to *C. trachomatis* during delivery can develop conjunctivitis soon after birth, whereas pneumonitis is seen first when the titer of transplacentally acquired maternal antibodies is declining (Schachter et al., 1979b; Kunimoto and Brunham, 1985).

Antichlamydial serum antibodies detected by complement fixation test do not correlate with resistance to primary and secondary rechallenge in experimental trachoma (Hanna et al., 1982). Recent qualitative analysis of antibodies against *C. trachomatis* antigens by immunoblotting has supported the concept that humoral immune response to the agent correlates with protection against ascending *C. trachomatis* infections in females (Brunham et al., 1987). The latter authors analyzed serum antichlamydial antibodies and the IgG class specificity in sera from women undergoing therapeutic abortion. Ten of these 52 women developed postabortal salpingitis. The risk of ascending *C. trachomatis* infection after therapeutic abortion was associated with low titers of serum antibodies to *C. trachomatis,* as was earlier found by Osser and Persson (1984). Such association has also been demonstrated in the absence of serum antibodies to chlamydial antigens with molecular weights of 29, 32, 75, and 100 kDa (Brunham et al., 1987).

In vitro, *C. trachomatis* is able to stimulate human B lymphocytes to proliferate and can induce differentiation of B cells to immunoglobulin-secreting plasma cells (Bard and Levitt, 1984). Elementary bodies of *C. trachomatis* induce umbilical cord mononuclear cells to proliferate and produce lymphokines and IgM antibodies (Räsänen et al., 1986). As neonatal cells lack previous contact with antigens, this finding suggests that *C. trachomatis* contains mitogenic components. The mitogenicity of *C. trachomatis* probably explains some features of chlamydial infections. Mitogens activate cells to produce a variety of antibodies, including autoantibodies. Autoantibodies have been detected in patients with chlamydial salpingitis (Anderson and Møller, 1982) and lymphogranuloma venereum (Lassus et al., 1970). Newborns with chlamydial pneumonia have peripheral blood B lymphocytosis, plasmacytosis, and hyperimmunoglobulinemia (Levitt et al., 1983). Dense infiltrations of plasma cells and lymphoid follicles in the stroma is a histopathological characteristic of chlamydial cervicitis and endometritis (Kiviat et al., 1988; Paavonen et al., 1986). All these phenomena suggest that *C. trachomatis* is also a polyclonal B-cell activator in vivo.

CELL-MEDIATED IMMUNE RESPONSE

Cell-mediated immunity (CMI) in chlamydial infection is still not well understood. Thus comparatively few studies have dealt with cell-mediated immunity in humans infected with *C. trachomatis*.

Skin tests with chlamydial antigen (Frei skin test) had traditionally been used to diagnose lymphogranuloma venereum (LGV) infection by *C. trachomatis* (serotypes L_1–L_3) (see also Chapter 21). The test was believed to detect delayed hypersensitivity to LGV agents (Fig. 21). However, the test remains negative in the majority of patients with LGV and often gives false-positive reactions (Schachter et al., 1969), which is why it cannot be recommended as a diagnostic tool. In trachoma patients, skin test positivity is associated with severe upper tarsal disease in adults, whereas children are generally negative (Sowa et al., 1965; Ballard, 1982; cf. Monnickendam and Pearce, 1983).

Reinfection and the host's immune response seem important in the development of severe inflammatory changes leading to blindness in trachoma. In all likelihood, cell-mediated immune reactions are not exclusively of a protective nature in trachoma. Cell-mediated immunity may be involved not only in the healing but also in the scarring process of that disease. The majority of cases of chlamydial conjunctivitis (paratrachoma) (i.e., cases infected with *C. trachomatis*, serotypes D–K) are skin test (Frei test) -negative (Barwell et al., 1967). Skin tests in the great majority of patients with isolation-positive, uncomplicated chlamydial genital tract infection are also negative (Barwell et al., 1967). A cell-mediated immune response can, however, be detected in compli-

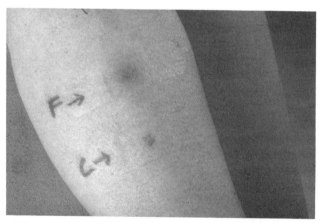

FIGURE 21. A positive skin test (Frei test) indicating delayed hypersensitivity to *C. trachomatis*. (Courtesy of Dr. D. Oriel.)

cated genital infections, such as salpingitis (Hallberg et al., 1985) (see also below).

Cellular immune response in chlamydial infection has also been tested by in vitro methods, such as the lymphocyte transformation test (LTT) (Hanna et al., 1979). Generally, results obtained by skin testing correlate well with those of in vitro tests for cellular immunity. However, chlamydial genital infections seem to be an exception, as positive LTT results are often seen in skin test-negative cases (Barwell et al., 1967; Brunham et al., 1981).

The LTT has been performed by culturing lymphocytes from patients in the presence of chlamydial antigen and tritiated thymidine. If the lymphocytes are sensitized, they respond by transformation into actively dividing blasts. The transformation and accompanying increased DNA synthesis have been assayed by measuring the uptake of tritiated thymidine with a liquid scintillation counter. Brunham and associates (1981) studied the optimal conditions of this assay in chlamydial infections.

An in vitro LTT with chlamydial antigen has been studied in patients with ankylosing spondylitis (Pattin et al., 1976), Reiter's disease (Schachter and Dawson, 1978), and lower (Brunham et al., 1981; Brunham et al., 1982a; Qvigstad et al., 1984) and upper (Hallberg et al., 1985) genital tract infections.

Chlamydia trachomatis-specific LTT response has been considered a specific marker for chlamydial infection, since patients with positive chlamydial culture and/or serological evidence of present or past chlamydial infection had higher LT stimulation indices (LTSI) than patients without such evidence (Brunham et al., 1981, 1982a). Brunham et al. (1981, 1982a) also found a positive correlation between LTSI and the chlamydial inclusion count in lower genital tract samples. They concluded that LTSI reflect the antigenic mass of organism present. No correlation was found between LTTs and antibody titer levels, degree of inflammatory changes, or localization of infection in female patients with cervicitis (Qvigstad et al., 1984) or in those with salpingitis (Hallberg et al., 1985).

Hallberg and co-workers (1985) demonstrated a more long-lasting response in LTTs in salpingitis patients with than without perihepatitis. This might indicate a cellular immune component in the pathogenesis of Fitz-Hugh–Curtis syndrome caused by *C. trachomatis*. A high LTSI was found to correlate more reliably with current infection than the serum antichlamydial antibody titers. After a chlamydial infection, antichlamydial antibodies persist longer than elevated LTSI (Brunham et al., 1982a).

Animal Models

In recent years animal models have been widely used to study different aspects of human (Table 10) and animal (Table 11) chlamydial infections (cf. Taylor-Robinson, 1986).

GUINEA PIGS

One of the first animal models used in chlamydial research was the guinea pig, in which eye, genital tract, and respiratory tract infections can be induced by the guinea pig inclusion conjunctivitis (GPIC) agent (cf. Murray, 1977; Barron et al., 1979, 1982, 1984; Rank et al., 1985). This agent is a member of the species *C. psittaci*.

In the guinea pig, GPIC infections are naturally acquired; they seem to spread via sexual transmission and induce genital infection. In general, intracytoplasmic chlamydial inclusions cannot be detected in clinical smears 20 days after infection with the GPIC agent. Such a spontaneous and rapid recovery from GPIC infection generally does not occur in many instances of human and other animal chlamydial infections.

The GPIC can cause nongonococcal urethritis (NGU) in male guinea pigs, and the infection can spread to female animals and cause cervicitis or vice versa. The target cell for the GPIC cervicitis is the stratified squamous epithelium of the endocervix (Barron et al., 1979). Hydrosalpinx was reported to develop as a consequence of salpingitis induced by the GPIC agent (Schachter et al., 1982c). The agent can also spread to the offspring of the guinea pig and cause conjunctivitis in the newborn animals.

The guinea pig model has also been widely used to study immunological aspects of chlamydial infections (Rank et al., 1979; Rank and Barron, 1983b; Batteiger and Rank, 1986). A short-lived immunity can be induced after both eye

TABLE 10. Animal Models for *C. trachomatis* Infections
(Including Immunological and Vaccine Studies)

Animal	Serotype	Organ system under study	Study [author(s) and year of publication]
Mice	A–C	Eye	Graham, 1965, 1967
		Respiratory	Kuo et al., 1982; Colley et al., 1986
	D–K	Genital	Graham, 1967
		Respiratory	Chen and Kuo, 1980; Williams et al., 1981; Kuo et al., 1982; Swenson et al., 1983; Swenson and Schachter, 1984
	L₁–L₃	Genital	Graham, 1967;
		Respiratory	Tuffrey and Taylor-Robinson, 1981; Kuo et al., 1982; Burnham et al., 1985a; Heggie et al., 1986; Tuffrey et al., 1982, 1984a,b, 1986a,b
Cats	A–C	Eye	Woodland et al., 1983
	D–K	Genital	
Rabbits	D–K	Genital	Smith et al., 1973
		Joints	
Monkeys			
Taiwan (*Macaca cyclopsis*)	A–C	Eye	Alexander and Chiang, 1967; Wang et al., 1967; Wang and Grayston, 1967; Gale et al., 1971
Owl (*Aotus trivirgatus*)	A–C	Eye	Murray et al., 1971
Cynomolgus (*Macaca fasicularis*)	A–C	Eye	Taylor et al., 1982a; Caldwell et al., 1987; Taylor and Prendergast, 1987
Grivet (*Ceropithecus aethiops*)	D–K	Genital	Ripa et al., 1979; Møller and Mårdh, 1980a,b, 1982; Møller et al., 1980, 1982; Møller, 1986
Pig-tailed (*Macaca nemestrina*)	D–K	Genital	Gale et al., 1977; Berger et al., 1984; Patton, 1985; Patton et al., 1982, 1983, 1986a, 1987a; Wølner-Hansen et al., 1986a
Marmoset (*Callithrix jacchus*)	D–K	Genital	Johnson et al., 1980, 1984
Rhesus (*Macaca mulatta*)		Genital	Smith et al., 1973
		Joints	Patton et al., 1987b
Chimpanzee (*Pan troglodytes*)		Genital	Jacobs et al., 1978; Taylor-Robinson et al., 1981
Baboon (*Papio cynocephalus*)		Genital	Darougar et al., 1977a
		Respiratory	Harrison et al., 1979a; DiGiacomo et al., 1975

TABLE 11. Models for Animal Chlamydial Infections

Animal	Chlamydial organism	Organ system under study	Study [author(s) and year of publication]
Guinea pigs	Guinea pig inclusion conjunctivitis (GPIC) agent	Eye Genital Respiratory	Barron et al., 1979 Rank et al., 1979, 1985 Rank and Barron, 1983a,b; Schachter et al., 1982c; Pasley et al., 1985a,b; Batteiger and Rank, 1986; Watkins et al., 1986
Mice	Mouse pneumonitis agent	Genital Respiratory	Kuo and Chen, 1980 Barron et al., 1981, 1984; Williams et al., 1981, 1982b; Swenson et al., 1983, 1986
Cats	Feline keratoconjunctivitis (FKC) agent	Eye Genital	Ostler, 1969 Darougar et al., 1977a; Woodland and Darougar, 1986

and genital challenge. Passive immunization, on the other hand, is not protective in recipient animals. Likewise, infection of pregnant animals does not convey immunity to the offspring.

Guinea pigs with GPIC agent infections of the conjunctival sac that had been infected with the agent previously are immune. The animals get a short-lived (12- to 48-hr) eye disease that is indistinguishable clinically and histologically from that observed after primary challenge. The same was true when Triton X-100-soluble extract of the agent was used for challenge. The findings were consistent with ocular delayed hypersensitivity. Such a hypersensitivity was also found when primary challenge was made at a remote site, i.e., the vagina or the intestinal tract (Watkins et al., 1986).

When cyclophosphamide is given, the guinea pig does not recover from the infection (Rank and Barron, 1983b). In experimentally infected guinea pigs given antithymocyte sera, no T-cell response was found. Delayed-type hypersensitivity to the GPIC agent could, however, be demonstrated (Rank and Barron, 1983a).

Estradiol given in high doses to gonadally intact guinea pigs resulted in a prolonged GPIC infection of the female genital tract. In addition, ascending genital and urinary tract infections (i.e., endometritis, cystic salpingitis, and cystitis) occurred more frequently than in controls. The antibody response to the GPIC agent was the same as that found in non-estradiol-treated animals (Barron, personal communication). However, the appearance of local antibodies in genital secretion was delayed. Prolonged infections were also observed in ovariectomized guinea pigs given doses of 10 μg estradiol per day (Pasley et al., 1985a).

MICE

In 1942 the mouse pneumonitis agent was isolated. Since then, very few (if any) strains of this agent have been reported as isolated. The mouse pneumonitis agent is classified as a *C. trachomatis* agent, and it produces inclusions in tissue cell cultures that stain with iodine.

The mouse pneumonitis agent disappears approximately 3 weeks after challenge. The immune response in the mouse is similar to that seen in experiments with the GPIC agent in the guinea pig. A strain-specific resistance to rechallenge occurs. This observation formed the basis for a subdivision of *C. trachomatis* (Alexander et al., 1967) before the micro-IF test was introduced (Wang and Grayston, 1970).

The mouse pneumonitis agent has been used experimentally in mice for the study of chlamydial genital (Barron et al., 1981, 1984; Swenson et al., 1983) as well as respiratory (Kuo and Chen, 1980; Williams et al., 1981a,b) tract infections.

The mouse pneumonitis agent can cause salpingitis, eventually involving tubal occlusion and formation of hydrosalpinx (Swenson et al., 1983). Recently, the effect of antibiotic treatment on the course of murine salpingitis and subsequent infertility was studied (Swenson et al., 1984, 1986). Tetracycline therapy had a protective effect on fertility when instituted before inoculation and, in most cases, one week after the challenge as well. However, when treatment was started two weeks after the inoculation, only marginal improvement of tubal pathology was seen, and there was no effect on the preservation of fertility.

Swiss-Webster mice become immune to rechallenge when infected vaginally with the mouse pneumonitis agent. A serum response with specific IgM antibodies occurred after 7 days, whereas IgG antibodies to the mouse pneumonitis agent were detected after 14 days. Antibodies in genital secretion occurred by day 20 postinfection. Delayed-type hypersensitivity developed 3 weeks after infection (Barron et al., 1984).

Both human oculogenital serotypes A–K and lymphogranuloma venereum serotypes L_1–L_3 of *C. trachomatis* have been used to produce ocular, lung, and genital infections in mice. Mice have been challenged with *C. trachomatis* and used in mouse toxicity prevention (neutralization) tests (Bernkopf, 1957; Wang and Grayston, 1963). Such tests were the first basis for a subdivision of the species into subspecies.

In the study of eye infections, ocular exposure to *C. trachomatis* serotype A resulted in sensitization as evidenced by early and delayed-type dermal reactivity and serotype-specific antibody formation against both live and irradiated EBs. This response can be transferred to unexposed mice via serum and lymphoid cells (Colley et al., 1986).

In the mice infected by *C. trachomatis,* patchy consolidations with luminal exudate and peribronchiolar cellular infiltrates were found. Chlamydial inclusions were detected in bronchiolar and alveolar cells. The inflammatory exudate consisted predominantly of lymphocytes and histiocytes (Graham, 1965; 1967).

White Swiss-Webster mice have also been used as models for the study of *C. trachomatis* pneumonitis (Chen and Kuo, 1980). The lung showed congestion and patchy consolidation. There were signs of interstitial pneumonitis with an extensive infiltration by neutrophils. The alveoli were filled with exudate. Chlamydial inclusions were present in the interstitium and bronchial epithelium. After 3 days, monocytic cells gradually became more dominant. The inflammation was not detectable after 10–14 days. Williams and co-workers (1982a) using *C57 black mice* obtained findings similar to those of Chen and Kuo (1980). The maximum inflammatory reaction, which was mild, appeared on days 7–10 and was dominated by lymphocytes. However, in contrast to the findings of Chen and Kuo (1980), little consolidation was found in the lungs. The early changes seen in the Swiss-Webster mice might have been attributable to a toxic, high-titer inoculum A humoral and cell-mediated immune response was first detected on day 7.

Strains of *C. trachomatis* were used to infect mice via the intrauterine route or into the ovarian bursa. Serotypes L_1 and L_2 did not produce inflammatory changes in the oviduct or the uterus. Endometritis and salpingitis did occur, however, when the mice were infected with serotypes D and E. The lesions occurred earlier in mice pretreated with progesterone. Susceptibility varied between different strains of mice. The lesions were more severe in *C3H mice* than in *T0 mice* (Tuffrey et al., 1986b).

Using both immunologically competent and nude mice, which they infected in the uterine cavity with a LGV strain, Tuffrey and Taylor-Robinson (1981) found progesterone to be a key factor in the development of *C. trachomatis* genital tract infections. This finding is in contrast to data derived in guinea pigs (Pasley et al., 1985b). Progesterone-treated *CBA mice* were rechallenged with a human strain of *C. trachomatis* in the uterine wall. The infection cleared significantly more quickly in previously infected animals than in controls. There was no difference in the susceptibility to infection between CBA mice with a distant past infection and low serum antichlamydial antibody titers, and recently challenged animals with high titers. Thus no protective effect of previous infection could be demonstrated.

Stephens and co-workers (1982b) used the mouse as a model to study the influence of corticosteroids on chlamydial infections. Mice have also been exposed to *C. trachomatis*, serotype L_2, in order to study this agent's possible oncogenic capacity in a cervical neoplastic model. No cervical abnormalities developed, which is in contrast to similar experiments conducted with cytomegalovirus (Heggie et al., 1986).

Mice have also been used as models for the study of systemic infections with serotypes L_1–L_3 of *C. trachomatis*. Pathological features resembled those of human lymphogranuloma venereum (LGV) infections. The infected animals developed resistance to reinfection on the basis of cellular immune mechanisms. Immune serum was not protective, whereas immune spleen cells were (Brunham et al., 1985a).

CATS

The cat has been used as a model for the study of eye and genital infections by the feline keratoconjunctivitis (FKC) agent. This agent is a member of the species *C. psittaci* (Ostler et al., 1969).

Feline keratoconjunctivitis genital infections can result in urethritis in male cats and in vaginitis in female cats. Urethritis in experimental infections continued for 4 weeks during which marked inflammatory urethral changes and discharge occurred. The vaginal infection is characterized by an increased discharge (Darougar et al., 1977a).

As stated above, cats have also been used as models for the study of eye infections (Woodland and Darougar, 1986). When the FKC agent was used in conjunction with cat streptococci, it produced more severe conjunctivitis than when used alone (Darougar et al., 1977a).

Chlamydia trachomatis has also been used to induce conjunctivitis in cats (Woodland et al., 1983).

MONKEYS

Inoculation of *C. trachomatis* in the cervix of *grivet monkeys* (*Ceropithecus aethiops*) can result in cervicitis (Møller, 1986) with a consequent spread of the agent to the endometrium and the fallopian tubes (Ripa et al., 1979; Møller and Mårdh, 1980a, 1982). Inflammatory signs were present in the tubes on day 3 postinfection. On days 7–21 a pronounced inflammatory reaction could be seen (Fig. 22). Thereafter, the lesions regressed. Tubal occlusion could be seen in some of the monkeys at follow-up. When the tubes were closed by ligature, salpingitis did not develop upon *C. trachomatis* inoculation in the cervix or the

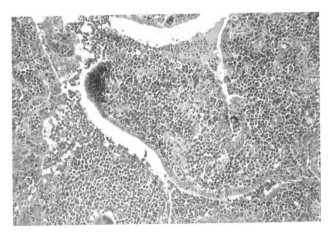

FIGURE 22. Section of a tube of a grivet monkey infected by *C. trachomatis*. (Courtesy of Dr. B. Møller.)

uterus (even after curettage), indicating a canalicular spread in chlamydial salpingitis (Møller and Mårdh, 1980a). Because salpingitis can result in tubal occlusion, it is tempting to believe that genital chlamydial infection plays a role in infertility.

The histological findings in the tubes of grivet monkeys were similar to those found in naturally acquired chlamydial infections in women. Thus a primarily polymorphonuclear cell response was found throughout the tubal wall. There was also a more or less complete destruction of the tubal cilia, and an inflammatory exudate in the tubal lamina (Møller and Mårdh, 1980a).

The grivet monkeys developed an antibody response with a conventional IgM and IgG switch. IgM antichlamydial antibody production was detected after 7 days, whereas IgG antichlamydial antibodies occurred after 10–21 days. The IgM antichlamydial antibody titers leveled off after 2–3 weeks and were not detectable 8 weeks postinoculation. The IgG antichlamydial antibody titer remained high during the study period (i.e., 12 weeks) (Ripa et al., 1979).

Grivet monkeys developed vasitis and epididymitis when injected in the vas deferens with *C. trachomatis* (Møller and Mårdh, 1980b). The infection caused a marked infiltration of polymorphonuclear leukocytes and lymphocytes throughout all layers of the spermatic cord (Fig. 23). Also, the ducts of the epididymis contained inflammatory cells (Fig. 24). These studies suggest a canalicular spread of chlamydiae in chlamydial epididymitis.

Berger (1984) used the *pig-tailed macaque (Macaca nemestrina)* as a prime model for chlamydial epididymitis. He also inoculated his animals through the spermatic cord and found a mononuclear perivascular inflammation in the area of the epididymis. The pig-tailed macaque has also been used as a model for

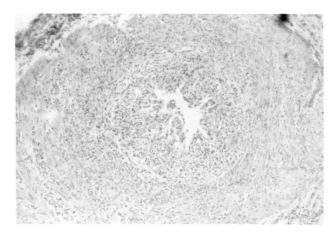

FIGURE 23. Section of the spermatic cord in a grivet monkey infected by *C. trachomatis* showing vasitis. (Courtesy of Dr. B. Møller.)

salpingitis (Patton et al., 1982, 1983, 1986a; Patton, 1987a; Wølner-Hanssen et al.,1986a).

Experimental primary infection of the fallopian tubes was produced by intratubal inoculation of *C. trachomatis,* serotypes E and F (Patton et al., 1982, 1983, 1987a). *Chlamydia trachomatis* was reisolated from both the endosalpinz

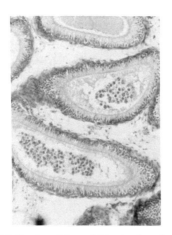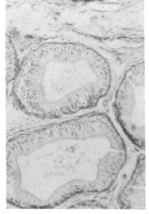

FIGURE 24. Section of the epididymis of a grivet monkey (to the left) and of a control animal (to the right) that, after infection with *C. trachomatis,* developed epididymitis. (Courtesy of Dr. B. Møller.)

and the endocervix 1 week after the inoculation. A moderate lymphocytic infiltration was detected in the submucosa by day 7. By days 14 and 21 the lymphocytic infiltration was heavy and extended into the submucosa. By day 35 the inflammatory cell response had spontaneously subsided, although epithelial cell injury persisted. The presence of *C. trachomatis* was demonstrated by immunofluorescence and immunoperoxidase staining with monoclonal antibody to *C. trachomatis*. Only secretory cells contained chlamydial inclusions.

Because a single inoculation of *C. trachomatis* caused self-limited tubal disease (Patton et al., 1982) and no residual tubal damage, the effects of repeated homologous and heterologous chlamydial inoculations were studied (Patton et al., 1987a). The fallopian tubes were infected with *C. trachomatis* for 4 consecutive months. Homologous reinfections produced the most severe scarring and adhesion formation. Thick, widespread adhesions involved the uterus, the bladder, the bowel, and the anterior abdominal wall. Heterologous reinfections produced widespread scarring but fewer adhesions. Thus repeated inoculations of live genital strains of *C. trachomatis* produced extensive tubal scarring, adhesion formation, and obstruction that were not apparent in primary chlamydial infection. The findings were similar to those for women with recurrent salpingitis.

The effect of repeated cervical infections with *C. trachomatis* after a single tubal inoculation of the organism was studied in the pig-tailed macaque by Wølner-Hanssen and associates (1986a). A severe salpingitis resulted.

The effect of preimmunization on distal tubal disease has also been studied in monkeys. Since no destruction of infected fallopian tubes was observed after chlamydial infection in organ cultures (Hutchinson et al., 1979)—which, however, is technically difficult to induce since, for example, tissue cell cultures cannot possibly be centrifuged as monolayer tissue cell cultures—it was thought that other microorganisms might be responsible for the adnexal scarring following *C. trachomatis* infection. Pig-tailed monkeys infected repeatedly in the cervix were given a single inoculation of *C. trachomatis* directly in the fallopian tubes. No visible salpingitis was produced after cervical inoculation, but severe tubal disease with extensive adhesions followed a single tubal inoculation. Histopathological studies of the tubes showed plasma cells scattered throughout the submucosal tissue. Patchy epithelial lesions showed extensive deciliation with altered tubal architecture. Myometritis was found in the uterus. These findings suggest that the host immune response to repeated chlamydial genital inoculations produces severe tubal disease with irreversible tissue damage, a disease process similar to ocular trachoma (Duke-Elder, 1965). Such a view is in accordance with the demonstration of a cell-mediated immune response to *C. trachomatis* in patients with acute salpingitis (Hallberg et al., 1985).

A subcutaneous pocket model for chlamydial salpingitis based on subcutaneous tubal transplants was developed by Patton and associates (1986a,

1987b, 1988). The advantage of this model is that several isolated pockets (up to 20) can be established as autografts in each animal and studied separately. The model allows for studies to define temporally related events of infection and histological alterations. In addition, immunocompetent cells involved in tubal infections can be investigated. The disadvantage is that the pocket model does not allow for studies of the natural history process and of macroscopic changes of the tubes in salpingitis, or the evaluation of possible relationships between cervical and tubal infections. Patton et al. (1986a) demonstrated that subcutaneously implanted fallopian tube transplants are susceptible to *C. trachomatis* infection. The microbiological and histopathological features were similar to those found in intact monkeys directly inoculated with *C. trachomatis* in the fallopian tubes (Patton, 1985). An acute inflammatory reaction occurred in the autograft during the first week of challenge. Thereafter chronic inflammatory changes were noted. The subcutaneous model can serve as a substitute for the intact monkey model. It is useful for the study of the immunopathology of tubal *C. trachomatis* infection, acquired immunity against *C. trachomatis,* and prevention of infection by immunization. The kinetics of the immune response can also be studied with this model, as can the influence of hormones on infection.

Marmoset monkeys (Callithrix jacchus) have been used for the study of chlamydial cervicitis. The animals were culture-positive for 2 to 5 weeks after infection. The infection cleared within a week in the case of previously infected animals. A mucopurulent cervicitis developed in some nonpreviously exposed animals, whereas other monkeys showed only minimal inflammatory changes. There was a predominance of polymorphonuclear leukocytes, but a few mononuclear leukocytes were also detected (A. P. Johnson et al., 1984).

Monkeys have also been used as models for the study of *C. trachomatis* eye infections. Wang and Grayston (1967) used *Taiwan monkeys (Macaca cyclopsis)* in experimental vaccine trials and for serological studies of trachoma (Wang and Grayston, 1971). Alexander and Chiang (1967) studied pregnant monkeys and their offspring after infection with TRIC agents.

Caldwell and co-workers (1987) used *cynomolgus monkeys (Macaca fasicularis)* to identify chlamydial antigen in tears. Tear IgA antibody specific for major outer membrane protein (MOMP) was detectable 14 days postinfection, whereas antichlamydial IgA antibodies specific for LPS or 60-kDa and 68-kDa polypeptide fragments were not detectable until day 21. The antibodies persisted for weeks after the peak of clinical disease, in contrast to tear antichlamydial IgG antibodies, which peaked 4 weeks postinfection when maximal inflammation was detected.

Owl monkeys (Aotus trivirgatus) have been used in vaccination trials with inactivated (irradiated) *C. trachomatis* organisms. Vaccine was applied topically to the eyes. The animals developed eye infection on rechallenge, although the infection had a prolonged course and produced more ocular discharge than in nonvaccinated controls. Antichlamydial antibody titers in serum and tears were 10 times higher in the vaccinated monkeys than in the controls (Murray et al., 1971).

Baboons (*Papio cynocephalus*) have been used as models for the study of *C. trachomatis*-induced pneumonitis. Subjects showed patchy and nodular areas of interstitial peribronchiolar and perivascular infiltrations with lymphocytes, plasma cells, eosinophils, and neutrophils. There were germinal centers within nodules. Plugs of inflammatory exudate were seen in airways within nodules. No chlamydiae could be reisolated from the baboons (Harrison et al., 1979a). The animals also developed nasopharyngitis. Baboons have also been used as animal models to study infections by human *C. psittaci* strains, i.e., IOL-207 (a TWAR strain). The infection produced urethritis and conjunctivitis (Darougar et al., 1977a).

KOALAS

Natural *C. psittaci* infections in koalas occur in certain areas of Australia. The infection causes salpingitis with tubal occlusion and is a cause of infertility. Under experimental conditions, the agent was found to be transmitted by sexual intercourse between koalas (Brown and Grice, 1986). This mode of transmission also seems to exist under natural conditions.

Diagnosis

Diagnosis of Chlamydial Infections

ISOLATION

Host–Parasite Interactions

Chlamydiae are obligate intracellular parasites and therefore require living (eukaryotic) cells to reproduce. The earliest methods used to isolate chlamydiae (i.e., laboratory animals and embryonated hen's eggs) were too insensitive, laborious, and expensive to be employed for large-scale use in routine diagnostic work. The first tissue cell culture used to recover *C. trachomatis* employed McCoy cells that were exposed to irradiation 5 days before use (Gordon and Quan, 1965). Irradiated cells are cumbersome to use, which limits their general application in clinical diagnostic laboratories.

The application of cytostatics rather than irradiation as a pretreatment of host cells for chlamydiae represented a simplification and a new possibility for routinely diagnosing chlamydial infections in the clinical laboratory. When using cells treated with the cytostatic drug cycloheximide (Ripa and Mårdh, 1977), which today is the most widely used drug for the isolation of *C. trachomatis,* fresh cells can be used. This is thought to increase the sensitivity of the culture technique. Employing other previously recommended cytostatic drugs, i.e., cytochalasin B (Sompolinsky and Richmond, 1974) and iodoxyuridine (IUdR) (Wenthworth and Alexander, 1974), meant that the cell treatment had to be performed at least 3 days in advance of infection.

Both irradiation and treatment with cytostatics reduce the metabolic turnover of the host cell, which is considered advantageous to the chlamydial parasite. The chlamydiae are "energy parasites," which by virtue of the cell treatment are believed to gain better access to high-energy compounds (ATP) stored by the host cell.

When using HeLa 229 cells (Kuo et al., 1972), treatment with the macromolecule DEAE-dextran enhances susceptibility to chlamydial infection. The DEAE-dextran treatment can be administered in conjunction with the infection. Today this method is used by comparatively few laboratories but has been employed with great success since the beginning of the 1970s.

DEAE-dextran treatment facilitates the initial contact between the parasite and the host cell; when this procedure is used, neither irradiation nor cytostatic treatment is required. The DEAE-dextran treatment is aimed at reducing the negative charge of the host cell surface. Treatment enhances the uptake of serotypes D–K, but not that of serotypes L_1–L_3.

A method involving irradiation of McCoy cells (i.e., irradiation from a Cobolt cannon or an X-ray machine) is described in detail in Table 12, and the cycloheximide treatment is described in Table 13.

Recently, Woodland and co-workers (1987) used mitomycin-C, a drug that acts on eukaryotic cells by producing crosslinks between strands of DNA, for pretreatment of McCoy cells to be infected by *C. trachomatis*. The authors found this method more sensitive than cycloheximide treatment. By the mitomycin-C method 28 of 321 genital samples were positive for *C. trachomatis*, as compared with 21 positives by the cycloheximide method. The authors also found that chlamydial inclusions in mitomycin-C-treated cells became larger than those in cycloheximide-treated cells. The cells were treated with mitocin C overnight before infection could take place. Thereafter they were trypsinized in order to produce cell monolayers in test tubes, which were infected by clinical samples after a cell sheet had been formed.

TABLE 12. Techniques for Isolation of *C. trachomatis*
in Irradiated McCoy Cells[a]

McCoy cells are cultured in Eagle's medium, containing 10% horse serum, 30 μg/ml glucose, 200 μg/ml ristocetin, and 100 μg/ml streptomycin.
↓
The cells are exposed to 5000 rad (γ radiation from a cobalt-60 cannon).
↓
Five days later, the cells are transferred to flat-bottomed tubes containing cover slips.
↓
A monolayer is formed after 2 days, when it is ready for inoculation.
↓
An 0.5 ml specimen is centrifuged at 1600 g for 1 hr onto the cell sheet.
↓
Incubation is made for 48 hr at 35°C.
↓
Cells are stained with iodine after being fixed in methanol.

---

[a]From Gordon and Quan (1965).

TABLE 13. Culture of *C. trachomatis* in Cycloheximide-Treated McCoy Cells

Culture McCoy cells in RPMI 1640 (Flow, Ltd.) supplemented with 10% fetal calf serum, 1% glutamine, 10 μg/ml gentamicin, and 2.5 μg/ml amphotericin B.

↓

Transfer 3- to 4-day-old cells (1 ml of 1.5×10^5 cells/ml) to flat-bottomed plastic tubes containing a cover slip or to microtitration plates.

↓

Incubate cell culture for 24 hr at 37°C.

↓

Remove culture medium and inoculate clinical specimen in equal volume with fresh culture medium (as above but with 0.5% (w/v) glucose and 100 μg vancomycin/ml).

↓

Centrifuge 3000–4000 g for 1 hr at 35°C.

↓

Remove medium and add 2 ml of the culture medium described above, i.e., with glucose and vancomycin but with the addition of 1–2 μg/ml of cycloheximide.

↓

Incubate cell culture for 72 hr at 35–37°C.

↓

Stain cover slips with iodine and mount them cell side down on slides, or stain with labeled monoclonal antibodies to *C. trachomatis*.

↓

Examine under a light (×1000–1250) or fluorescent microscope (×400) for chlamydial inclusions.

Cell Lines and Comparison of Cell Treatments

McCoy cells (L cells) are currently used by the vast majority of laboratories for the isolation of *C. trachomatis*. The McCoy cell line that is used today for the isolation of chlamydiae cannot be distinguished from the tumor mouse fibroblast cell line L929 (Blyth and Taverne, 1974). It is thought that the McCoy cells originally used for the isolation of chlamydiae were human synovial cells, and the story goes that the McCoy cells were at some time exchanged (due to contamination) for L cells in one of the laboratories that first used McCoy cells for isolating chlamydiae.

Baby hamster kidney (BHK) 21 cells (Blyth and Taverne, 1974) have also been used by some laboratories, while others have employed or still employ Buffalo Green monkey (BGM) cells (Hobson et al., 1982a; Wills et al., 1984). Such cells treated with DEAE-dextran seem to be as susceptible as cyclohexi-mide-treated McCoy cells to infection by *C. trachomatis*.

As mentioned, some laboratories have worked with HeLa 229 cells for the isolation of chlamydiae (Kuo et al., 1972).

Croy and co-workers (1975) compared 11 cell lines for their susceptibility to infection by chlamydiae. They found HeLa 229 to be the most susceptible cell line when used in conjunction with DEAE-dextran treatment. It seems, however, that cycloheximide-treated McCoy cells have advantages over dextran-treated HeLa 229 cells for routine diagnostic laboratories.

In comparative tests using different treatments of McCoy cells, cycloheximide treatment rendered cells most susceptible to infection by *C. trachomatis* (as indicated by the number of inclusion formation units (IFU) found in experimentally infected cell cultures). Cycloheximide, cytochalasin B, IUdR, emetine, hydrocortisone, irradiation, and no treatment were employed (Evans and Taylor-Robinson, 1979). Assigning an index of 1.000 to the result of the cycloheximide treatment, the other treatments gave indices of 0.140, 0.119, 0.480, 0.125, 0.180, and 0.110, respectively.

Oyelese and associates (1987) recently described a modified culture method using HeLa 229 cells treated with cycloheximide. In this modified method, freshly trypsinized HeLa cells (in suspension) are used. Of 1085 clinical specimens, 84 were positive by both the standard (cycloheximide-treated McCoy cells in monolayer) and modified (HeLa 229) techniques. Two samples were positive only in the standard method and 21 only in the suspension method ($p <$ 0.001). The mean IFU in the 86 specimens by the monolayer method was $\log_{10}$ 2.99 ± 0.95 per coverslip and in the 105 specimens positive by the suspension method $\log_{10}$ 3.25 ± 1.09 per coverslip. Of the 19 specimens detected as positive by the suspension method, only 11 were positive for *C. trachomatis* by ELISA (Oyelese et al., 1987). There are, however, conflicting results regarding the benefit of using trypsinized cells for the detection of *C. trachomatis* infection (Kordova and Witt, 1980). Thus McCoy cells used in monolayer cultures have been found to be at least as sensitive as trypsinized McCoy cells (Hipp et al., 1983). The trypsinization was done with the aid of a 0.5 mg/ml suspension of trypsin added to the culture for 4 min at 35°C. Inactivation of the trypsin was achieved by adding fresh growth medium and certain additives to the culture.

The use of nontreated cells for the culture of *C. trachomatis* has been reported by single groups to be successful in the case of BHK 21 cells (Blyth and Taverne, 1974) and McCoy cells (Hobson et al., 1974). Many other groups that have used such a procedure could not report the same positive outcome.

Both HeLa 229 and McCoy cells have been used to isolate TWAR chlamydiae. Some researchers have claimed the former cell type to be more susceptible than the latter to TWAR infection, whereas others have found the two cell types to be equally useful. A combination of DEAE-dextran and cycloheximide treatment as well as centrifugation have made isolation possible or have increased the recovery rate (Kuo et al., 1986b, 1988) (see also Chapter 36).

Tissue Culture Medium

Eagle's Minimum Essential Medium (MEM) was previously used by most laboratories as a tissue culture medium for *Chlamydia*. However, the use of

RPMI 1640 medium (Flow Laboratories, Ltd.) has been found to increase the sensitivity of the cycloheximide method, and RPMI now seems to be employed by many laboratories as the standard culture medium for the isolation of chlamydiae (Mårdh, 1984).

In order to obtain optimal culture results, the use of combinations of antimicrobials that can inhibit bacterial and fungal overgrowth is important (Wentworth, 1973; Yoder et al., 1986; cf. Mårdh, 1984). In recent years, a combination of gentamicin, amphotericin, and vancomycin often has been used for this purpose.

Centrifugation

Except for when DEAE-dextran treatment is used, all techniques described for the isolation of *C. trachomatis* involve centrifugation of cell cultures in order to increase infectivity. Centrifugation has been found to be essential for the recovery of all serotypes of *C. trachomatis* with the exception of L_1-L_3. However, centrifugation may indeed enhance the yield of these three serotypes as well. Usually centrifugation by at least 3000–4000 g for 1 hr is recommended (Reeve et al., 1975). The centrifugation must be done in a centrifuge that allows regulation of the temperature, which should not exceed 37.0°C, at which point the host cell/chlamydiae interaction is maximal. Centrifugation at 36°C is often preferred. At above 38°C the chlamydiae will die rapidly.

In the method involving HeLa 229 cells and DEAE-dextran treatment (Kuo et al., 1972), centrifugation is not needed for *C. trachomatis,* because the macromolecule promotes the absorption of chlamydiae to the cell sheet.

Vials/Microtiter Plates

Some workers have used plastic vials with flat bottoms on which glass cover slips are laid to culture cells for infection by chlamydiae (Fig. 25). Today many laboratories prefer to culture the cells in microtiter plates (Yoder et al., 1986), which are centrifuged after inoculation with clinical samples. Standard microtiter plates with 96 wells have been found to be less sensitive than plates with fewer wells because each of the small wells in the 96-well plate holds too few cells.

The use of multiwell plates poses a potential specificity problem owing to the possibility of samples becoming mixed. This problem should be considered by every laboratory employing multiwell plates for culture.

Sampling Sites

The choice of sampling site(s) can influence the likelihood of recovering *C. trachomatis.* The use of both urethral and cervical cultures increases the recovery rate of *C. trachomatis* from the female genital tract by as much as 10–20% as

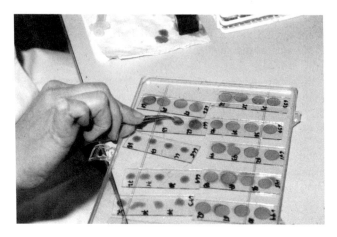

FIGURE 25. Isolation of *C. trachomatis* in cycloheximide-treated McCoy cells. Infected cells grown on cover slips for 72 hr were stained with iodine for detection of chlamydial inclusions.

compared with cervical sampling only. Rectal cultures add little to the recovery rate except for homosexual men. Neither does the study of pharyngeal swabs increase the percentage of culture-positive chlamydial conjunctivitis cases, nor sampling from the clinically nonaffected eye in cases of unilateral conjunctivitis (see also under "Diagnosis" of each disease entity).

The detection of genital chlamydial infections by culture depends not only on the number of sites sampled (e.g., urethra, cervix, and rectum) but also on the number of samples collected from each site. For example, the second and even the third consecutively collected cervical sample is often more positive than the first specimen sampled.

Blind Passages

In cultures using microtiter plates, the use of blind passages has been found by some workers to increase the sensitivity of the chlamydial culture method. Jones and associates (1986a) found an increase of 18% of endocervical, 28% of female urethral and 29% of male urethral cultures when using one passage. In tests of 221 samples subjected to five serial passages, 83 were positive; 29 (35%) only after two or more passages. The endocervical samples that were positive without passage often produced a great number of inclusions. The authors used 96-well microtiter plates. Other investigators (Stephens et al., 1982c; Stamm et al., 1983) used one blind passage. Their studies showed a less significant increase (1% to 3%) in the positivity rate by passaging. Some studies (Schachter,

1985; Schachter and Martin, 1987) using test tubes and glass slides showed that the vial system is more sensitive than culture in plates and that the effect of blind passages was negligible when vials were used.

Detection of Chlamydial Inclusions

For the detection of chlamydial inclusions in tissue cell cultures, Giemsa staining (Fig. 26) has been used by some laboratories, particularly those using the HeLa 229 culture system, whereas iodine staining (Fig. 27) has often been used by laboratories employing McCoy cells. During recent years, however, iodine staining has been exchanged for staining with labeled monoclonal anti-chlamydial antibodies in many laboratories (Fig. 28); the new method is thought to be more sensitive than iodine staining. The use of monoclonals rather than iodine is advantageous in that the cultures are less tiring to read, particularly when a large number of samples must be processed. Staining with labeled mono-clonals also accelerates the reading and is therefore time and labour saving. A disadvantage of using monoclonals is that a good fluorescence microscope is needed, which is expensive to purchase as are antibody preparations.

The monoclonal antibody used for detection of growth can explain differences in the detection rate of *C. trachomatis*. Thus a genus-reactive mono-clonal antibody might be less efficient than a MOMP-specific monoclonal antibody.

Immunoperoxidase staining can also be used (Fig. 29). This latter technique has the advantage of not requiring a fluorescence microscope. However, it has

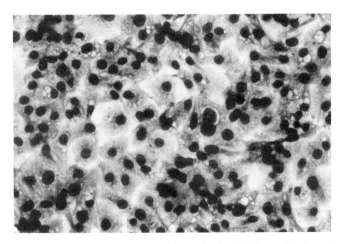

FIGURE 26. Giemsa-stained chlamydial inclusion in a McCoy cell culture (×400).

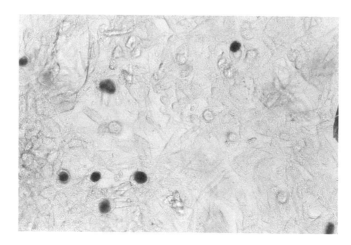

FIGURE 27. McCoy cells stained with Lugol's solution (iodine), demonstrating intracytoplasmic inclusions of *C. trachomatis* (×400). A color version of this figure appears following p. xvi.

not yet been widely used, partly because inclusions are more difficult to detect with immunoperoxidase than with labeled monoclonals.

Independent of which staining method is used, the experience of the microscopist in reading chlamydial tests is important. Artifacts mimicking chlamydial inclusions are commonly found in clinical samples (see below).

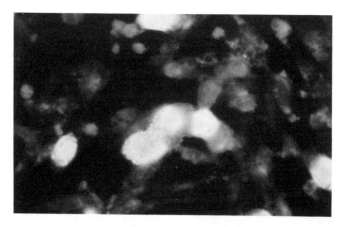

FIGURE 28. McCoy cells stained with fluorescein-labeled monoclonal antibodies showing chlamydial inclusions (×400). A color version of this figure appears following p. xvi.

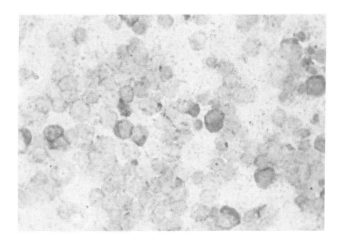

FIGURE 29. Chlamydial inclusions in McCoy cells stained with immunoperoxidase (×400). A color version of this figure appears following p. xvi.

Incubation

By current tissue cell culture techniques, incubation at 37°C for 48–72 hr is required for diagnosing *C. trachomatis* infections. Whether 2 or 3 days incubation should be used depends on the technique used to read the cultures and the time requirements for culture diagnosis, along with other factors.

Some workers state that the incubation period for tissue cell cultures can be reduced from 72 to 48 hr without reducing the sensitivity of the method, if monoclonal rather than iodine staining is used. Others feel that such a shortened incubation time decreases sensitivity too much to be acceptable. Data have also been published that favor increased sensitivity with a short (48 hr) incubation time (Thomas et al., 1977).

For the isolation of TWAR chlamydiae, using HeLa 229 cells, a three-day incubation at 35°C was found to be better than 37°C (Kuo and Grayston, 1988).

Sensitivity of Culture

Chlamydial culturing—as compared to direct-specimen antigen detection tests (see below)—is still the most sensitive technique in current use for the diagnosis of *C. trachomatis* infection in the genital tract of both males and females (Stamm et al., 1984a; Lipkin et al., 1986) as well as of the eyes and the nasopharynx of both neonates and adults (Stenberg and Mårdh, 1987).

Although culturing is the most sensitive diagnostic method available, one will probably still miss up to one-fifth or one-fourth of all chlamydial infections in cases subjected to testing. The situation is even worse when using direct-specimen antigen detection tests (see also section on diagnosis of chlamydial infections by direct analysis of clinical samples). However, the use of these tests in areas where cultures are not possible represents progress. In laboratories that used optimized culture techniques, the change to direct-specimen antigen detection tests most likely meant a decrease in the quality of diagnostic performance.

FACTORS INTERFERING WITH ISOLATION OF CHLAMYDIA TRACHOMATIS

Toxic Sampling Swabs

The type of sampling swab used for collecting specimens is important to the sensitivity of the detection method, as many swabs have proved toxic for chlamydiae (Mårdh and Zeeberg, 1981). Swabs tipped with calcium alginate are particularly toxic, although certain cotton-tipped wooden sticks can also be rather toxic. In one study of 14 different swabs in experiments with laboratory strains of C. trachomatis, only 7 of the swabs gave a 50% recovery rate as compared to the most optimal swab (Mahony and Chernesky, 1985). These latter authors also found swabs provided by commercial companies for collection of ELISA samples to be toxic for McCoy cells.

In order to increase the recovery rate of chlamydiae, brushes primarily used for the sampling of cervical specimens for cytological smears were recently recommended for chlamydial sampling (Trimbos and Arentz, 1986). Such brushes are believed to be more effective than cotton-tipped swabs because they supposedly provide more cells and therefore more chlamydiae in the sample

TABLE 14. Comparison of Results of Cultures for C. trachomatis when Sampling Swab Was Shaken (and Discharged Thereafter) or Maintained in Transportation Medium

Sex	Type of sampling swab used	Sampling swab in transportation medium	Number of patients	Number of culture-positive patients(%)	Number of inclusions
Males	ENT	Maintained	69	17 (25)	3423
	Inolex type 1	Shaken		19 (28)	5086
Females	ENT	Maintained	49	6 (15)	3268
	Torrent sterile applicator	Shaken		6 (15)	7376

TABLE 15. *C. trachomatis,* Immunotype
E, in Cycloheximide-Treated McCoy Cell
Cultures Inoculated with Specimens
Stored in Plastic Test Tubes for 48 hr in
the Presence of Various Sampling Swabs

Sampling swab used	Percent inclusions[a]
Inolex	
I	12.5
II	0.0
IV	8.3
Ultrafine	15.4
Medical wire, ENT	63.5
Torrent	7.5
Pure wraps	4.0

[a]As compared to controls.

obtained. Comparative tests, however, have given contradictory results. The cytological brush sampling technique seems advantageous if it is used after a cotton-tipped swab has been introduced into the cervical canal to clear away pus and cervical secretion. The possible increased risk of inducing an ascendance of a cervical chlamydial infection by the use of cytological brushes must also be evaluated before general use can be recommended.

In order to reduce the toxic effect of sampling swabs, experiments were performed in which the infected swab was vigorously shaken in the test tube before withdrawal from the transport medium. These experiments (Mårdh and Zeeberg, 1981) indicated that the toxicity of the swabs (Table 14) could be partly avoided by such a procedure, but the culture result was dependent on how effective the shaking had been before the swab was discarded (Table 15). It was believed that in a doctor's office lacking facilities for mechanical shaking (e.g., a table mixer) and with a busy practice that does not permit a lengthy manual shaking of test tubes, it is better to leave the swab in the test tube during transport to the laboratory. Furthermore, the local laboratory has to check whether the swabs used in their catchment region for sampling for chlamydiae are suitable for the purpose (nontoxic, etc.) (Mahony and Chernesky, 1985).

Inhibitory Body Fluid Constituents

To obtain optimal isolation results, cultures should preferably *not* be made from the first sample taken from the cervix. The first swab seems to absorb too much mucopurulent cervical secretion, which either contains fewer chlamydial particles (EBs) or is more toxic than subsequently (second or third) collected specimens.

Not only female but also male genital secretion (i.e., seminal fluid) is toxic for *C. trachomatis* serotypes D–K as well as serotypes L_1–L_3 (Mårdh et al., 1980a). Whether dilution of certain types of samples (in transport medium or tissue culture medium) in conjunction with the sampling will increase the recovery rate is not known.

In experimental infections of cycloheximide-treated McCoy cells, the presence of seminal fluid reduced the chlamydial inclusion count even when present in dilutions up to 1 : 1000 (Mårdh et al., 1980a). Analyses of constituents of seminal fluid for their possible antichlamydial effect showed that spermine, spermidine, zinc, and magnesium ions inhibited the formation of chlamydial inclusions. At high concentrations ($>1 : 64$), seminal fluid had a cytopathogenic effect. Inhibition of chlamydial growth by seminal fluid (Hanna et al., 1981) and constituents thereof (Greenberg et al., 1985) was also shown by others (see Chapter 9).

It has been stated that cycloheximide-treated McCoy cells should be somewhat more susceptible than IUdR-treated McCoy cells to the toxic effect of body fluids and to bacterial contamination. This is also the case when calf serum is added to the tissue cell culture medium (Schachter, 1984).

Toxic Glass and Plastic Wares

The test tube in which samples are sent to the laboratory can also contain substances (e.g., metal ions) that reduce the inclusion count or even completely hinder the detection of a chlamydial infection. Under experimental conditions, storage and culture of chlamydiae in acid-washed glass tubes has been found to give better results than the use of certain plastic tubes (Mårdh, unpublished data). Test-tube washing fluids can contain concentrations of certain metal ions that exceed even that of seminal fluid (see above).

Transport and Storage Conditions

In the temperate zones of the world, variations in transport temperature seem to play a minor role in the isolation of *C. trachomatis* (Kallings and Mårdh, 1982).

The sample should preferably be inoculated on tissue cell cultures on the same day that it was made, or at the latest the next day. Thus Mahony and Chernesky (1985) found a loss of 8% of positive results after overnight storage of 4°C in experiments using urethral and cervical samples. Further storage (in the refrigerator) decreased the isolation rate of *C. trachomatis* even more markedly.

The freezing of clinical samples marginally decreases the recovery rate and reduces the inclusion count in positive samples. Thus freezing can make the diagnosis of genital chlamydial infections impossible if the specimen contains just a small number of elementary bodies (EBs). Tjiam and co-workers (1984) found a 4% loss of positive genital specimens by freezing.

In some instances freezing might even enhance the recovery rate of *C. trachomatis* as indicated by in vitro experiments (Kallings and Mårdh, 1982). Tjiam and co-workers (1984) found 4% of genital samples to be positive only after freezing. The freezing is thought to result in cell lysis and liberation of intracellularly localized chlamydiae. A similar positive effect on the sensitivity of the isolation method was found by the same authors after storage of genital samples at 4°C for more than 48 hr.

When stored in 2-SP medium, the viability of TWAR chlamydiae was rapidly lost at room temperature but was relatively well preserved at 4°C (Kuo and Grayston, 1988).

Microbial Superinfection

Viral infections and bacterial superinfections of tissue cell cultures in patient samples can destroy the cell layer and thereby the possibility of detecting chlamydiae (Yoder et al., 1986). Viral infections—mainly herpes virus hominis infections—may cause cytolysis and thereby interfere with the isolation of chlamydiae. With currently used combinations of antimicrobials added to transport media and to tissue cell culture media used for the isolation of chlamydiae, breakthrough of bacterial growth (superinfection) is not common. Bacterial toxins and other compounds of bacterial origin may have a cell lytic effect.

Recently, infection by *Trichomonas vaginalis* and herpes simplex virus has been demonstrated as a cause of cell lysis in chlamydial cultures of genital specimens. Thus Colaert and co-workers (1987) found that of 1797 cell cultures, 5.3% resulted in cell lysis. Of the lytic cultures, 16.7% were infected by *T. vaginalis* and 12.5% by herpes simplex virus.

DIAGNOSIS OF CHLAMYDIAL INFECTIONS BY DIRECT ANALYSES OF CLINICAL SAMPLES

Introduction

Until recently, a definitive diagnosis of chlamydial infection usually depended on isolation of the organism. Efforts have been made to complete or replace isolation by demonstration of chlamydial particles, chlamydial antigens, or chlamydial nucleic acid directly in clinical samples in order to speed up the diagnostic procedure. The direct-specimen antigen detection tests have certain advantages over culture. They eliminate many problems concerning adequate specimen storage and transport, since chlamydial particles that are no longer viable or infectious can also be detected. Furthermore, the quality of clinical specimens can be assessed by microscopic techniques (content of cells versus secretion); samples sent for isolation, ELISA, and hybridization tests escape this control step. The technical procedures used in some direct-specimen antigen detection tests are usually quicker and simpler to perform than culture. However, one of these tests (i.e., the immunofluorescence test) requires considerable expertise and is laborious. False-positive reactions in immunofluorescence tests is with staphylococci (Krech et al., 1985; Francis and Abbas, 1985) and in enzyme immunoassays (ELISA tests) with *Acinetobacter* (Saikku et al., 1986a) and with some other bacteria have been stressed.

Recently, the restricted sensitivity of direct-specimen antigen detection tests as compared to culture has been highlighted (Taylor-Robinson et al., 1987) (see section on general remarks concerning the clinical value of "rapid" diagnostic tests).

Detection of Chlamydial Particles by Staining Procedures

Giemsa Staining

When Halberstaedter and von Prowazek demonstrated inclusion bodies in Giemsa-stained epithelial conjunctival scrapings from experimentally infected monkeys in 1907, it was the first time laboratory methods could support a clinical diagnosis of infection, which later proved to be caused by chlamydiae. Later that year, the same method was used to diagnose chlamydial "ophthalmia neonatorum." Since then, Giemsa staining has been one of the standard methods used to demonstrate chlamydial inclusions in clinical samples (Fig. 9). The presence of intracytoplasmic inclusions is pathognomonic for chlamydial ocular infections (Schachter, 1978), but inclusions are only infrequently found in scrapings from genital *C. trachomatis* infections. With Giemsa staining both *C. psittaci* and *C. trachomatis* inclusions can be detected, which is not the case with iodine staining (see next section). In bright-field illumination, chlamydial inclusions in epithelial cells appear as intracytoplasmic round or helmet-shaped structures consisting of reddish purple stained EBs and bluish purple reticulate bodies (RBs). "Pseudoinclusions" (cell structures and bacteria) resembling chlamydial inclusions may be seen. In dark-field illumination, inclusions show up as bright golden fluorescing structures. Although Giemsa staining is simple to perform, it is not a sensitive detection technique. In ocular infections, its sensitivity ranges from 22% to 56% (Rowe et al., 1979; Sandström et al., 1982). In genital infections it is even lower (Schachter and Dawson, 1978). Microscopy of Giemsa-stained smears is too fatiguing and time consuming for large-scale use.

Iodine Staining

Iodine staining (with Lugol's solution), which selectively stains glycogen, has been widely used for detection of *C. trachomatis* inclusions in cell cultures. The inclusions appear as a reddish brown granular mass in yellow cells, whereas *C. psittaci* and TWAR inclusions, which do not contain glycogen, remain unstained. Iodine can also be applied for direct demonstration of *C. trachomatis* inclusions in scrapings. Iodine staining is easy and quick to perform, and the microscopic reading of the smears is simpler than that for Giemsa. However, the sensitivity is low; in genital infections it is only 24–30% (Schachter and Dawson, 1978). Cells of urogenital origin contain glycogen and may therefore cause unspecific staining.

Papanicolaou Staining

Gupta and co-workers (1979) suggested that chlamydial infections can be detected in routine Papanicolaou-stained (Pap) cervical smears (Fig. 10). Typical findings associated with *C. trachomatis* infection include diffuse and focal intracytoplasmic coccoid bodies, inclusions, and perinuclear vacuolation. Multinucleation of the cells also occurs. Later studies unanimously disproved these results. Pap smear cytology is now considered unsensitive and subject to misinterpretation in the diagnosis of genital chlamydial infections (Paavonen and Purola, 1980; Dorman et al., 1983; Clark et al., 1985). However, its accuracy can be improved by combining it with immunofluorescent staining with monoclonal antibodies (see below and Chapter 3) (Kiviat et al., 1985b).

Immunoperoxidase Staining

In addition to chemical stains, immunological reactions have been employed for direct demonstration of chlamydiae in clinical samples. Immunoperoxidase staining of inclusions was found to be more sensitive than Giemsa staining (Woodland et al., 1978). The technique has also been used to detect inclusions in infected tissue cell cultures. Care is needed in the interpretation of immunoperoxidase-stained smears. In this test, inclusions are made visible by peroxidase–antiperoxidase staining with suitable substrates preceded by allowing antigenic sites in inclusions to react with hyperimmune rabbit antiserum and antirabbit serum. Erythrocytes and other cells containing endogenous peroxidase can cause false-positive reactions. True inclusions can be differentiated from false ones by their different morphology.

Immunofluorescence Tests

Immunofluorescence (IF) staining, by either the direct [fluorescein isothio-cyanate (FITC)-conjugated antiserum] or the indirect (FITC-conjugated second antiserum) method, has proved to be the most sensitive microscopic approach for the demonstration of chlamydial particles in clinical samples. The quality of the reagent (especially of the detecting antiserum) is a critical factor. By the indirect IF method using *polyclonal antisera,* only inclusions can be identified reliably. The method is not sensitive enough to resolve other structures. In IF tests using *polyclonal sera,* typical *C. trachomatis* inclusions are sharply defined intra-cytoplasmic masses with yellow–green fluorescence. Tests using polyclonal sera are of value only in the diagnosis of acute ocular chlamydial infections, where inclusions can frequently be found. Fluorescein isothiocyanate-conjugated *monoclonal* antibodies against *C. trachomatis* species-specific MOMP (Tam et al., 1984; Uyeda et al., 1984; Krech et al., 1985) or chlamydial genus-specific lipid polysaccharide (LPS) (Alexander et al., 1985) can also detect EBs. This is important because only 5–20% of genital smears studied by direct tests contained chlamydial inclusions (Tam et al., 1984; Kiviat et al., 1985a). The morphology of the chlamydial inclusions in IF- and Giemsa-stained smears is similar. Micros-copy of IF-stained specimens is relatively easy to perform, but the presence of leukocytes, keratinized epithelial cells, pigment granules, and bacteria other than chlamydiae can cause false fluorescent reactions. These organisms can be differ-entiated from true inclusions by location and morphology. Immunofluorescence staining is more sensitive and specific than Giemsa and iodine staining.

In addition to bright inclusions (which are uncommon in clinical samples), the detection of EBs and RBs is considered diagnostic. Elementary bodies stained with FITC-conjugated monoclonal antibody against MOMP appear as distinct, sharply outlined, apple green, disk-shaped particles (Fig. 30). Reticu-late bodies are about three times larger than EBs, having a peripheral fluorescing halo (Tam et al., 1984). All other fluorescing particles of varying size, intensity, and color should be considered as artifacts. Using the genus-specific stain, a large number of smaller, brightly fluorescing particles can be seen in addition to the spherical and uniformly sized EBs (Alexander et al., 1985). Such staining, which might represent reaction with chlamydial LPS (genus-specific antigen) outside the EBs, can obscure the vision of EBs. The number of chlamydial organisms required for diagnosis is under investigation, but has something to do with the experience of the microscopist. Usually 10 EBs per sample is the lower limit for positivity indicated by manufacturers.

Tests that require fatiguing microscopy are best handled by laboratories that process a small number of chlamydial specimens daily.

Fluorescein-labeled monoclonal antibodies, now commercially available

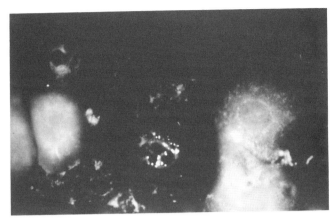

FIGURE 30. Smears of genital secretion stained with fluorescein-labeled monoclonal antibodies showing elementary bodies (EBs) (×1000). A color version of this figure appears following p. xvi.

from many sources, offer a possibility for culture-independent diagnosis of chlamydial infections. The sensitivity of the direct IF test in comparison with isolation has been indicated as 69–99% and the specificity 83–99% (Table 16). The lowest percentages have presented in screening tests of asymptomatic persons (low-risk groups), which calls to question the use of these tests in groups with low prevalence of *C. trachomatis* infections. The microscopist must be well trained regarding the sensitivity and specificity obtained by IF tests. High-prevalence populations are more suitable for direct IF testing than low-prevalence groups, but the sensitivity of such tests is still considerably lower than that of culture (Lipkin et al., 1986).

As is the case with genital specimens, the direct-specimen antigen detection tests have high specificity but low sensitivity when applied to conjunctival samples. Mårdh and associates (1987) used cycloheximide McCoy cell cultures and two monoclonal immunofluorescent antibody tests, i.e., Microtrak® (Syva) and Chlamyset® (Orion), to diagnose chlamydial conjunctivitis in 137 patients (66 adults and 71 neonates). Of these patients, 29 and 28 were positive in the two IF tests, respectively. Twenty-eight of the 137 cases studied were culture-positive. No difference between newborns and adults was found. The rapidity by which an answer can be obtained by IF tests, as compared to culture, can make such tests attractive in cases where there are differential diagnostic problems between gonococcal and chlamydial ophthalmia.

TABLE 16. Reported Sensitivity and Specificity of Tests Using Fluorescent Chlamydial Monoclonal Antibody for Direct Detection of Chlamydial Particles in Genital Specimens Compared with the Isolation of *C. trachomatis* in Cell Culture

Test and reference	Study group(s)	N	Prevalence of *C. trachomatis* (%)	Criterion of positivity	Sensitivity (%)	Specificity (%)
MIKROTRAK®						
Tam et al., 1984	STD,[a] contacts	926	23	≥ 10 EBs[c]	93	96
Thomas et al., 1984	STD, contacts	235	28	≥ 1 EBs	97	97
Uyeda et al., 1984	Asymptomatic females	401	7	≥ 2 EBs	96	99
Stamm et al., 1984	STD, contacts	1171	19	≥ 2 EBs	91	98
	Pregnant females	225	13	≥ 2 EBs	86	99
Stary et al., 1985	Asymptomatic prostitutes	700	13	≥ 1 EBs	75	99
Teare et al., 1985	STD, contacts	182	57	n. st.[d]	99	83
Foulkes et al., 1985	STD	137	14	≥ 10 EBs	89	87
Quinn et al., 1985	STD	536	12	≥ 5 EBs	97	98
	Asymptomatic females	704	15	≥ 5 EBs	88	99
Lipkin et al., 1986	Asymptomatic females	864	12	≥ 10 EBs	69	95
	Salpingitis patients	104	20	≥ 10 EBs	76	92
Chernesky et al., 1986	STD, OBGYN[b]	479	18	≥ 10 EBs	82	98
Smith et al., 1987	Asymptomatic females	1059	10	≥ 10 EBs	71	96
Hipp et al., 1987	STD, OBGYN, students	2030	15	≥ 10 EBs	73	99
Phillips et al., 1987	OBGYN	527	4	≥ 5 EBs	70	98
MAGEN®						
Alexander et al., 1985	STD	250	16	≥ 10 EBs	90	97
CHLAMYSET®						
Väänänen et al., 1985	STD	381	22	n.st.[d]	89	99

[a]STD = patients seen in a clinic for sexually transmitted diseases.
[b]OBGYN = patients seen in a clinic for obstetrics and gynecology.
[c]EBs = elementary bodies.
[d]n. st. = not stated.

Detection of Chlamydial Antigen

Enzyme Immunoassays

Tests based on enzyme immunoassay (EIA) represent another mode for the diagnosis of chlamydial infections without requirement of cell culture facilities. Caldwell and Schachter (1983) described a solid phase immunoassay system using an antigen capture principle capable of detecting *C. trachomatis* MOMP. Their assay could detect 0.5–1.0 ng purified MOMP and $5 \cdot 10^3$ EBs, but it was not applied to the study of clinical specimens. Recently, enzyme immunoassay kits for the rapid detection of chlamydial antigen, particularly geared for testing of genitourinary samples, have become commercially available. One of these test kits uses sensitized polystyrene beads (Chlamydiazyme®) whereas another uses microtiter plates coated with chlamydial genus-specific monoclonal antibodies (IDEIA®). In both systems the captured antigen is visualized with enzyme-antibody conjugates reacting with substrates, giving a colored product.

Recently, Mabey and co-workers (1987) used an ELISA technique whereby the samples were boiled for 15 min to extract chlamydial antigen. The assay was carried out with 200 microliters of extract in each well of the microtiter plate. Monoclonal antibody bound to a prepared enzyme immunoassay tray captures the chlamydial antigen from the extract. The antigen is detected with an alkaline phosphate-labeled monoclonal antibody. The phosphatase cleaves NADP and the resulting NAD enters a redox cycle of NAD/NADH coupled to an electron donor bound to a tetrazolium indicator. NADP cleaves red formazan, which is detected spectrophotometrically. The method is claimed to be more sensitive than conventional ELISA techniques.

Enzyme immunoassay kits have been reported to have a sensitivity of 62–96% and a specificity of 86–99% in comparison to cell culture (Table 17). As an automatable method, EIA might be more suitable for laboratories without access to the cell culture technique and that handle large numbers of specimens. Due to possible cross-reactions between chlamydiae and other bacteria (Saikku et al., 1986a), and due to the low specificity and sensitivity of the methods in the testing of low-risk populations for chlamydial infections, caution is advised in interpreting EIA results.

Chlamydiazyme® was shown to react with *Acinetobacter* (Saikku et al., 1986a). Under experimental conditions EIA was able to detect 10^3–10^5 bacteria per milliliter (Saikku et al., 1986a). In addition, some strains of *E. coli, G. vaginalis, N. gonorrhoeae,* and group B streptococci were reported to have given false-positive reactions in the Chlamydiazyme® test (Taylor-Robinson et al., 1987). In patients with cultures positive for *Acinetobacter* but negative for *C. trachomatis,* no false-positive Chlamydiazyme® test results were reported (Puolakkainen et al., 1987b). Possibly the amount of the bacteria in clinical

TABLE 17. Reported Sensitivity and Specificity of Enzyme Immunoassays (EIAs) for Detection of Chlamydial Antigen in Genital Specimens Compared with the Isolation of C. trachomatis in Cell Culture

Test and reference	Study group(s)	N	Prevalence of C. trachomatis (%)	Sensitivity (%)	Specificity (%)
CHLAMYDIAZYME®					
Jones et al., 1984	STD[a]	416	16–20	81–86	90–98
Hambling and Kurtz, 1985	Females	225	20	89	86
Mumtaz et al., 1985	STD	140	27	92	97
Amortegui et al., 1985	OBGYN[b], legal abortion	514	9	82	98
Howard et al., 1986	STD, OBGYN	1640	21	86	97
Moi and Danielsson, 1986	STD (males)	1011	20	86	95
Chernesky et al., 1986	STD, OBGYN	479	18	89	97
Hipp et al., 1987	STD, OBGYN, students	2030	15	83	97
Smith et al., 1987	Asymptomatic females	1059	10	62	94
Danielsson et al., 1987	STD	307	19	85	96
	OBGYN	329	5	93	97
IDEIA®					
Caul and Paul, 1985	STD	191	35	96	99
Pugh et al., 1985	STD	312	31	92	99
Tjiam et al., 1986	STD	596	11	66	94
PHARMACIA CHLAMYDIA EIA®					
Danielsson et al., 1987	STD	307	19	83	96
	OBGYN	329	5	80	98

[a]STD = patients seen in a clinic for sexually transmitted diseases.
[b]OBGYN = patients seen in a clinic for obstetrics and gynecology.

samples is too small (smaller than has been used in the in vitro experiments) to interfere with the EIA test in routine diagnostic work.

Recently, a quick and easily performed EIA test (Testpack TM Chlamydia), which does not need specialized equipment, has been introduced for detection of *C. trachomatis* antigen in endocervical samples (Coleman *et al.*, 1988). A test increasing the specificity of Chlamydiazyme® known as a confirmatory test (Chlamydiazyme Confirmatory Test, ® Abbott) has recently become available.

Other Immunoassays

Detection of *C. trachomatis* antigen by radioimmunoassay (RIA) and time-resolved fluoroimmunoassay (TR-FIA) has been described (Terho and Matikainen, 1981; Caldwell and Schachter, 1983; Matikainen, 1984). So far these tests have not been applied in clinical trials. Immune dot-blot tests have been applied to detect *C. trachomatis* antigen. With this method, antigen is trapped on nitrocellulose membrane and detected with autoradiography with monoclonal antibody (Richmond *et al.*, 1988). Compared to isolation, this dot-blot test showed promising results when testing ocular and genital samples.

Electron Microscopy

Electron microscopy (EM) has been applied directly to the detection of *C. trachomatis* EBs in clinical samples (Ashley et al., 1975; Martinov et al., 1985). In one study (Martinov et al., 1985), clinical samples were fixed in glutaraldehyde, centrifuged for 90 min at 15,000–20,000 rpm, fixed in 1% osmium, and dehydrated in alcohol or propylene oxide. After embedding the samples in Epon, ultrathin sections were prepared, put on grids, and studied under an electron microscope (Fig. 31). Hyperimmune rabbit antichlamydial antiserum and ferritin-conjugated antirabbit serum have also been used to visualize chlamydial inclusions (Ashley et al., 1975). The EM technique is time consuming and therefore rather unsuitable for large-scale clinical use. It has, however, been used to study genital samples (Dimitrov et al., 1984) and synovial fluid (Martinov et al., 1987).

Detection of Chlamydial Nucleic Acid

Recent advances in recombinant DNA technology have made it possible to use nucleic acid probes for detection of specific chlamydial DNA sequences. The tests are based on the tendency of complementary DNA strands to reassociate under appropriate conditions. Consequently, DNA can be detected by a radioactively (or otherwise) labeled probe. One drawback of the DNA probe technique is that pretreatment of clinical samples is required to reduce background activity.

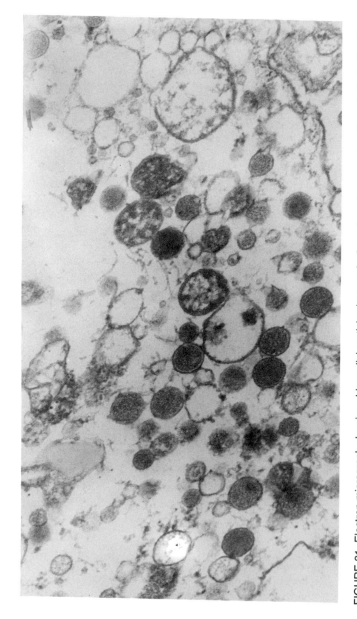

FIGURE 31. Electron micrograph showing chlamydial particles in a urethral specimen from a male with urethritis ($\times 20,000$). (Courtesy of Dr. S. Martinov and Prof. G. Popov.)

Diagnostic hybridization tests have been introduced for several microbes (Kaper et al., 1981; Moseley et al., 1982; Stålhandske and Pettersson, 1982), including *C. trachomatis* (Hyypiä et al., 1985; Palva, 1985). Spot hybridization (Hyypiä et al., 1985; Palva, 1985) and sandwich hybridization (Palva et al., 1984) techniques have been used for the detection of *C. trachomatis* DNA.

In directly testing for chlamydial DNA in clinical specimens, the reported sensitivity was 10^5 genomes for the spot hybridization test and 10^5-10^6 genomes for the sandwich technique (Palva et al., 1984; Palva, 1985). Approximately one-fourth of chlamydial culture-negative specimens gave a positive signal in spot hybridization tests of clinical specimens, whereas one-fourth of culture-positive samples remained negative.

The desired sensitivity might be achieved by enzymatically amplifying [polymerase chain reaction (PCR)] the chlamydial target DNA before employing the hybridization method (Saiki et al., 1985). Several studies have presented data regarding apparent detection of chlamydial infection cases by DNA hybridization but not by culture (Palva et al., 1984, 1987; Horn et al., 1986; Pao et al., 1987). The probes used have been carefully controlled not to cross-react with the nucleic acids of other microorganisms that are often encountered in genital tract infections (Palva et al., 1984). Using chlamydial culture as the reference method, the specificities of the in situ, slot-blot, and sandwich hybridization tests were 80% (Horn et al., 1986), 95% (Pao et al., 1987), and 85% (Palva et al., 1987), respectively. In a recent study (Puolakkainen et al., 1987), the hybridization test was compared with the optimized culture and direct-specimen antigen detection methods. No chlamydial DNA-positive cases were detected that were negative in culture or direct-specimen antigen detection tests.

General Remarks on the Clinical Value of "Rapid" Diagnostic Tests

As mentioned earlier, and as can be seen in Tables 15 and 16, the sensitivity of the direct-specimen antigen detection tests does not reach that of *C. trachomatis* isolation in tissue cell cultures. Most of the samples that remain negative in the direct tests (EIA, IF, and hybridization tests) but are positive in isolation show only a few inclusions in tissue cell culture (i.e., they contain only a few chlamydial organisms). On the other hand, the sensitivity of the isolation techniques is approximately 70–80% (Schachter, 1985), and the sensitivity of the direct tests is even lower. The small number of chlamydial organisms and consequent low concentration of antigen and DNA is one reason for discrepant results between culture on the one hand, and EIA and hybridization tests on the other. Both EIA, IF, and hybridization tests detect true positives that, due to long storage or transport time, no longer contain infectious EBs. The category of false positives detected by the new "rapid" tests includes specimens that inadvertently lower the specificity of the test under evaluation.

Isolation of *C. trachomatis* in tissue cell culture does not constitute a "golden standard" with a 100% specificity and sensitivity. However, if performed under optimal conditions, it is still more sensitive than the newer diagnostic tests and it is specific. The differentiation of true positives from false positives resulting from nonspecificity of the test under evaluation is difficult. The problem of selecting an appropriate reference method has partially been solved by the evaluation of several different methods simultaneously.

In a study conducted by Chernesky and co-workers (1986), the sensitivity of both IF (MikroTrak®) and EIA (Chlamydiazyme®) was 70% in tests of male urethral specimens, but higher in tests of female cervical specimens (88 and 98%, respectively). Taylor-Robinson and co-workers (1987) compared EIA (Chlamydiazyme®), IF (MikroTrak®), and isolation in tissue cell culture (cycloheximide-treated McCoy cells). On the male specimens the EIA had a sensitivity of 58% and a specificity of 99%. The corresponding figures in female specimens were 67 and 89%, respectively. The latter workers found only a marginal improvement in sensitivity and specificity if the comparison was made by isolation in tissue cell culture. If samples tested by IF (MikroTrak®; detecting MOMP of *C. trachomatis*), EIA (Chlamydiazyme®; detecting LPS, the genus-specific chlamydial antigen), and isolation are positive in both IF tests and EIA, but negative by isolation studies, they are most likely true positives (Howard et al., 1986). In a study by Chernesky and co-workers (1986), seven such specimens were identified among 479 specimens with a positivity rate (by isolation) of 18.4%.

The quality of the specimens (i.e., the representativeness of material for assay) is critical to the test result. The number of organisms in the specimens has been suggested to be lower in asymptomatic than in symptomatic patients (Smith et al., 1987). In addition, the type of swab used, the sampling technique, and possibly sequential swabbing can affect the quality of the specimens. In males, especially, sequential swabbing might produce unequal specimens for comparison (Phillips et al., 1987). Since *C. trachomatis* shows a preference for columnar cells, the number of such epithelial cells in the sample reflects its quality. This quality test can only be performed in specimens requiring microscopy (e.g., IF tests). The sensitivity of the direct-specimen antigen detection tests is strongly affected by sample quality. For instance, in a study using IF tests (MikroTrak®) on cervical specimens taken from females with a low prevalence of *C. trachomatis,* the sensitivity of IF tests was 92%, if only samples with five or more columnar epithelial cells were included for calculation. However, the sensitivity was 40% for slides containing fewer than five columnar epithelial cells (Phillips et al., 1987).

The prevalence of *C. trachomatis* in the study population is strongly related to the predictive values of positive and negative testing. In low-prevalence settings the predictive value for a positive test will be unexpectedly low, although the sensitivity and the specificity of the test might be acceptable. For example, only 50% of positive test results will be true positives (a predictive value of a positive test of 50%) if the prevalence of *C. trachomatis* infection is 5% and the test under evaluation has a sensitivity and a specificity of 95%. However, if the prevalence is 25%, 86% of the positive test results will also be positive by the reference method. Therefore, diagnosis of sexually transmitted infections by *C. trachomatis* in a low-prevalence population should not be made by ELISA tests in order to avoid false-positive results that may cause unnecessary anxiety among patients and their partners, unless confirmatory tests are performed.

SEROLOGY

Complement Fixation

Complement fixation (CF) is an insensitive tool for diagnosing genital, eye, and certain other infections caused by *C. trachomatis*. It detects antibodies to the chlamydial genus-specific antigen; consequently, the detection of antibodies to this chlamydial lipopolysaccharide antigen cannot differentiate between *C. trachomatis* and *C. psittaci* infections. Both IgG and IgM are detected by the CF test. In cases of lymphogranuloma venereum (LGV), antibodies are usually detectable by CF tests, but few other deep-sited *C. trachomatis* infections can be diagnosed this way (e.g., infections of the upper genital tract in both males and females will not be detected). Complement fixation tests are also of no value in infant chlamydial infections; polysaccharides induce poor antigen stimulation in small children (Robbins, 1978). Recent results suggest that the CF test is also too insensitive to be useful for detection of antibodies to TWAR agents (see under each disease entity). Psittacosis/ornithosis (*C. psittaci* infections) can be diagnosed by CF tests.

Microimmunofluorescence

Microimmunofluorescence (micro-IF) was first adapted by Wang and Grayston (1970) for immunological classification of *C. trachomatis* strains; it was later adapted for detection of chlamydial antibodies in human and animal sera (Wang, 1971; Wang and Grayston, 1974, 1984). In the micro-IF test, purified chlamydial EBs, either produced from yolk sac infection of embryonated hen's egg or from cell cultures, are used as antigens. The antigens are applied on a glass slide with the aid of a pen (Fig. 32). Originally antigens from EBs of each of the serotypes of *C. trachomatis* were included in the test along with EBs from a few *C. psittaci* strains. However, it was cumbersome and time

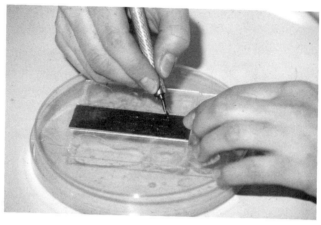

FIGURE 32. Application of antigen with the aid of a pen on a glass slide to be used in microimmunofluorescence tests.

consuming to screen and titrate sera against such a large selection of antigens. Efforts have been made to simplify this test. The number of chlamydial antigens has been reduced by pooling antigens of closely related serotypes (Wang et al., 1975, 1977). In addition, combinations of antigens of serotypes causing similar diseases, such as A–C, D–K, L_1–L_3 (Treharne et al., 1977), or even a mixture of all 15 serotypes of *C. trachomatis* (McComb et al., 1979), have been employed. Thomas and others (1976) used a single broadly reactive EB (from serotype L_2) as antigen. Yong and associates (1979) found RBs of serotype C to show broad reactivity in micro-IF tests.

The micro-IF test can be used to detect type-specific antibodies (i.e., antibodies formed against the type-specific determinants on the chlamydial particles). Consequently, it allows differentiation between *C. psittaci* and *C. trachomatis* as well as between different serotypes.

Micro-IF serology has played an important role in epidemiological studies of chlamydial infections. It has proved to be a sensitive and specific test to measure antichlamydial antibodies not only in serum but also in local secretions (e.g., in tears). It allows determination of the antibodies to different Ig classes (IgG, IgM, IgA). However, the laborious preparation of the antigens and the subjective and difficult interpretation inherent in all fluorescence tests are obstacles to its wider spread; relatively few laboratories use micro-IF tests currently.

Inclusion Immunofluorescence

To simplify the production of IF antigens, Richmond and Caul (1975) prepared a test employing cell-grown, whole inclusions of *C. trachomatis*, serotype E (I-IFAT). Similarly, Saikku and Paavonen (1978) used serotype L_2. The I-IFAT test detects antibodies directed against species- and genus-specific antigenic structures, since both types of antigen are present in inclusions. The inclusion immunofluorescence test can be used to detect antibodies in secretions and to determine their immunoglobulin class.

Enzyme Immunoassays

In recent years many serological tests employing the enzyme immunoassay principle for detection of chlamydial antibodies have been described (Lewis et al., 1977). Although EIA is a sensitive method, its applicability depends on the antigen used. Different antigens have been employed, i.e., EBs (Levy and Mc-Cormack, 1982; Jones et al., 1983; Finn et al., 1983; Mahony et al., 1983), RBs (Saikku et al., 1983; Jones et al., 1983), purified genus-specific antigen (Evans and Taylor-Robinson, 1982), and purified major outer membrane protein (Puolakkainen et al., 1984). Determination of immunoglobulin class specificity is possible with EIA tests. However, highly purified antigens might be more suitable for this latter purpose (Puolakkainen et al., 1985).

Other Tests

An indirect hemagglutination test (IHA) (Benedict and O'Brien, 1958), a neutralization test (NT) (Hahon and Cooke, 1965), a radioisotope precipitation (RIP) test (Gerloff and Watson, 1967), gel diffusion tests (Collins and Barron, 1970; Lycke and Peterson, 1976), and immunoelectrophoresis tests (Caldwell et al., 1975b; Caldwell and Kuo, 1977) have been applied to the detection of chlamydial antibodies. However, their sensitivities and specificities have been found to be too low, or the tests have otherwise been found unsuitable for routine use in chlamydial serology. Newer approaches in chlamydial serology include radioimmunoassay (RIA) (Meurman et al., 1982), enzyme-linked fluorescence immunoassay (ELFA) (Numazaki et al., 1985), and immunoperoxidase assay (IPA) (Piura et al., 1985), but their diagnostic value when used under routine conditions must be further evaluated.

Occurrence of Antichlamydial Antibodies, and General Remarks on the Interpretation of Serological Chlamydial Tests

Chlamydial serology, as studied by micro-IF tests, has proved an efficient tool in seroepidemiological studies (Table 9). Serological studies have also given clues regarding chlamydial etiology in a number of syndromes (Wang and Grayston, 1982).

In the diagnosis of human chlamydial infections, antibody assays (serology) have usually played only a complementary role to isolation and direct-specimen antigen detection tests. Micro-IF tests also offer a presumptive possibility for diagnosing chlamydial infections in cases where it is difficult, impossible, or rather inconvenient to collect adequate samples for culture studies (e.g., in arthritis, carditis, epididymitis, salpingitis, and infant pneumonitis).

Uncomplicated genital mucosal chlamydial infections usually do not induce a readily detectable antibody response. Such infections, as well as deep-sited genital infections, may be asymptomatic or produce only few symptoms, that is, the disease can have been long-standing before the patient attends (if ever). Therefore only stationary or declining antichlamydial IgG antibody titers can be detected in many PID cases. Antichlamydial serum IgG antibodies may persist, even in adequately treated infections, for years (Puolakkainen et al., 1986). The high prevalence of antichlamydial IgG antibodies in the population is another factor diminishing the value of chlamydial serology as a diagnostic tool.

Antichlamydial IgM antibodies are only inconsistently found in most clinical syndromes asssociated with *C. trachomatis* infection. IgM antibodies can also be spurious and can form as a result of polyclonal B-cell stimulation (Persson and Bröms, 1986).

Antichlamydial IgA antibodies can be detected in serum and various other body fluids in patients infected with *C. trachomatis*. Mucosal antichlamydial antibodies, mainly of the IgA class, have been suggestive of an active, ongoing *C. trachomatis* infection of the cervix (McComb et al., 1979). The diagnostic significance of the demonstration of IgA antibodies, however, is restricted due to the low sensitivity of such antibody determination. The persistence of urethral IgA antibodies for several years (Terho and Meurman, 1981) and the high prevalence of local antibodies (S-IgA) in STD clinic populations (Schachter et al., 1979a) further diminishes the diagnostic value of such antibody determinations. The presence of IgA in cervical secretion correlates with the isolation of *C. trachomatis* from the cervix (Treharne et al., 1978a). The correlation between the occurrence of local and serum antichlamydial antibodies has been shown to be much stronger than that between the presence of local antibodies to *C. trachomatis* and the isolation of the agent from cervical secretion (Richmond et al., 1980). The detection of antichlamydial S-IgA antibodies in cervical secretion, according to Brunham and co-workers (1983), correlates inversely with the quantitative recovery of *C. trachomatis* from the cervix. This might reflect an inhibitory effect of local IgA antibodies on recovery from *C. trachomatis* infections; the antibodies might hinder the uptake of the organism in tissue culture cells.

Much of the seroepidemiological data on the prevalence of antichlamydial antibodies must now be reevaluated because of the recent knowledge (or awareness) of cross-reactions between TWAR antibodies and antigens of other chlamydiae. However, in micro-IF tests, reactions of *C. trachomatis* antibodies with *C. psittaci* and TWAR chlamydiae antigens can be differentiated. This is not the case when complement fixation tests are used. Some workers, but not others, have found cross-reactions between *Chlamydia* on the one hand, and *Legionella* and *Coxiella* spp. on the other (cf. Gray et al., 1986).

An unspecific B-cell stimulation may be one explanation for the demonstrated antibody activity to *C. trachomatis* in some cases (cf. Gray et al., 1986), where serological tests suggest exposure to the organism but other evidence of infection is lacking (as in many children). Such B-cell stimulation might be the result of infection with, say, group A streptococci, *M. pneumoniae, S. pneumoniae, H. influenzae,* or *Staphylococcus aureus,* as these agents are known to be B-cell mitogens. Serological characteristics in different chlamydial syndromes are discussed under each disease entity.

IV

Antibiosis and Vaccines

Antibiotic Susceptibility Testing

T'ang and co-workers (1957), who had adapted Cox's method (1938) for the growth of rickettsiae in embryonated hen's eggs in order to isolate chlamydiae, also studied the susceptibility of *C. trachomatis* to certain antibiotics. They found chlamydiae to be resistant to aminoglycosides and susceptible to tetracyclines. It is noteworthy that one of the first observations made in the experimentally infected hen's eggs was that penicillin affected the growth of chlamydiae. Two other chlamydial research pioneers, Gordon and Quan, also used embryonated hen's eggs for antibiotic susceptibility studies in 1962. In order to improve the isolation technique for tissue cell cultures, they were able to demonstrate that such drugs as bacitracin, nystatin, and polymyxin had no antichlamydial effect and could be used to suppress bacterial overgrowth in chlamydial cultures.

Shiao and co-workers (1967) reported certain strains of *C. trachomatis* to have a decreased susceptibility to tetracycline, penicillins, and sulfonamides in experimental infections in embryonated hen's eggs. However, it has been claimed that the eggs can metabolize certain antibiotics with varying efficiencies, making the results of susceptibility tests obtained in embryonated eggs uncertain (Ghione et al., 1967).

Several methods have been described for determining the antibiotic susceptibility of chlamydiae using tissue cell cultures (Ridgway et al., 1976; Alexander et al., 1977; Kuo et al., 1977; Lycke, 1982). In one method of determining minimum bactericidal (i.e., chlamydiacidal) concentration (MBC), the antibiotic compound being tested is added to the tissue cell culture 1 hr after infection and remains present during the entire test period, including when, if ever, the test strain is passed to fresh tissue cell cultures. Such passage may be necessary to obtain stable endpoints. This method is thought to correspond with techniques used to determine the minimum bactericidal concentration of antimicrobials in MBC tests of eubacteria (Fig. 33). A variant of the procedure for determinating MBC(2) is to add the drug to the culture 2 days postinfection. In both MBC and

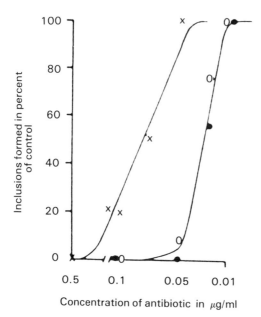

FIGURE 33. Antibiotic susceptibility testing of *C. trachomatis* against tetracyclines. (From E. Lycke, 1982.)

MBC(2) tests, inhibition of growth is established by passage of the test cell in the absence of the drug. In order to determine the minimum inhibitory concentration (MIC), the drug and the chlamydiae must be added to the tissue cell culture simultaneously. Generally, the MBC and MIC values are similar, whereas the difference between MBC(2) and MIC probably reflects the difference between what is known as the cidal and static concentrations of an antibiotic in tests of eubacteria.

Webberley and associates (1987) recommended the use of labeled monoclonal antibodies for reading antibiotic susceptibility tests. They found that this procedure yielded twofold higher values for MIC and MLC (minimum lethal concentration). Other authors had previously used monoclonals for the same purpose (Cevenini et al., 1986c). In principle, these results agree with claims that labeled monoclonals yielded better detection of *C. trachomatis* in clinical tissue cell cultures than did iodine.

Currently under debate is the length of time that should elapse between infection and reading of the cultures in antibiotic susceptibility tests. The reproductive cycles of various serotypes or even of strains within a given serotype may vary with different antibiotics, e.g., penicillins.

Inclusions with aberrant morphology are found in the presence of β-lactam antibiotics (Fig. 34A and B). Very small inclusions can be found in the presence

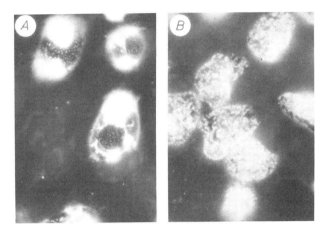

FIGURE 34. Formation of L-form-like cells of *C. trachomatis* under influence of penicillin (A) and control (B). (Courtesy of Dr. T. Krech.)

of sulfonamides. Thus antimicrobials can induce morphological alterations that can make reading of susceptibility tests difficult or uncertain.

In order to test interlaboratory differences in the performance of chlamydial antibiotic susceptibility tests, four U.S. microbiological laboratories tested the same 40 strains of *C. trachomatis* for their susceptibilities to clindamycin, erythromycin, and tetracycline. The MIC ranges for the three drugs were 0.5–0.8 µg/ml, 0.032–1.02 µg/ml, and 0.032–1.02 µg/ml, respectively. The differences between laboratories were greater than the differences between isolates. The results of this study (involving only laboratories with reputations for quality performance) mean that *C. trachomatis* antibiotic susceptibility values from individual laboratories must be interpreted accordingly. Thus there is an urgent need for standardized methods of *C. trachomatis* antibiotic susceptibility testing.

Susceptibility of Chlamydiae to Different Antimicrobials

OVERVIEW

Chlamydiae are susceptible to a number of antibiotics (Table 18). Considered particularly useful are certain drugs that interfere with chlamydial protein synthesis, e.g., tetracyclines and erythromycin.

Antibiotics that are most active against *C. trachomatis* include tetracyclines, erythromycin, sulfonamides, and rifampicin (Table 18). Clindamycin also appears to be active against *C. trachomatis* with a minimum inhibitory concentration of <2.0 μg/ml (Harrison et al., 1984) and has been used in the therapy of salpingitis, for example (Gjønnaess et al., 1982a). Penicillins are not regarded as highly active against *C. trachomatis* in vitro, although they may inhibit the growth of the organism in vivo (Bowie et al., 1982; Bowie, 1982). Cephalosporins, aminoglycosides, and nitroimidazoles have virtually no activity against *C. trachomatis* (Sweet et al., 1983; Sanders et al., 1986). Sulfonamides alone or in combination with trimethoprim have been found effective against *C. trachomatis* in clinical trials (Paavonen et al., 1980).

Tetracycline treatment of cases of chlamydial urethritis and cervicitis has been found in short-term follow-up studies to be as efficient as penicillin treatment of uncomplicated cases of gonorrhea caused by susceptible, non-β-lactamase-producing strains of *N. gonorrhoeae*. Thus the treatment is believed to be efficient in more than 95% of cases. However, long-term (several months) follow-up studies to evaluate the therapeutic effect of antibiotic treatment of genital and other chlamydial infections are virtually nonexistent.

TABLE 18. Antibiotic Susceptibility of *C. trachomatis*: Overview of Results of in Vitro Studies of MIC for Certain Drugs

Group of antibiotic	Drug	MIC (μg/ml)	Group of antibiotic	Drug	MIC (μg/ml)
Sulfonamides	Sulfamethoxazole	0.5	Macrolides	Erythromycin	0.032–1.05
	Trimethoprim/sulfamethoxazole	1.0		Rosaramycin	0.015–4.0
	Trimethoprim	20.0		Spiramycin	0.5
				Roxithromycin	0.05–0.8
				Azithromycin	0.11
Penicillin	Benzylpenicillin	1.0			
	Phenoxylmethylpenicillin	1.0			
	Methicillin	100	Spectinomycin	Spectinomycin	128–256
	Ampicillin	10.0			
	Amoxicillin	1.0			
	Carbenicillin	1.0	Rifampins	Rifampicin	0.007
	Mecillinam	10			
			Quinolones	Ofloxacin	0.5–1.0
				Difloxacin	0.125–0.25
				Ciprofloxacin	0.125–2.0
Cephalosporins	Cephaloridine	100			
	Cefuroxime	>100			
	Cefoxitin	>100	Aminoglycosides	Kanamycin	> 50
				Gentamicin	> 50
Tetracyclines	Oxytetracycline	0.032–1.02			
	Doxycycline	0.2	Nitroimidazoles	Metronidazole	>500
	Minocycline	0.015–0.03			
	Lymecycline	0.1	Various drugs used in transport and tissue culture media to suppress growth of bacteria and fungi	Colistin	>500
				Vancomycin	>100
				Sopramycin	>200
Chloramphenicol	Chloramphenicol	1.0–5.0		Nystatin	>500
				5-Flurocytocine	> 50
	Lincomycin	256–512			
	Clindamycin	0.5–1.0			

SULFONAMIDES

The two species of the genus *Chlamydia* differ in their susceptibility to sulfonamides in vitro; *C. trachomatis* is more susceptible than *C. psittaci*. This fact was one criterion responsible for the subdivision of the genus into two species (see also Chapter 2).

A number of sulfonamides, e.g., sulfathiazole, sulfadiazine, and sulfasoxazole, have been used to treat chlamydial infections such as lymphogranuloma venereum (Schachter and Dawson, 1978). One advantage of using sulfonamides in cases of genital lesions is that they will not mask a concomitantly acquired infection with *T. pallidum*. In earlier days, sulfonamides were also used to treat trachoma. Today they are not recommended as the first choice treatment of chlamydial infections.

Combinations of trimethoprim and various sulfonamides, e.g., sulfamethoxazole, have been found to be comparatively effective for the treatment of chlamydial urethritis (Bowie et al., 1977a; Johanisson et al., 1979). Trimethoprim-sulfa can be an alternative for treatment of chlamydial infections in patients with drug allergies. It is also a therapeutic alternative in chlamydia-infected persons in whom syphilis cannot be ruled out, since this drug combination will not mask a concomitant treponemal infection.

Trimethoprim alone is ineffective against *C. trachomatis*. It proved ineffective in half of a series of male patients with chlamydial urethritis, who remained culture-positive 2 weeks after finishing treatment; many of the patients still had dysuria and/or urethral discharge at that time. Patients who failed to respond to trimethoprim were successfully cured by subsequent treatment with oxitetracycline (Nielsen et al., 1984).

PENICILLINS

Chlamydiae are considered to lack the peptidoglycan structure found in the cell wall of eubacteria; nevertheless, these organisms have been claimed to have penicillin-binding proteins. Both *C. trachomatis* (see below) and *C. psittaci* (Matsumoto and Manire, 1970) are affected by β-lactam antibiotics.

Penicillin can affect the formation of intracytoplasmic inclusions in tissue cell cultures. It has been claimed that L-form-like chlamydial cells can be formed under the influence of penicillin (Fig. 34A and B). Abnormal initial bodies (IBs) of *C. trachomatis* are produced that fail to mature into elementary bodies (EBs) (Johnson and Hobson, 1977). A similar effect has been seen under the influence of other β-lactam antibiotics.

Great variation (10^4-fold) in the MIC between various β-lactams has been reported in tests using McCoy tissue cell cultures (Hobson et al., 1982b). Thus the following concentrations of penicillins inhibit normal inclusion formation in McCoy cell cultures: phenoxymethyl penicillin 0.01 μg/ml, benzylpenicillin 0.1 μg/ml, and methicillin 10 μg/ml.

Treatment with amoxicillin was generally found to eradicate *C. trachomatis* from the urethra of men with nongonococcal urethritis and in women with mucopurulent cervicitis (Bowie et al., 1981; Paavonen et al., 1988b). Other workers have also studied the therapeutic effect of amoxicillin on genital chlamydial infections, with variable results. Hobson and co-workers (1982b) found 11 (79%) of 14 patients with salpingitis to be "permanently" culture-negative for *C. trachomatis* at 5 to 14 days treatment with either ampicillin or amoxycillin. A more recent study (Møller et al., 1985) reported a good therapeutic effect of pivampicillin in uncomplicated genital chlamydial infections, i.e., with a daily dose of 3.0 g for 10 days. However, when the dose or length of treatment was decreased, the curative effect was markedly reduced, which limits the value of this drug for more general use in the treatment of chlamydial infections.

The use of some parenteral β-lactam antibiotics in the treatment of pelvic inflammatory disease (PID) has been evaluated in relation to a chlamydial etiology of the condition. A combination of such a drug and a tetracycline (or a macrolide) has been recommended in PID therapy to broadly cover the most frequently encountered etiological agents of PID (Wølner-Hansen et al., 1986b).

CEPHALOSPORINS

Cephalosporins are generally less active against *C. trachomatis* in vitro than penicillins. Thus higher concentrations of cephalosporins than penicillins are generally needed to inhibit the formation of normal chlamydial inclusions in tissue cell cultures, i.e., generally at least 100 μg/ml with the exception of cephaloridine (1.0 μg/ml), cephradine (10.0 μg/ml), and ceftriaxone (10.0 μg/ml) (Hobson et al., 1982b).

Cephalosporins, e.g., ceftriaxone (1 g/day intramuscularly), have been found ineffective in the treatment of chlamydial urethritis in males and chlamydial PID in women (Stamm and Cole, 1986; Sweet et al., 1983).

TETRACYCLINES

Most of our information regarding antibiotic therapy of chlamydial infections has been obtained by treatment with different tetracycline drugs (Bowie, 1982). The curative effect (at least as indicated by control cultures after short-term follow-up studies) is approximately 95% in uncomplicated genital chlamydial infections in both males and females when using standard regimens of tetracycline and most of its analogs, i.e., provided a course of at least 10 days is given. Some doctors prefer to prescribe a 7-day course. In complicated genital infections, 14 days of tetracycline treatment is usually recommended.

Some studies (Forslin et al., 1982) have shown that the use of certain tetracycline analogs, when given in standard doses (i.e., tetracycline 500 mg four times daily, oxytetracycline 250 mg four times daily, doxycycline 200 mg stat followed by 100 (SIC!) mg daily, and minocycline 100 mg twice daily) can result in low tissue levels in the upper female genital tract. Acceptable levels were considered to be achieved by the use of lymecycline 300 mg twice daily. It was therefore also proposed that the standard dose (100 mg daily) of doxycycline recommended in many countries should be increased to 200 mg daily during the entire treatment of genital chlamydial infections. In the United States, 200 mg doxycycline per day has long been recommended. Apart from the pharmacokinetic data mentioned, there are other factors influencing the choice of tetracycline drug to be used in the therapy of chlamydial infections, such as photosensitization (a risk associated with the use of most tetracycline analogs, with the exception of lymecycline), occurrence of esophageal lesions (capsule preparation), effect on the gastrointestinal flora (e.g., the efficiency of intestinal adsorption of the drug), other side-effects (e.g., dizziness), and, finally, the price of the drug.

No resistance of *C. trachomatis* to tetracyclines has been reported so far.

MACROLIDES

The therapeutic effect of erythromycin on genital chlamydial infections in both men and women has often been considered so good as to render the drug an acceptable alternative to tetracyclines. On the other hand, others have reported an unacceptably high failure rate with erythromycin, i.e., up to one-fourth of all cases treated. The recommended standard regimen has been 500 mg erythromycin stearate twice daily for 7–10 days (Oriel et al., 1977; Lassus et al., 1979; Johannisson et al., 1979, 1980; Hunter and Sommerville, 1984). With some erythromycin analogs a better adsorption from the gut is obtained when the drug is taken with milk.

Chlamydial strains with a reduced susceptibility to erythromycin have been recovered from patients in the San Francisco area (Mourad et al., 1980). However, there is no indication that such strains create any therapeutic problems.

Erythromycin is the drug of choice for treatment of chlamydial infections in pregnant and lactating women (Chow and Jewesson, 1985), in infants, and in young children (under 7 years of age).

For newborns with chlamydial conjunctivitis, it is important to institute general, not just local, erythromycin therapy because usually the nasopharynx is colonized as well. The dose given must be high enough, i.e., 50 mg/kg body weight twice daily, since lower doses will result in an unacceptable number of therapeutic failures. Therapy for infant chlamydial infections should continue for at least 2 weeks (Sandström, 1987).

The new macrolide roxithromycin is active against *C. trachomatis*. MICs between 0.05 and 0.8 μg/ml have been reported. The MIC and MBC for this drug were found to be identical (Stamm and Suchland, 1986). Its clinical value remains to be established, although preliminary reports seem positive as regards its clinical usefulness.

Of the new macrolides, azithromycin differs from erythromycin by virtue of its prolonged half-time. Azithromycin has been claimed to have an extremely high tissue affinity. In tests of six strains of *C. trachomatis*, an MIC_{50} of 0.075 μg/ml and an MIC_{90} of 0.11 μg/ml for azithromycin were found, as compared to 0.024 μg/ml and 0.042 μg/ml for erythromycin (Slaney et al., 1987).

Another new macrolide, miocamicin, was considered to have cured 25 of 30 cases of genital chlamydial infection when used in a dose of 600 g three times daily (Longhi, 1987).

RIFAMPINS

Rifampicin and rifapentine have a pronounced effect against *C. trachomatis* in in vitro tests (Nabli, 1971). MIC values lower than those found for tetracyclines have been reported. In most countries the use of rifampicin or its analogs is restricted to mycobacterial infections, such as pulmonary tuberculosis. Thus these drugs should not be used as a standard treatment of chlamydial infections.

QUINOLONES

Quinolones, i.e., synthetic derivatives of nalidixic acid possessing a 6-fluoro substitute, are active against a number of bacterial species, including penicillin-resistant gonococci and some other agents that cause genital infection. Therefore quinolones are of potential interest for the treatment of genital chlamydial infections, since concomitant genital infections by multiple agents are common in such patients.

The in vitro activity of different quinolones varies (Rettig et al., 1986) (Table 17). Low MICs, i.e., 0.125–0.25 g/ml, have been found for one of the new carboxyquinolones, difloxacin (Liebowitz et al., 1986). Ofloxacin has been found by some investigators (Stamm and Suchland, 1986) to be one of the most active quinolones in vitro against *C. trachomatis* with an MIC of 0.5 to 1.0 μg/ml. However, Bischoff (1986) found only a 20% cure rate at short-term follow-up after a 5-day course with 200 mg ofloxacin twice daily in patients with genital chlamydial infection.

Negative results have been reported with regard to the curative effect of both norfloxacin and ciprofloxacin on genital chlamydial infections in cases of concomitant gonorrhea when treatment with the quinolones was given as a single dose. Norfloxacin was not effective against *C. trachomatis* in men with NGU (Bowie et al., 1986a). In another study, norfloxacin cured only 23 of 42 *Chlamydia*-infected men with urethritis (Longhi, 1987). Ciprofloxacin had a poor clinical result when the dosage was 500 mg given orally twice a day for 7 days. Thus half of the men in a series of nongonococcal, nonchlamydial cases still had signs of urethritis at follow-up (Arya et al., 1986).

CLINDAMYCIN

Clindamycin (6-chlorolincomycin) has a moderate activity in vitro against *C. trachomatis;* an MIC of 1.0 μg/ml has been reported (Harrison et al., 1984). When 600 mg of clindamycin was given orally three times daily for 7 days to men with NGU, an initial clinical response was often seen. However, approximately 40% of men initially culture-positive for *C. trachomatis* had urethritis one and a half months after initiation of treatment. There was no apparent relationship between the demonstrated in vitro susceptibility of *C. trachomatis* and the ultimate clinical response (Bowie et al., 1986b).

Gjønnaess and associates (1982a) used 300 mg clindamycin orally daily to treat PID patients, half of whom were *Chlamydia* culture-positive from the cervix and 65% of whom had antibodies to *C. trachomatis*. A good clinical response (98%) was found in the vast majority of cases.

The reported MIC of lincomycin for *C. trachomatis* is considerably higher (MIC 256–512 μg/ml) than that of clindamycin (1.0 μg/ml).

DRUGS WITH POOR ACTIVITY AGAINST *C. TRACHOMATIS*

A number of drugs have poor effects on *C. trachomatis* (Table 18). These include the aminoglycosides, e.g., gentamicin and kanamycin. Therefore gentamicin is often added to tissue cell culture media used for the isolation of chlamydiae just to suppress growth of eubacteria. Vancomycin also possesses a low antichlamydial activity, and is often added to tissue cell culture media to suppress microbial overgrowth.

Some antimicrobials with poor activity against *C. trachomatis* are used in transport media for chlamydial samples (see Chapter 6).

Thiamphenicols also have a poor clinical effect on genital chlamydial infections, which should be considered in relation to their widespread use in the treatment of gonorrhea in many parts of the world. Spectinomycin, which is used to treat Hemophilus ducreyi aud penicillinase-producing (PPNG) strains of *N. gonorrhoeae,* also has poor activity against *C. trachomatis* (Alexander et al., 1977).

Other drugs with poor effect against *C. trachomatis* are nitroimidazoles (e.g., metronidazole and tinidazole), which are frequently used to treat trichomoniasis, bacterial vaginosis, and anaerobic infections of the genital tract.

Body Fluid Constituents with Antichlamydial Activity

Several constituents of seminal fluid have an antibacterial effect (Mårdh and Colleen, 1975) as well as antichlamydial activity (Mårdh et al., 1980; Hanna et al., 1981). Among the seminal fluid constituents that can inhibit chlamydial inclusion formation in tissue cell cultures are various metal ions, e.g., Zn^{2+} (Mårdh et al., 1980; Greenberg et al., 1985). Zinc occurs in high concentrations in seminal fluid (Colleen et al., 1975). The presence of chloride sulfate and oxide salts of zinc throughout the entire culture procedure was necessary to demonstrate the antichlamydial effect in McCoy, HeLa 229, and primary prostatic epithelial cells (Greenberg et al., 1985). The Cu^{2+} ion has also been demonstrated to possess antichlamydial activity (Mårdh et al., 1980).

Polyamines, e.g., spermine, inhibit *C. trachomatis* inclusion formation in tissue cell cultures in a concentration-dependent fashion. Whether the effect of spermine is mediated by a toxic effect on the host cell or on the chlamydial cell, or both, is not known (Mårdh et al., 1980a). A dose-related decrease in the number of chlamydial inclusions in McCoy cells was demonstrated in the presence of methylamine and monodamyl cadaverine (Söderlund and Kihlström, 1983).

Lysozyme concentrations of 8.5–58.0 mg/liter have been demonstrated in seminal fluid (Colleen and Mårdh, 1974). Lysozyme, which affects the peptidoglycan of eubacteria (resulting in cell lysis), had no effect on chlamydial reproduction as indicated by the formation of inclusions in experimentally infected McCoy cell cultures. If anything, lysozyme enhanced inclusion formation in McCoy cell cultures (Fig. 35) when added at a concentration of 5 to 100 µg/ml tissue culture medium (Mårdh et al., 1980a). A biphasic dose–response effect was demonstrated. Antichlamydial activity of tears (Elbagir et al., 1988a)

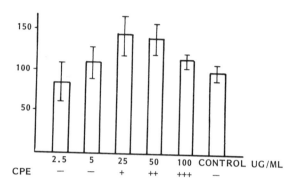

FIGURE 35. Effect of lysozyme on *C. trachomatis* inclusion formation in McCoy cell cultures.

and of amniotic fluid (Wølner-Hanssen and Mårdh, 1982d; Elbagir et al., 1988b; Thomas et al., 1988) has also been demonstrated.

Sueltenfuess and Pollard (1963) found a duck strain of *C. psittaci* to be susceptible to interferon (IFN). Later studies (Rothermel et al., 1983a) indicated γ-interferon (γ-IFN) to be the factor in lymphokine that activated human macrophages to inhibit intracellular *C. psittaci* replication. Rothermel and co-workers (1983b) found murine fibroblast interferon to inhibit RB replication and *C. trachomatis* inclusion formation. Interferon reduced intracellular development of *C. trachomatis* by 90%, whereas growth of *C. psittaci* was unaffected. Purified human γ-IFN added to HEp-2 tissue cell cultures (derived from a human carcinoma of the larynx) reduced the EB yield of *C. trachomatis*, serotype L_2. The interferon influenced the maturation of RBs to EBs. High concentrations (>350 IU/ml) of interferon inhibited inclusion formation (Shemer and Sarov, 1985).

Persistence, Relapses, and Reinfections of Chlamydial Infections

Chlamydial infections can remain clinically silent for a considerable period of time. Both human beings and animals can be carriers of *C. trachomatis* and *C. psittaci* for years.

Latency generally means persistence without multiplication of the agent. The term has mainly referred to viral infections. Latency in that sense is not known to take place in chlamydial infections. "Chronic" or "persistent" infection are probably better terms to use in connection with chlamydial infections.

In human beings, persistent chlamydial infection has been best documented in relation to trachoma, i.e., in infections by *C. trachomatis* serotypes A, B, B_a, and C. Paratrachoma cases persisting for several years have been described; i.e., one case continued for more than five years (Bialasiewicz and John, 1987.) The persistence of genital infections by *C. trachomatis,* serotypes D–K, for up to at least one year has been documented in newborns infected at birth (Rees et al., 1977a, 1977b; Bell et al., 1986). As with many other infections, differentiating between relapse and reinfection is often difficult.

Human *C. psittaci* infections persisting for more than 10 years have been documented anecdotally (Meyer and Eddie, 1953). In experimental infections in animals, *C. psittaci* can persist for years. Thus, as an example, Gale and co-workers (1971) found an ocular infection persisting in a Taiwan monkey for over 10 years.

Chlamydial serum antibodies probably do not prevent mucosal reinfection, but they may play a role in limiting the extent of chlamydial disease. There is an inverse correlation between the number of *C. trachomatis* organisms that can be recovered from the cervix and the presence of S-IgA antibodies to the agent in cervical secretion (Brunham et al., 1983). Epidemiological data suggest that prior genital chlamydial infection may provide some protection against reinfection. Jones and Batteiger (1986) evaluated 2546 men and 1998 women with and without a history of exposure to *C. trachomatis*, serotypes D–K. The isolation rate of *C. trachomatis* was lower at the index visit in those with rather than without a known exposure to the organism. In both men and women the isolation rate was significantly lower when the documented prior infection occurred 6 months before the index visit than when longer time had passed. This might suggest that the protective immunity is relatively short-lived. The frequent recurrence of chlamydial infections in a sexually active population also supports the hypothesis that the protection is short-lived. Barnes and co-workers (1986) used monoclonal antibodies to type isolates from patients who had had at least two episodes of chlamydial infection separated by an intervening negative culture. All their patients had received chemotherapeutic agents known to be effective in vitro against *C. trachomatis*, suggesting that type-specific immunity is not always conferred after mucosal chlamydial infection or that natural chlamydial infection does not always prevent further infection even with the same serotype of *C. trachomatis* (Barnes et al., 1986).

In the vast majority of controlled studies on the treatment of genital chlamydial infection in men and women with short-term follow-up, the persistence of *C. trachomatis* was negligible (Bowie et al., 1981b; Brunham et al., 1982c; Sanders et al., 1986). However, Oriel (1986), Mårdh (1987), and others have criticized the previous studies on the basis of lack of long-term follow-up. A conventional one-week course of antibiotic therapy can result in inapparent treatment failure with persistent chronic infection. Persistence or late recurrence of cervical and endometrial chlamydial infection might account for many cases of chronic or subchronic pelvic inflammatory disease. A comparison of short-term versus long-term tetracycline therapy with prolonged follow-up (6 to 12 months) is thus needed to further assess the optimal dosage and duration of therapy in genital and other chlamydial infections.

Persistent infections in tissue cell cultures by both *C. psittaci* and *C. trachomatis* can be demonstrated (Morgan and Bader, 1957; Manire and Galasso, 1959; Lee and Moulder, 1981). Cryptic cell forms of *C. psittaci* have been reported to occur in tissue cell cultures (Lee and Moulder, 1981), whereas no such cell forms of *C. trachomatis* have been described.

The EBs of *C. trachomatis* can leave the host cell without the cell rupturing (Todd and Caldwell, 1985). This allows a continuous production of infectious chlamydial particles (EBs) at perhaps a very low rate through the life span of the host cell. This may be the basis of a persistent chlamydial infection.

It has been demonstrated in experimentally infected tissue cell cultures that depression of chlamydial infection can be effected by a culture medium deficient in certain amino acids. ''Reactivation'' of the replication by cytostatic treatment (i.e., by cycloheximide) of the host cells has also been described (Hatch, 1975; Moulder et al., 1980).

It is possible that subinhibitory concentrations of antibiotic might produce a "latentlike" chlamydial infection in vivo. Homologous specific secretory IgA antibodies might also play such a role.

When staining *Chlamydia*-infected cells with dyes, the chlamydiae will not stain during certain stages of their replication cycle and at those times are "nondetectable," i.e., they have a superficial similarity to viruses in their eclipse phase. This might be one reason that chlamydiae were once believed to be viruses. The DNA of the chlamydiae can, however, be detected in the host cell throughout their whole reproduction cycle.

Cytokines might activate host cells such that productive chlamydial infection is inhibited, but intracellular chlamydial viability is maintained (Taylor et al., 1987a; Byrne et al., 1988) (see also Chapter 9).

Subclinical chlamydial infections can exacerbate, and clinically silent infections can become overt. Although few data support the idea, it seems that certain infections can trigger a latent chlamydial infection. Gonorrhea may be one such infection. That is, if a chlamydial urethritis appears several weeks after an episode of gonorrhea, the urethritis might not be the result of a second infection acquired at the same time as the gonococcal infection but rather of an exacerbation of a previously acquired chlamydial infection.

Worthy of consideration is the possibility that the lack of certain triggering factors might render chlamydial strains unable to produce infection, which can result in a false-negative culture diagnosis.

11

Vaccines

The development of chlamydial vaccines is generally considered desirable since *C. trachomatis* and *C. psittaci* are common pathogens and chlamydial infections can result in severe complications. The prospectives for such vaccines from a molecular standpoint have recently been discussed by Ward and associates (1988). Until recently, *C. trachomatis* vaccine studies and trials mainly focused on prevention of trachoma. Some of these study groups progressed to human field trials (Grayston et al., 1964; Guerra et al., 1967; Soldati et al., 1971; Grayston, 1971; Nichols and Snyder, 1971; Bietti et al., 1972; Collier, 1972). However, because the results were not promising, trachoma prevention is now being approached mainly by other means, i.e., by education and treatment.

Different laboratory animals have been used in trachoma vaccine research, e.g., mice (Soldati et al., 1970), guinea pigs, and monkeys. Mice infected intraperitoneally with purified trachoma agents developed a cellular immune response. A similar response was demonstrated in volunteers vaccinated with a purified killed lyophilized suspension of elementary bodies (Soldati et al., 1970).

Infection with *C. trachomatis* is associated with both humoral and cell-mediated immunity. Vaccination studies on Taiwan monkeys revealed a partial protective effect against *C. trachomatis* conjunctivitis with homologous, but not heterologous, strains (Wang et al., 1967). Animals infected with heterologous strains developed more severe conjunctivitis than nonvaccinated animals.

A *C. trachomatis* vaccine aimed for oral use has also been tested in other monkey models. The monkeys were enterically immunized with killed and live *C. trachomatis* organisms (Whittum-Hudson et al., 1986). The animals were then challenged ocularly with *C. trachomatis* and the local immune response in the conjunctiva was analyzed. In immunized animals, the ratio of T helpers and suppressor/cytotoxic T lymphocytes was closer to 1 than in nonimmunized monkeys. Also, subepithelial, extrafollicular B lymphocytes were dominant in the vaccinated monkeys. Furthermore, more IgA- and IgG-bearing, but fewer

IgM-bearing, cells were detected. However, no correlation between the cellular changes and resistance to chlamydial infection was noted (Whittum-Hudson et al., 1986). Taylor and Prendergast (1987) used *C. trachomatis* LPS recombinant vaccine in ocularly challenged cynomolgus monkeys without protective effect.

Owl monkeys have also been used in vaccination studies that employed topical application of a vaccine consisting of irradiated *C. trachomatis* organisms (McDonald et al., 1984).

In trachoma vaccine studies some protective immunity against trachoma following vaccination has been noted. However, in U.S. studies the effectiveness of the trachoma vaccine was low. At late follow-up no difference in the ocular condition between vaccinated subjects and controls could be demonstrated (Grayston and Wang, 1978).

Italian investigators used partially purified elementary bodies as antigen in their vaccine, which was administered intradermally to volunteers who were blind for reasons other than trachoma. The volunteers were infected by the trachoma serotypes of *C. trachomatis*. However, there was difficulty in evaluating the protective effect of the vaccine. Thus, as in many other vaccine trials, behavioral changes induced by the trial and improvements in living standard during the study period, i.e., changes induced in the natural course of the trachoma disease, interfered with the evaluation. It was also believed that the vaccination caused a worsening of the pathological changes in the eyes, which might have been due to an anamnestic response to previous ("natural") exposure to *C. trachomatis* (Guerra et al., 1967; Soldati et al., 1970).

Trials in various animal models (see Chapter 5) also pointed to the risk of side effects of vaccination when using the guinea pig inclusion conjunctivitis (GPIC) agent, the mouse pneumonitis agent, and *C. trachomatis*, respectively.

Identification of chlamydial antigens with protective and hypersensitivity-inducing properties would be important in future *C. trachomatis* vaccine production. Serotype-specific protection might be induced without development of serotype-specific hypersensitivity. Developments in gene technology might assist in solving these problems.

To be protective, the *C. trachomatis* vaccine must have a high particle content (Grayston et al., 1971) and include the infecting serotype(s) (Wang et al., 1967). Such vaccines have so far been expensive to produce in large quantities and have provided only brief protection (Grayston, 1971). Besides the fact that poor results may follow administration of vaccines with insufficient antigenic mass or containing heterologous serotypes (Grayston et al., 1971), the disease can be more serious in a vaccinated subject than in a nonvaccinated one.

Chlamydia psittaci vaccines have been evaluated in various animal models. In a study in cattle of a vaccine against the bovine abortion agent, the route of challenge proved to be important in terms of protection. In subcutaneously or intramuscularly challenged animals, no protection could be noted. However, intradermally challenged animals were protected (McKercher et al., 1973). Intradermal challenge, where the agent is introduced through the skin, probably more resembles the natural course of infection in cattle. In skin, the cellular protective mechanisms interact with the *C. psittaci* agent; by other routes, however, the infecting agent may escape dermal immunological events.

Also studied were enteric *C. psittaci* vaccines for protection against ocular and genital tract infection in guinea pigs. The guinea pigs were conjunctivally and vaginally challenged with the inclusion conjunctivitis (GPIC) agent. Less severe clinical disease developed and fewer infected cells were observed at the challenge sites in immunized animals, indicating that some protection had been conferred (Nichols et al., 1978).

In cats, the effect of vaccination with the feline pneumonitis agent (a *C. psittaci* species) following respiratory and ocular infection with *C. psittaci* has been studied. Reports on the effect of the vaccination vary widely, i.e., from protection to no protection at all (cf. Wills et al., 1987). However, the immunization and challenge routes have varied from one study to another, which may partially explain the noted discrepancies. In a recent study, Wills and co-workers (1987) vaccinated cats subcutaneously and challenged them ocularly. Conjunctivitis of reduced severity was noted in the immunized animals. However, no difference was observed between immunized and nonimmunized animals in the shedding of the agent or in the transmission of the infection from the gastrointestinal or genital tracts.

V

Chlamydia trachomatis Infections

Trachoma

EPIDEMIOLOGY

Hundreds of millions of people are affected by trachoma, a conjunctival and corneal infection caused by *C. trachomatis,* mainly of serotypes A, B, B_a, and C (Grayston and Wang, 1975). Certain "genital" serotypes (e.g., D) of *C. trachomatis* have also been recovered from the eyes of some trachoma patients. In principle, trachoma occurs throughout the world. Infection by *C. trachomatis,* serotype A, has been demonstrated in the Middle East and North Africa, but not the United States or the Far East (Wang and Grayston, 1982). The disease is a major public health problem in many rural areas of the developing world, particularly hot and dry regions. It is estimated that about 2 million persons are blind and even a greater number of persons are suffering from partial loss of vision as a result of trachoma (Fig. 36).

For now, *blinding* trachoma constitutes a health problem in the so-called trachoma belt, i.e., an area reaching from North Africa and the sub-Saharan region, through the Middle East, to the dry regions of the Indian subcontinent and Southeast Asia. There are also pockets of blinding trachoma in certain regions of Latin America and in the Pacific (Dawson et al., 1981). *Nonblinding* trachoma can be found in all the above-mentioned areas as well as in most dry subtropical and tropical countries (Dawson et al., 1981).

In most areas of Sudan, trachoma is hyperendemic and is still the main cause of blindness followed by onchocerciasis. In rural areas up to 60–80% of the population have been or are presently infected. The rate of blindness has been estimated at 4.1–4.2%. In the Khartoum (capital of Sudan), the trachoma rate is only 20–30%. There the disease is nonblinding, possibly as a result of both easy access to treatment and a higher awareness of trachoma in the population of the capital city than in the rural areas. Interestingly, the intensity of the disease and the complication rate of trachoma in certain areas of Sudan increases by distance

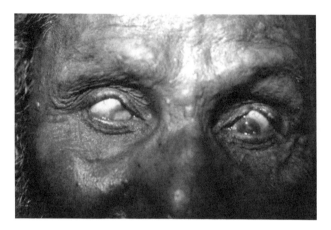

FIGURE 36. A man blinded by trachoma.

from the main roads (highways), which is attributable to the decreasing ease with which individuals can receive medicine and counsel. The rate of blindness is thought to relate strongly to bacterial superinfection, such as those of streptococci, staphylococci, *H. influenzae,* or measles.

Trachoma is still common in many rural areas in Egypt. The 1937 study of Attiah and El Tobgy stated that 97% of the population suffered from trachoma. In 1974, 48% of school children from rural areas had the clinical diagnosis of trachoma (Mordhorst and Hegazy, 1974). In 1982, Schachter and Dawson reported that 25% of Egyptian children in villages had moderate or severe trachoma. In a recent study (Barsoum et al., 1987), 26% of 777 primary school students had active trachoma, and the overall prevalence of the disease ranged from 16 to 35%. Of 312 patients with ocular complaints, 39% had trachoma.

Although trachoma is still endemic in many rural areas in Egypt, its prevalence is declining there and in many other places, e.g., Tunisia (Dawson et al., 1976) and southern Iran (Jones, 1975). In Saudi Arabia some decades ago, a milder trachoma was generally seen in town sites than in rural areas, including oasis (Nichols et al., 1967). The antibody response in Saudi Arabian children with trachoma was studied by McComb and Nichols (1970).

Trachoma is a common disease (Darougar et al., 1971b) in Iran. It is of interest that in studies of genital chlamydial infections in Iranian prostitutes, antibodies to *C. trachomatis* serotypes D–K were present in 94.2% and to serotypes A–C in 2%. Only 6.9% had a positive culture for *C. trachomatis.*

In South Africa, in areas where active trachoma was recently common, *C. trachomatis* has been recovered less often from persons with nongonococcal genital infection than in persons in whom trachoma is uncommon. In other areas of South Africa where trachoma has been rare, persons with nongonococcal genital infection are often *C. trachomatis* culture positive. Antibodies to the agent have been found in the former rather than the latter group of individuals (Ballard, 1982).

Earlier trachoma had been a significant clinical problem in Australia, particularly in the Northern Territories. In 1957, its prevalence in the aboriginal population was 63–69%, with a blinding rate of up to 7%. In western Australian schools in the late 1950s, the incidence of trachoma was 30%. During the 1960s, trachoma accounted for 2.2% of all cases of blindness in Australia (cf. Howard, 1966).

The disease of trachoma also occurred among North American Indians (Hoshiwara et al., 1971), from whom *C. trachomatis* serotype B_a was isolated.

Grayston and co-workers (1977) isolated the first trachoma organism from a Taiwan patient in 1958. Thereafter, this group conducted several studies in Taiwan concerning the natural history of trachoma and the effects of trachoma vaccines and antibiotic treatment. In 1960–1961, WHO performed an island-wide prevalence survey in Taiwan which revealed that up to 40% of individuals at any age had active trachoma (Assaad and Maxwell-Lyons, 1967). Woolridge and co-workers (1967) examined approximately 900 incoming first grade school-children (age 5 years) and noted that 23% of them had active trachoma. During 6 years of school, 43% of those with normal eyes at entry developed trachoma, and one-third with trachoma at entry reverted to normal eyes. It was concluded from this study that in the early 1960s virtually all persons in Taiwan had contracted trachoma during their lifetimes, but many healed spontaneously without sequelae (Woolridge et al., 1967). The tendency to spontaneous healing of trachoma was further supported by a study by Grayston and co-workers (1977), whereby family households that had both members with normal eyes and members with active trachoma were followed from the early 1970s to 1980. Most households showed evidence of single serotype infection only (Grayston et al., 1977).

The incubation time of trachoma is 1–3 weeks (in experimentally infected volunteers), whereas the blinding process can take decades. Transmission with infected material occurs either by direct (eye-to-eye) or by indirect (hands, clothing, and flies) contact. Children in endemic areas are often infected very early in life. Intrafamiliar spread appears important. Better sanitary conditions and other improvements leading to a higher standard of living have doubtless contributed to a reduction or even disappearance of trachoma in many areas.

IMMUNOPATHOLOGY

Halberstaedter and von Prowazek were the first to demonstrate a possible association between a probable infectious agent and trachoma. In 1907 they could demonstrate intracytoplasmic inclusions in conjunctival scrapings from trachoma patients (Fig. 9). However, the first successful isolation of chlamydiae from the eyes of a trachoma patient was not accomplished until 1957 when T'ang used embryonated hen's egg for that purpose.

In experimentally infected monkeys, chronic chlamydial infection has been shown to persist for up to 10 years (Gale et al., 1971).

Trachoma is a chronic keratoconjunctivitis that usually affects both eyes. The first symptoms of the disease may be minimal and go unnoticed. Watering, mucopurulent discharge, foreign body sensation, and ptosis may occur. Clinical signs involve the eyelids (swelling and redness), the conjunctivae [edema, diffuse infiltration, papillary and follicular responses (Fig. 37), and scars (Fig. 38)], and cornea (lesions, punctate keratitis, and scars).

One factor known to escalate nonblinding trachoma to blinding trachoma is bacterial conjunctivitis. This infection often causes corneal ulceration, which has been called acute ophthalmia. Corneal ulceration may also occur as a result of trichiasis and entropion that results from mechanical damage caused by the inturned eyelashes (Fig. 39). The lesion may be followed by scarring. Corneal vascularization rarely involves the visual axis during the acute stage of trachoma and thus does not affect vision. Trachomatous conjunctival inflammatory disease in the upper fornix may lead to defective lid closure. Also, defective tear secretion may favor traumatic and secondary infective damage of the cornea. Defective tear production implies a disappearance or reduction of the washing effect and antibacterial activity (e.g., of lysozyme) of the tears. Corneal lesions include inflammatory alterations of the epithelium and anterior stroma. Superficial neo-

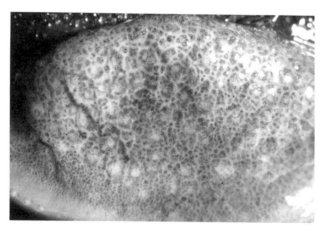

FIGURE 37. Tarsal follicles and papillae in an early case of trachoma. (Courtesy of Dr. J. Treharne.)

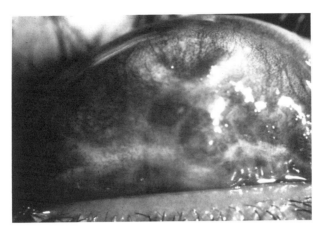

FIGURE 38. Scarring of the upper tarsal conjunctiva in a case of trachoma. (Courtesy of Dr. J. Treharne.)

vascularization (vascular pannus) may be seen. The pannus is usually more pronounced at the superior limbus. Pannus also develops in experimentally infected monkeys (Wang and Grayston, 1967). Patients with corneal vascularization and central corneal scarring may be seen after superinfection, malnutrition, and poor social conditions. Corneal vascularization and connective tissue infiltration may also be present all around the limbus and extend over the cornea leading to opacity and blindness (Fig. 36). Lymphoid follicles of the limbus may

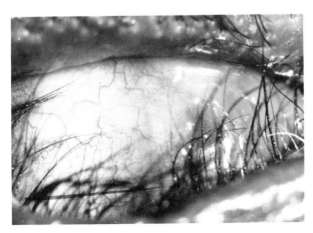

FIGURE 39. Trichiasis and entropion in a case of trachoma. (Courtesy of Dr. J. Treharne.)

resolve but leave characteristic depressions. These have been called Herbert's pits. They are also occasionally seen after paratrachoma (caused by *C. trachomatis,* serotypes D–K) (see also Chapter 3).

The process from primary infection to blinding sequelae may take up to 25 or 30 years. Reinfections and other ocular infections contribute to the blinding process (Taylor et al., 1982a,b; Grayston et al., 1985a). In milder cases there may be spontaneous resolution of the inflammatory phase, whereas more severe cases may progress to blindness.

STAGING AND CLINICAL DIAGNOSIS

A diagnosis of classical trachoma requires at least two of the following clinical signs: follicles on the upper tarsal conjunctiva, limbic follicles, typical conjunctival scarring, and vascular pannus most marked at the superior limbus (Dawson et al., 1981).

Trachoma can be clinically classified by stages or by the intensity of the inflammation in the tarsal conjunctiva, which is considered to be representative of the trachomatous inflammation of the whole eye. MacCallan's classification describes the evolution of trachoma (MacCallan, 1936; Dawson et al., 1981). Thus it neither classifies according to intensity of inflammation nor identifies individuals at risk of sight loss. Therefore it has no prognostic value. The MacCallan classification is presented in Table 19.

Another classification of trachoma was created by Dawson and co-workers (1975, 1981) based on the presence of inflammatory changes in the upper tarsal conjunctiva. In this classification, lymphoid follicles and papillary hypertrophy

TABLE 19. Staging of Trachoma[a]

Stage	Alterations
I	Early infective trachoma
	Immature follicles
	No conjunctival scarring
II	Established trachoma
	Follicles with papillary hypertrophy
	No conjunctival scarring
III	As stages I and II, but conjunctival scarring
IV	Conjunctival inflammation resolved
	Scar tissue eventually progressing
	Noninfectious

[a]After MacCallan (1936).

TABLE 20. Staging of Trachoma Based on Scoring of Lymphoid Follicles
and Papillary Hypertrophy[a]

Intensity of trachoma	Follicles	Papillae
Trivial	Not present or sparse	Normal, or minimal or moderate hypertrophy
Mild	Present, but only in areas close to the lid margin	Same as trivial
Moderate	Present abundantly in the whole upper eyelid	Moderate hypertrophy, prominent papillae
Severe	Same as moderate	Pronounced hypertrophy, conjunctivae thickened and opaque

[a]After Dawson and associates (1975, 1981).

are clinically scored from 0 to 3, where 0 corresponds to next-to-normal findings and 3 to pronounced changes. Based on this scoring, an intensity scale for trachoma is obtained. The intensity-based scale includes four classes: trivial, mild, moderate, and severe (Dawson et al., 1981) (Table 20).

In 1987 (Thylefors et al., 1987), a simplified scheme for easy and reliable grading of trachoma was presented by WHO. The scheme was designed for assessment of trachoma prevalence and intensity, and of signs predictive of visual loss at the community level. The grading system is based on the recording of the presence or absence of five selected key signs inherent to trachoma. These signs include medium trachomatous inflammation in the conjunctiva with follicular inflammation (TF), intense trachomatous inflammation with diffuse thickening of the conjunctiva (TI), scarring of tarsal conjunctiva (TS), corneal opacity (CO), and inturned eyelashes (trichiasis; TT). This grading scheme has been tested in Burma and Tunisia (Thylefors et al., 1987) as well as Tanzania (Taylor et al., 1987b), and good reproducibility, both intraobserver and interobserver, has been noted. In addition, it is easily learned by ophthalmologists and ophthalmic nurses, rendering it suitable for widespread application in trachoma field studies (Taylor et al., 1987b).

CLINICAL FINDINGS

The clinical features of trachoma were recently reviewed by Dawson (1986). In the infectious stages, distinct follicles with intense infiltration and papillary hypertrophy in the conjunctiva (Fig. 37), particularly in the upper tarsal conjunctiva, can be seen. Later, cicatrization of the conjunctiva appears as fine linear and small stellate scars in mild cases and as broad confluent or synecchial scars in more severe cases (Fig. 38). At this stage there may be spontaneous resolution. Progression of scarring may lead to entropion (inward deviation of the eyelashes) and trichiasis (misdirection of the eyelashes) (Fig. 39). Inturned eyelashes may cause corneal lesions. The intensity of the conjunctival inflammatory changes forms the basis for clinical classification of the disease (Dawson et al., 1981) (Table 19).

LABORATORY DIAGNOSIS

Laboratory tests can be used to confirm the clinical diagnosis of trachoma, to monitor the effect of therapy, and to support epidemiological studies.

Chlamydial inclusions can be detected in samples scraped with a metal spatula from the upper tarsal conjunctiva with firm, even strokes across the tarsal surface (WHO, 1975; Jones, 1974). The material obtained is evenly spread on clean glass slides, and then fixed and stained with Giemsa (WHO, 1975). Each Giemsa-stained smear (Fig. 9) requires 30–40 min of careful examination. Conjunctival smears can also be stained by fluorescent monoclonal antibodies. Immunofluorescence staining with monoclonal antibodies is more rapid than Giemsa staining, i.e., 5–10 min is required for microscopy. However, recent studies indicate that tests using labeled monoclonal antibodies have a low sensitivity (Wilson et al., 1986). Immunofluorescence tests using polyclonal labeled antichlamydial antibodies have an even lower sensitivity in mild trachoma (Dawson et al., 1976). Dawson and co-workers (1976) used Giemsa and polyclonal antibody immunofluorescent antibodies to stain chlamydiae. They studied Tunisian children with mild trachoma, in whom only 4% were chlamydiae positive. The tests performed much better in patients with moderate and severe trachoma, i.e., the tests were positive in 20 and 56% of the cases, respectively. Nichols and associates (1967), also using polyclonal immunofluorescence tests, detected chlamydiae in only 2.8% of children with mild trachoma living in town sites in Saudi Arabia. In Saudi Arabian children with more severe trachoma living in oasis, the test was positive in 41.5%.

It is best to use samples swabbed from the conjunctiva for the isolation of chlamydiae. Culture studies are more sensitive than microscopy of Giemsa-stained smears (Darougar et al., 1979). In active trachoma, *C. trachomatis* has been isolated in 7–82% of cases; it is isolated more frequently with increasing severity of the trachoma (Darougar et al., 1971a, 1977b; 1979).

In monkeys experimentally infected with the trachoma serotypes of *C. trachomatis,* the organism could only be demonstrated by culture within 8 weeks of challenge (Taylor et al., 1981). This suggests the difficulties of diagnosing trachoma by culture, except in the very early stages of disease.

More than 90% of children with mild trachoma have negative cultures and cytological examinations (Giemsa stains). The same is true for 25% of children with florid clinical signs of trachomatous inflammation.

Recently, Mabey and associates (1987) tested 172 patients with mild, 30 with moderate, and 26 with severe trachoma and 997 individuals with no disease. Of the samples, 20.3, 46.7, 26.9, and 5.0% had positive ELISA tests, respectively, while by isolation, 12.4, 33.3, 36.8, and 3.3% were positive in the four groups. Thus chlamydial antigen was demonstrated in 49 subjects without trachoma.

In field studies, culture and direct-specimen antigen tests, i.e., immunofluorescence and ELISA tests, are unsuitable for the diagnosis of trachoma. Rather, cytological studies of Giemsa-stained smears have traditionally been used for diagnosis. The method has high specificity and low sensitivity, particularly in mild trachoma (see also above).

The direct-specimen antigen detection tests done so far seem to underscore the overall prevalence of trachoma in a population; the less severe the disease, the more this statement applies.

Microscopic techniques (not requiring a fluorescent microscope) might become suitable for trachoma field studies in certain areas, i.e., when techniques based on immunoperoxidase staining of monoclonal antibodies are more developed. Clinical experience with these tests, however, is still scant and their value in trachoma field studies has not been evaluated. Wilson and associates (1986) used fluorescent monoclonal antibody tests for the diagnosis of trachoma. In their test series of 475 children, 114 (25%) had inflammatory trachoma. Of these, nine had positive IF tests. In five of nine samples more than 100 EBs were found, whereas in the remaining cases only 10–20 EBs could be detected per sample. The authors used no other diagnostic method for comparison.

In a study of Egyptian rural patients with clinical signs of trachoma, staining with labeled monoclonal antibodies exposed twice as many *Chlamydia*-positive cases (63%) as staining with Giemsa (32%) (Barsoum et al., 1987).

Micro-IF tests can detect antibodies against the trachoma serotypes (A, B, B_a, and C of *C. trachomatis*) in both sera and tears. CF antibody titers of sera tend to be low. Serum micro-IF IgG antichlamydial antibodies are often found, whereas IgM antibodies are not. Possibly antichlamydial serum IgM antibodies occur infrequently as a result of reinfection by a new trachoma serotype. In recent years, trachoma associated with "genital" serotypes has been detected in locations previously known as trachoma areas (Harrison et al., 1985).

Tears can be collected by placing filter paper strips or cellulose sponges in the lower conjunctival fornix (WHO, 1975). A correlation between the presence of chlamydial tear IgG antibody with the isolation of *C. trachomatis* from the conjunctiva has been found (McComb and Nichols, 1969; Hanna et al., 1973; Treharne et al., 1978b).

PREVENTION AND TREATMENT

A WHO program involving local intermittent tetracycline treatment has improved the trachoma situation in many countries. For example, in the four northernmost provinces of Sudan, where the program began in 1962, there has been a clear drop in the incidence of trachoma.

The topical trachoma treatment recommended by WHO is a twice-daily application of tetracycline ointment for 5 consecutive days once a month for 6 months (WHO, 1975). The effect of this treatment is short-lived, and a major drawback of local treatment is that *C. trachomatis* also occurs at extraocular sites, such as the nasopharynx (Malaty et al., 1981). In addition, prevention of trachomatous blindness cannot be achieved by use of topical antibiotics alone, which is why systemic treatment is recommended.

Educational programs (e.g., by UNICEF) on eye hygiene are believed to be an important epidemiological tool, comparable to the distribution of soap. In some villages, the schoolmaster or another individual is sometimes expected to fulfill the program by administering eye ointment on a scheduled basis.

Doxycycline has been successfully used in the treatment of mild, chronic, nonblinding trachoma in American Indians (Hoshiwara et al., 1971). Because children are the major target group for treatment of trachoma, tetracycline was never considered the drug of choice. However, there have been recent arguments pointing out the advantage of tetracycline for treatment of children. The optimal dose regimen for tetracycline or other drug treatment of trachoma has not yet been established. As in all antibiotic treatments, the blood levels achieved and the length of therapy are essential to the outcome (Dawson and Schachter, 1985).

Oral erythromycin is considered a therapeutic alternative in trachoma, possibly in conjunction with local treatment by the same drug. Whether the new macrolides, e.g., roxithromycin, are also effective in trachoma therapy remains to be established.

Sulfonamides have previously been used in the treatment of trachoma, but have not been recommended since the late 1950s because of their potential side effects.

Genital and Associated Infections in the Male

INTRODUCTION

C. trachomatis causes a number of infectious conditions in the male genital tract, including infections of the accessory genital glands (Tables 1 and 21).

NONGONOCOCCAL URETHRITIS (NGU) AND POSTGONOCOCCAL URETHRITIS (PGU)

Epidemiology

In Western countries the incidence of nongonococcal urethritis (NGU) currently exceeds that of gonococcal urethritis (GU)—in some areas by as much as 5–10 times. In most industrialized countries today, NGU is the most common manifestation of venereal disease in males. It may have important consequences when complicated, for example, by epididymitis. Up to 50–60% of NGU cases have been shown to be caused by *C. trachomatis* (Dunlop et al., 1972; Oriel et al., 1972; Holmes et al., 1975; Schachter et al., 1975b; Alani et al., 1977; Ripa et al., 1978a; Terho, 1978; Thelin et al., 1980; cf. Bowie, 1984).

Some studies suggest that gonococci are more infectious than chlamydiae. The attack rate of gonorrhea is greater than that of chlamydial genital infection, although the latter is still not well defined.

Most (50–75%) sex partners of chlamydial NGU cases have positive genital cultures for *C. trachomatis* (Oriel et al., 1972; Holmes et al., 1975; Terho, 1978; Paavonen et al., 1978; Thelin and Mårdh, 1982; Bowie, 1984), indicating that the infection is transmitted sexually.

TABLE 21. Clinical and Laboratory Criteria for *C. trachomatis* Infections in Men[a]

	Clinical criteria	Laboratory criteria	
		Presumptive	Diagnostic
Nongonococcal urethritis (NGU)	Discharge, dysuria; clear or yellow urethral discharge on examination	Urethral Gram stain with ≥4 PMNs/×1000 field; pyuria on first visit urine	Positive culture or direct-antigen test
Acute epididymitis	Fever, testicular pain, evidence of urethritis, epididymal tenderness on examination	As for NGU	As for NGU; positive culture on epididymal aspirate
Proctitis	Rectal pain, discharge, bleeding; mucopurulent discharge; spontaneous or induced bleeding on anoscopy	Rectal Gram stain with >1 PMN/1000× field	Positive culture or direct-antigen test
LGV proctocolitis	Severe rectal pain, discharge, bleeding; markedly abnormal anoscopy with anal lesions extending into colon; fever, lymphadenopathy	Rectal Gram stain with >1 PMNs/1000× field	Positive culture or direct-antigen test; CF antibody titer ≥1/64

[a]PMN = polymorphonuclear leukocyte; LGV = lymphogranuloma venereum; CF = complement fixation.

Several culture studies have shown chlamydial urethritis to be less common in homosexual than heterosexual men. The study by Stamm and associates (1984b) indicated that chlamydial infection could be detected by culture studies in only 5% of homosexual men. However, serological studies demonstrate the presence of antibodies to *C. trachomatis* equally often in homosexual and heterosexual groups of men (Persson, 1986). The last author also found roughly every second man attending a VD clinic to have antichlamydial antibodies, regardless of sexual preference.

Figure 40 shows the number of cases of venereal urethritis—of both gonococcal and chlamydial origin—diagnosed in genitourinary medical outpatient clinics in Great Britain. Marked socioeconomic and racial differences in susceptibility to gonococcal and nongonococcal urethritis have been claimed to exist in U.K. patients (McCutchan, 1984).

Diagnosis of Urethritis

The diagnosis of urethritis is usually based on the demonstration of an increased number of polymorphonuclear leukocytes (PMLs) in smears of urethral

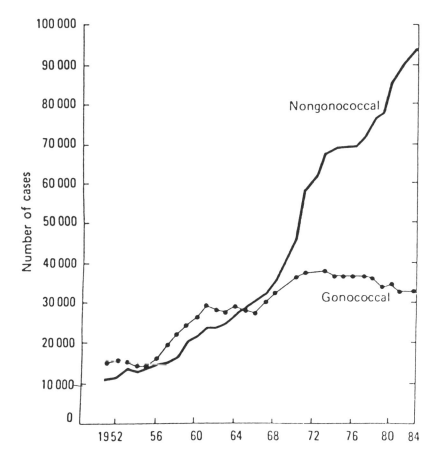

FIGURE 40. Reported cases of nongonococcal and gonococcal urethritis in England and Wales 1951–1984. (Source: WHO.)

discharge. It has been recommended that the cutoff level of the number of leukocytes per high-power field, i.e., between a normal and pathological urethral smear, be decreased from 10 to four cells (Bowie, 1978). However, it should be remembered that the number of leukocytes shed can vary greatly during a 24-hr period in the same individual.

In a study (Arya et al., 1984) of 236 consecutive male STD clinic patients who were sexually active, four polymorphonuclear leukocytes per high-power field in a Gram-stained urethral smear were a useful cutoff point for separating men with and without gonorrhea. The cutoff point also correlated well with the occurrence of *C. trachomatis*. However, the value of Gram-staining in the diagnosis of urethritis was limited in therapeutic decision making when the patient was first seen (Laudis et al., 1988).

In NGU, intracellular diplococci can*not* be seen in methylene blue-stained urethral smears, a finding that is the basis for the "spot" diagnosis of chlamydial urethritis (Fig. 41).

In a study of almost 600 men presenting to an STD clinic in Seattle, 12% were culture-positive for *C. trachomatis,* while approximately half had micro-IF antichlamydial antibodies to the agent. Of the men with *C. trachomatis* urethral infection, approximately one-fourth had no signs or symptoms of urethritis and approximately one-third had a normal number of leukocytes in urethral Gram stain. Clinicians appropriately treated 91% of gonorrhea patients on their initital visit (before culture results were available), versus 51% of patients with chlamydial urethritis (Stamm et al., 1984c). This and other studies indicate that screening for chlamydial urethritis is warranted in male high-risk populations.

Wiedner et al. (1986) found *C. trachomatis* in 47% of 74 men with cytologically proven NGU, i.e., 4 PMLs per high-power field and/or 15 PMLs per high-power field in a sediment of 3 ml of first voided urine (VB1). In 13 men with cytologically proven NGU, *C. trachomatis* was found in 36.1%.

In a study of asymptomatic urethritis cases, pyuria correlated better with infection than urethral Gram stain (Stamm and Cole, 1986). The study also concluded that chlamydial urethritis can remain asymptomatic for at least a month and a half.

In a series of adolescent males, examination of first catch urine for the diagnosis of urethritis, i.e., sediments from the initial 15 to 20 ml of voided

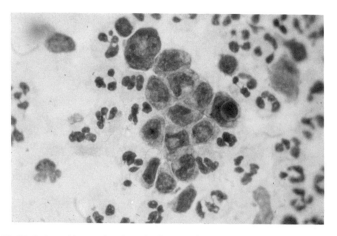

FIGURE 41. Methylene blue-stained urethral smear from a male with NGU showing numerous polymorphonuclear leukocytes in the absence of diplococci (×1000).

urine, had a sensitivity of 95% and a specificity of 93%. The predictive value of such a positive test was 91% (Adger et al., 1984). Thus 21 of 23 (93%) males with more than 10 leukocytes per high-power field had gonorrhea or chlamydial infection, as compared to only 1 of 27 (4%) of men with a negative sediment examination.

The urinary leukocyte esterase dipstick test was evaluated for its diagnostic performance in urethritis in 435 asymptomatic, sexually active, adolescent males aged 13–19 years who had provided a first catch urine sample followed by sampling for culture for *C. trachomatis* and *N. gonorrhoeae* (Shafer et al., 1987). The test has a five-point color scale. The sensitivity was 72%, the specificity 93%, the predictive value of a positive finding (PV+) was 58%, and PV of a negative result (PV−) was 96%. No difference in the performance of the leukocyte esterase test was found with regard to time of sampling before the last micturition. The test picked up 28 cases that were culture-negative. All together 66 (15%) were positive in the esterase test, while 53 (12%) were culture-positive for either *C. trachomatis* (9%) or *N. gonorrhoeae* (3%). The test is thus used as a screening test for male urethritis but requires additional diagnostic procedures, such as culture, for definitive etiological diagnosis.

Perera and co-workers (1987) also used the leukocyte esterase test and found it to be a rapid and sensitive screening test in the diagnosis of NGU.

Clinical Findings

The incubation period for NGU is 1–3 weeks and that for gonococcal urethritis 2–8 days. Patients of both types present with dysuria and urethral discharge (Fig. 42). It is usually not possible on the basis of clinical criteria alone to differentiate NGU from gonorrhea. The discharge in NGU may vary from watery to purulent, although it is most often watery. In gonorrhea the discharge is usually more profuse and more purulent than in chlamydial urethritis. Itching is another symptom seen more often in chlamydial than in gonococcal urethritis (Ripa et al., 1978a). Asymptomatic chlamydial urethritis cases are seen frequently, i.e., asymptomatic cases are more common than symptomatic cases. Many symptomatic cases of NGU become asymptomatic within 3 weeks. However, the percentages of untreated NGU patients who will become carriers, experience relapses, and develop complications are still poorly defined. Approximately one-fourth of all cases of NGU will clear spontaneously within 3 weeks, although most will do so within 2 months. Many cases become culture-negative for *C. trachomatis* within a few weeks. How often this represents spontaneous healing is not known. Neither is it known whether immune mechanisms will hinder the demonstration of a persistent chlamydial infection by culture studies.

Johannison and co-workers (1982) found that only 14 of 27 men with *Chlamydia*-positive NGU were still positive after 2 weeks. Terho had earlier

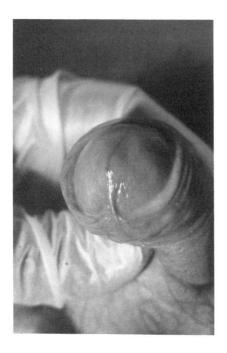

FIGURE 42. Urethral watery discharge in the urethral meatus of a man with chlamydial urethritis. A color version of this figure appears following p. xvi. (Courtesy of Dr. D. Oriel.)

reported similar findings in 2 of 13 patients studied 1 to 4 weeks after therapy. Other studies showed that a urethral chlamydial infection can persist for months or, in some cases, years. However, the influence on the course of infection of reexposure to consorts that are still carrying chlamydiae has not been evaluated in such cases.

The role of mycoplasmas and ureaplasmas in both chlamydial and non-chlamydial urethritis remains unclear (Taylor-Robinson et al., 1979; cf. Taylor-Robinson and McCormack, 1980; Taylor-Robinson et al., 1985).

Postgonococcal urethritis (PGU) is defined as urethritis not caused by *N. gonorrhoeae*, occurring after adequate treatment of gonorrhea (Holmes et al., 1967b), e.g., generally 1-day treatment with a β-lactam antibiotic or a single dose of spectinomycin. Obviously, PGU represents a consequence of mixed urethral infection by *N. gonorrhoeae* and the organism(s) responsible for NGU. In NGU cases signs of urethritis can persist or, more commonly, reappear soon after therapy for gonorrhea. *Chlamydia trachomatis* can be recovered from 45% to 81% of PGU cases; it is thus the most frequent cause of this type of urethritis (Richmond et al., 1972; Holmes et al., 1975; Oriel et al., 1975; Vaughan-Jackson et al., 1977; Terho, 1978; Johannison, 1981). PGU patients may have acquired both *N. gonorrhoeae* and *C. trachomatis* simultaneously, but since the incubation period of chlamydial urethritis is longer, the chlamydial infection often does not manifest itself until after the gonorrhea has been diagnosed and treated. Up to one-third of men with gonococcal urethritis have also been found to harbor *C. trachomatis* in the urethra (Johannisson et al., 1982). As mentioned, the risk of contracting gonorrhea has decreased in many industrialized countries during recent years. Therefore the percentage of chlamydial urethritis cases also infected by gonoccoci has decreased markedly in these countries.

Some men first become culture-positive for chlamydiae after treatment of their gonorrhea. This need not only result from the gonococcal infection that was acquired first (resulting in a "postgonococcal" infection); rather, it can result from the chlamydial infection having been acquired first and then being exacerbated by the gonococcal infection. Thus the gonorrhea might "trigger" the chlamydial infection (see also Chapter 10).

Diagnosis of Chlamydial Urethritis

Chlamydial urethritis can be detected by isolating the agent from a urethral sample. A nontoxic (Mårdh and Zeeberg, 1980) swab is introduced 3–4 cm into the urethra, turned three-fourths of a turn, and withdrawn. (For a discussion of toxic sampling swabs, see also Chapter 6.)

Direct demonstration of chlamydial antigen in smears of urethral secretion by immunofluorescence or ELISA has been claimed in some studies to be as efficient as culture for the diagnosis of chlamydial urethritis. However, other recent studies found direct-specimen antigen detection tests to have a low sensitivity in both low- and high-risk groups for chlamydial urethritis, i.e , the diagnosis is missed in one-fourth of all culture-positive cases (Taylor-Robinson et al., 1987).

The use of urine sediments for the diagnosis of chlamydial urethritis has been evaluated by both culture and ELISA (Chlamydiazyme®, Abbott). *Chlamydia trachomatis* was isolated from 20 of 190 men studied. Of the ELISA-positive cases, 94.5% were also positive in culture with a specificity of 93.8%. In asymptomatic cases, the sensitivity and specificity of the ELISA (Chlamydiazyme®) test were 88.8 and 97.1%, respectively (Lewis et al., 1987).

DNA probes covalently labeled with biotin have also been used to diagnose chlamydial urethritis in males, but their relative value in the diagnostic battery remains to be established.

Nucleic acid sandwich hybridization has proved a rather insensitive means of diagnosing chlamydial urethritis in male STD clinic patients. Its sensitivity in a series of 100 cases of assumed chlamydial genital infection was only 53%, although a specificity of 100% was found (Puolakkainen et al., 1987b).

Serology is not a useful diagnostic tool in chlamydial urethritis. Non-gonococcal urethritis is a superficial mucosal infection that generally does not induce an antichlamydial antibody response as detected by currently commercially available antigens.

Treatment

The standard treatment for chlamydial urethritis is tetracyclines or erythromycin for 7–10 days. As in all infections, the dose of antibiotic used and the duration of therapy are essential. A daily administration each of 200 mg of doxycline, 600 mg of lymecycline, 2 g of tetracycline or oxytetracycline, or 2 g of erythromycin seems to result in acceptable antibiotic levels provided it is divided into at least two doses per day. Bowie (1982) reviewed a number of dose regimens that did *not* prove effective against NGU.

The optimal length of therapy in NGU has been a matter of discussion (Holmes et al., 1967a). Ten days seems marginally more effective than one week. Less than a week of either tetracycline or erythromycin seems definitely inappropriate. Some physicians prefer to give a 2-week course, claiming better results than that of a 10-day course. Some studies (John, 1971) suggest that 3 weeks of treatment is better than 2, whereas other studies (Helmy and Fouler, 1975) did not show this to be the case.

In general, tetracycline analogs seem to have a slightly better effect than erythromycin. However, the reported effectiveness of some of the new macrolides, e.g., roxithromycin, might reduce the claimed difference in efficiency between the two groups of drugs.

In order to prevent the development of PGU, a course of tetracycline following standard gonorrhea treatment (by penicillins, cephalosporins, or spectinomycin) is now recommended for the treatment of urethritis regardless of the culture result. For PGU patients who still have signs or symptoms after a standard course of treatment, an extended treatment period of 3 weeks with tetracycline has been recommended regardless of the result of culture for *C. trachomatis*.

Short-term follow-up studies (Møller et al., 1985) indicate that certain β-lactam antibiotics, e.g., pivampicillin, may be therapeutic alternatives in chlamydial urethritis. However, when the treatment period is shortened to less than 10 days or the daily dose decreased to less than 1 g, the effectiveness of the treatment is reduced to unacceptable levels.

Partners of NGU and PGU patients should be examined and treated; otherwise reinfection of the index case is likely to occur. The evaluation of treatment effectiveness in NGU and PGU requires long-term follow-up studies. Astonishingly few such studies exist. With few exceptions, most therapeutic studies of NGU have involved clinical examination and possibly laboratory testing a few weeks after completion of the antibiotic course. How often the treatment results only in suppression of the urethral infection with disappearence of symptoms and signs for some time until a later recurrence (even after months have passed) remains to be determined.

Sequelae

Urethral stricture may complicate urethritis in the male. In the Western industrialized countries in the preantibiotic era, this complication was seen in up to 5% of patients infected with *N. gonorrhoeae*. The stricture usually occurred in the bulbar part of the urethra. Urethral stricture was seen less often in NGU patients. Today urethral stricture is thought to occur in less than 0.1% of urethritis cases. A history of urethritis is found in approximately every third case subjected to urethral stricture operation. In developing countries, i.e., in Africa, urethral stricture has remained a common clinical problem and has been reported in up to 4% of men with gonorrhea.

So far the incidence of urethral stricture in documented cases of chlamydial urethritis is low. A patient who developed stricture 2½ years after an acute episode of chlamydial urethritis has been described (Colleen and Mårdh, 1982) (Fig. 43).

Approximately 0.5–3.0% of all NGU cases are complicated by epididymitis (Kaufman and Wiesner, 1974). A similar percentage of epididymitis cases oc-

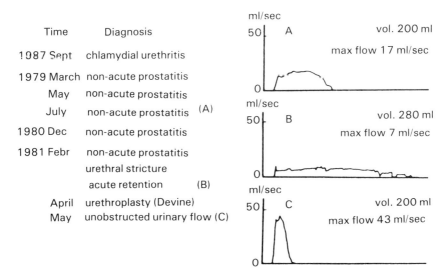

FIGURE 43. Development of urethral stricture in a 23-year-old man whose culture-proven *C. trachomatis* urethritis was diagnosed in September 1978. A symptomatic chronic nonbacterial prostatitis was diagnosed in March 1979. Urinary flow was unobstructed in July 1979 (A); acute retention occurred in February 1981. Preoperative urinary flow measurement indicates stricture (B). After urethroplasty, the patient's supernormal voiding ability indicates that the detrusor has been hypertrophied (C). (From Colleen and Mårdh, 1982.)

curred in *Chlamydia*-positive and -negative NGU cases (Terho, 1978). Sometimes the preceding NGU episode was asymptomatic. Infertility only rarely results from chlamydial epididymitis, but few, if any, prospective studies have been published on this topic.

EPIDIDYMITIS

Epidemiology

Currently, the majority of cases of epididymitis in young (<35 years), sexually active males in the United States was caused by *C. trachomatis* (Harnisch et al., 1977; Berger et al., 1978, 1979, 1980; Berger, 1984). Similar results were obtained in Scandinavia by Colleen and Mårdh (1982) as well as by Scheibel and co-workers (cf., Colleen and Mårdh, 1982). In the Scandinavian studies cited, 30 (39%) of 76 men under 35 years of age with epididymitis were culture-positive for *C. trachomatis*, whereas only 1 of 34 men with epididymitis who were older than 35 were culture-positive. In a more recent study from Leeds in the U.K. by Mulcahy and co-workers (1987), *C. trachomatis* infection was diagnosed in 13 of 29 (45%) men with epididymitis who were less than 35 years of age. Four of these 13 men also had gonorrhea. Chlamydial infection was rare in men over 35.

Epididymitis is rarely STD-associated in elderly men. When instrumentation and urological disease precede epididymitis, enterobacteria are often the causative agents. However, chlamydial infection can also occur in this population, a fact generally not known.

As indicated by experimental infections in monkeys (Møller and Mårdh, 1980b), the chlamydial infection is thought to spread from the urethra canalicularly via the spermatic cord (Fig. 23) to the epididymis (Fig. 24). However, invasion of the epididymis by lymphatic routes might also be a possibility. In infected monkeys the testicles doubled in size. The epididymis and spermatic cord remained swollen for 1–2 weeks. Urethral discharge and an increased number of leukocytes in urethral smears were seen.

Clinical Findings

Acute chlamydial epididymitis generally manifests itself as scrotal pain, tenderness, swelling, and sometimes abdominal pain and fever. It is almost always unilateral (Fig. 44). A urethral discharge can be demonstrated in some cases even if the patient denies urethral symptoms. Erythema and redness of the scrotum are seen in chlamydial epididymitis, but are less pronounced than in gonococcal epididymitis. The "spermatic cord" is often inflamed and swollen in

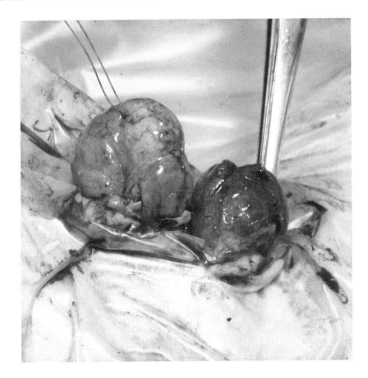

FIGURE 44. Chlamydial epididymitis in an experimentally infected grivet monkey showing the inflamed epididymis to the right and the noninfected organ to the left. A color version of this figure appears following p. xvi. (Courtesy of Dr. B. Møller.)

chlamydial epididymitis, suggesting a canalicular spread of the infection from the urethra to the epididymis.

Symptoms usually develop rapidly (within 2–24 hr). Chlamydial epididymitis can debut without a history of urethral symptoms. This was the case in 12 of 16 Danish epididymitis patients 19 to 42 years of age. Ten of these were infected by *C. trachomatis* and four by *N. gonorrhoeae* as well (Kristensen and Scheibel, 1984).

In an English study of 148 men presenting with a painful, swollen, and tender epididymis or with testicular or scrotal pain and who had not been given antibiotic treatment, epididymitis was *not* diagnosed in 108 patients, 23 (21%) of whom had urethritis. All epididymitis cases were unilateral. Of those men less than 35 years old (the cutoff age used in the first publication on chlamydial epididymitis by Berger and co-workers, 1978), half had chlamydial urethritis. Of those 35 years or older, only two (15%) had chlamydial urethritis (Hawkins et al., 1986). Urinary tract abnormalities usually do not accompany chlamydial epididymitis; nor does bacteriuria. Dysuria, on the other hand, occurs in less than half of all cases of chlamydial urethritis.

Diagnosis

For diagnosis of chlamydial epididymitis, culture of *C. trachomatis* and *N. gonorrhoeae* should be made from the urethra, whereas culture for bacteria should be made from the urine. If possible, a needle aspirate of the epididymis performed under local anesthesia should be obtained for culture studies.

Elevated titers of serum IgG antichlamydial antibodies can generally be found in micro-IF tests in patients with chlamydial epididymitis (Colleen and Mårdh, 1982; Wang and Grayston, 1982).

Chlamydial epididymitis can mimic torsion of the testis and testicular malignancy. Surgical exploration must be offered to patients in whom the testis cannot be delineated by palpation or in patients with previous episodes of scrotal pain. The patient with torsion is generally under 20 years of age.

Treatment

Tetracyclines or erythromycin for 10–14 days is the recommended treatment for chlamydial epididymitis. Such therapy eradicated *C. trachomatis* from all of 11 epididymitis cases (Holmes, 1979). Of 14 young men with acute epididymitis given antibiotic therapy, 11 showed a good clinical response (Nilsson and Fischer, 1979). It must be remembered that sexual partners of patients with chlamydial epididymitis must also be investigated and treated accordingly.

If there is even the slightest suspicion that the patient with chlamydial epididymitis has also acquired gonorrhea, treatment should include a β-lactam-resistant penicillin or cephalosporin to cover for infection either with or without a PPNG strain of *N. gonorrhoeae*.

Postgonococcal epididymitis may be seen when penicillin therapy is given to patients assumed to have gonococcal epididymitis who also have a chlamydial infection.

Therapy of chlamydial epididymitis should also involve symptomatic treatment, including bed rest and elevation of the scrotum to provide maximal lymphatic and venous drainage. Bed rest should continue until the scrotum is no longer tender. If symptoms recur, continued bed rest should be recommended.

Sequelae

Transient oligospermia has been reported in association with epididymitis following NGU (Tozzo, 1968), but its precise relationship to subsequent involuntary childlessness has not been determined. However, it is possible that a transient subfertility follows an episode of acute chlamydial epididymitis.

PROSTATITIS

Acute prostatitis and chronic bacterial prostatitis are relatively rare conditions that are associated with urinary tract infection, usually caused by enterobacteria (Drach et al., 1978). In the common condition nonbacterial prostatitis, a chlamydial etiology has not been established on the basis of cultures from either the urethra or expressed prostatic fluid (Mårdh et al., 1978). However, chlamydial urethritis can be diagnosed by culture in approximately 10% of all nonbacterial prostatitis cases.

As is the case with analyses of urethral secretion, expressed prostatic fluid, and seminal fluid, culture studies of prostatic biopsies have not indicated that *C. trachomatis* is an etiological agent of nonbacterial prostatitis (Vinje et al., 1983).

Direct-specimen antigen detection tests (ELISA and IF) of urethral and epididymal samples of patients with prostatitis have not indicated chlamydial etiology. Such tests are of interest because prostatic fluid and semen contain constituents with antichlamydial activity, e.g., spermine, spermidine, and high concentrations of certain ions, such as Zn^{2+} (Mårdh et al., 1980a).

Grant and co-workers (1985) based their belief of the etiological role of *C. trachomatis* in nonbacterial prostatitis on the fact that three of nine patients were culture-positive for the agent. The authors do not state the type of sample from which the organism was recovered, nor do they mention the culture technique used. They report a stationary titer of antichlamydial serum antibodies. Poletti and co-workers (1985) also studied ''nonacute abacterial'' prostatitis cases using cycloheximide-treated McCoy cells according to the procedure of Hobson and associates (1974), i.e., no centrifugation of the cultures was done (see Chapter 6). They isolated *C. trachomatis* from prostatic cells in 10 of 30 patients subjected to transrectal prostatic biopsy. They also noted that even when the specimens from the patients were diluted 1 : 2, the same nonspecific cytotoxic effect was observed. Rectal contamination was not ruled out.

Attempts to establish prostatitis by transperitoneally injecting *C. trachomatis* in the prostate of three grivet monkeys failed (Møller and Mårdh, 1982). The monkeys did, however, subsequently develop urethritis, vasitis, and epididymitis (Møller and Mårdh, 1982).

Patients who have had an STD often have symptoms suggestive of prostatitis (Kaufman and Wiesner, 1974; Chandiok, 1985). The clinical symptoms of prostatitis include perineal discomfort, urethral discharge, dysuria, increased frequency of urination, pain on ejaculation, and reduced libido. Some patients report lower abdominal pain and pain radiating down along the thighs. Obstructive symptoms, such as reduced urinary flow and postmicturition dribbling, are also seen. Posterior urethritis is a common manifestation of prostatitis. Leukocytosis in expressed prostatic fluid is an objective finding in prostatitis.

The complex interaction between somatic and psychological factors in prostatitis with factors of aquiring STDs has been highlighted by Nilsson and associates (1975).

Serological tests for *C. trachomatis* in the diagnosis of prostatitis have limited value, as indicated by micro-IF tests of serum and expressed prostatic fluid (Mårdh et al., 1978).

If *C. trachomatis* is recovered from a prostatitis patient, treatment with tetracycline or an analog for 2–3 weeks should be administered. Sexual partners should also be treated (cf. Colleen and Mårdh, 1984).

PROCTITIS

Strains belonging to serotypes D–K of *C. trachomatis* can be isolated from rectal samples of both heterosexual and homosexual men (Munday et al., 1981). Of 1429 homosexual men, 8% had gonococcal rectal infection, 5% had chlamydial infection, and 1% had both types of infection. Rectal chlamydial infection was strongly related to age, occurring most frequently in adolescents. The majority of rectal infections by chlamydiae and gonococci are asymptomatic (Rompalo et al., 1986). Cell cultures from the rectum yielded *C. trachomatis* in 6.5% of 51 unselected homosexual and bisexual men. The inclusion count in the positive chlamydial cultures was low, as was the number of EBs in immunofluorescence tests (Sulaiman et al., 1987). In comparison, *C. trachomatis* was isolated from the urethra of 9.3% and from the pharynx of 4.3% of the 51 men.

Rectal shedding of *C. trachomatis* serotypes D–K might be associated with very mild symptoms. Asymptomatic infections also occur (Stamm et al., 1982). Symptoms of chlamydial proctitis include rectal bleeding, mucous discharge, and diarrhea.

In one study, about 15% of all cases of proctitis among homosexuals was thought to be caused by *C. trachomatis*. Hemorrhagic proctitis can be a sign of *C. trachomatis* infection (Christopherson et al., 1985). This condition may be misdiagnosed as bleeding hemorrhoids. The distal gastrointestinal tract, including the rectum, can be engaged in the classical, tropical form of lymphogranuloma venereum (caused by *C. trachomatis*, serotypes L_1–L_3) (see also Chapter 24).

In U.S. patients, LGV strains of *C. trachomatis* have been isolated from rectal lesions (Quinn et al., 1981b; Schachter, 1981). The clinical manifestation of LGV infection in these patients is ulcerative proctitis rather than the classical form of LGV.

Granulomas consisting of giant cells can be seen in rectal biopsies of patients with LGV proctitis. The histological findings may resemble those seen in the intestinal tract of patients with Crohn's disease (Rodaniche et al., 1943).

Genital Tract and Associated Infections in the Female

INTRODUCTION

The spectrum of clinical manifestations of *C. trachomatis* infections in the female is shown in Tables 1 and 22.

Of all lower genital tract infections in women caused by *C. trachomatis*, approximately 70% are asymptomatic. On the other hand, most infections of the female genital tract produce a variety of overlapping symptoms, including vulvar pruritus, dysuria, dyspareunia, increased or altered vaginal discharge, low abdominal pain, irregular bleeding, low back pain, etc. Since many genital pathogens alone or in combination can cause identical signs and symptoms, it is impossible to establish an etiological diagnosis solely on the basis of symptomatology. Therefore physical examination and laboratory testing play key roles in the diagnosis of infectious genital conditions.

The prevalence of *C. trachomatis* in nonpregnant women seen in STD clinics has ranged from 1% to over 30% (Holt et al., 1967; Hilton et al., 1974; Burns et al., 1975; Oriel et al., 1978; Johannison et al., 1980; Thelin et al., 1980; Stamm and Holmes, 1984; Mumtaz et al., 1985). In pregnant women in various settings the prevalence has varied from 2% to 26% (Hammerschlag et al., 1979; Mårdh et al., 1980b; Hardy et al., 1984; Harrison et al., 1984; Stamm and Holmes, 1984; Khurana et al., 1985; Sweet et al., 1987; Lefévre et al., 1988). Handsfield and associates (1985) studied approximately 1000 women seen in a family-planning clinic setting and defined the simple demographic and clinical criteria that best predicted the presence of *C. trachomatis*. It was most common in young women aged 15 to 21, and declined strikingly thereafter. In addition to age, significant risk factors were the history of a new male sex partner, the presence of yellow mucopurulent endocervical exudate, cervical mucosal bleeding induced by swabbing, and the use of a nonbarrier birth control

TABLE 22. Clinical and Laboratory Criteria for *C. trachomatis*
Infections in Women[a]

	Clinical criteria	Laboratory criteria	
		Presumptive	Diagnostic
Mucopurulent cervicitis (MPC)	Mucopurulent endocervical discharge, cervical erythema, edema, and induced mucosal bleeding	Cervical Gram stain with >10 PMNs/×1000 field	Positive culture or direct-antigen test
Acute urethral syndrome (AUS)	Dysuria–frequency syndrome in young, sexually active women	Pyuria, no bacteriuria	Positive culture or direct-antigen test (cervix or urethra)
Pelvic inflammatory disease (PID)	Lower abdominal pain; adnexal tenderness on pelvic exam; evidence of MPC	As for MPC; cervical Gram stain positive for ICGND; Plasma cell endometritis on endometrial biopsy	Positive culture or antigen test (cervix, endometrium, tube)
Perihepatitis	Right upper quadrant abdominal pain; evidence of PID	As for MPC and PID	As for PID; high-titer IgM or IgG antibody to *C. trachomatis*

[a]MPC, mucopurulent cervicitis; PMN, polymorphonuclear leukocyte; AUS, acute urethral syndrome; ICGND, intracellular gram-negative diplococci; PID, pelvic inflammatory disease.

method (Table 23). For clinicians seeing patients in adolescent clinics, family-planning clinics, gynecological outpatient clinics, and STD clinics, it is important to emphasize these simple risk factors, particularly when resources are limited and screening for *C. trachomatis* must be selective and effective. In a study by Handsfield and co-workers (1985), the overall prevalence of *C. trachomatis* infections was surprisingly high (9%) given that the population studied was a family-planning clinic. They calculated that a screening program that tested all women with two or more of these risk factors (which is only 65% of the total number of women seen) would detect 90% of all *C. trachomatis* infections.

A suggested approach for the diagnosis of *C. trachomatis* infections in women is given in Table 22.

ACUTE URETHRAL SYNDROME

Epidemiology

The most common STD agents producing acute urethral syndrome (AUS) in women are *C. trachomatis, N. gonorrhoeae,* and herpes simplex virus (HSV).

TABLE 23. Variables Shown by Stepwise Multivariate
Logistic-Regression Analysis to Be Independently
Associated with Chlamydial Infection in Women
Attending Family-Planning Clinics[a]

Variable	Odds ratio (95% confidence interval)	P value
Age ≤24 yr	3.3 (1.8–6.1)	<0.001
New sex partner in the preceding 2 months	3.4 (2.0–5.6)	<0.001
Purulent or mucopurulent endocervical exudate	3.0 (1.8–5.4)	<0.001
Endocervical bleeding induced by swabbing	2.3 (1.2–4.3)	<0.05
Use of contraception or a nonbarrier method	2.2 (1.0–4.8)	<0.05

[a]From Handsfield et al. (1986).

These agents also cause cervicitis, and thus patients with acute urethral syndrome frequently manifest cervical infection as well (Komaroff, 1984). Yeasts and *T. vaginalis* primarily cause vaginitis but may also be isolated from the urethra, where they cause (Komaroff, 1984) acute urethral syndrome. *Chlamydia trachomatis* is the major cause of the acute urethral syndrome in patients with pyuria (also called dysuria–pyuria syndrome). In their landmark study, Stamm and colleagues (1980) isolated *C. trachomatis* in 10 of 16 (63%) patients with the urethral syndrome who had sterile bladder urine and pyuria.

Clinical Findings

Patients with vaginitis usually complain of external dysuria whereas patients with urethritis usually complain of internal dysuria, i.e., dysuria felt deeper inside the body. The increased frequency, increased urgency, and hematuria primarily associated with bladder infections in women are usually caused by *E. coli*, *Proteus* spp., or *Staphylococcus saprophyticus*. The presence of an altered vaginal discharge or genital odor in a patient with internal or external dysuria suggests cervicitis or vaginitis. Acute onset and short duration of symptoms favor the diagnosis of cystitis, whereas a history of gradual onset and long duration of symptoms suggest chlamydial infection. Suprapubic or bladder tenderness is also suggestive of cystitis.

The urethra usually appears normal in women with chlamydial urethritis. Urethral lesions and severe inflammation obviously suggest HSV infection. Women with cervical and urethral chlamydial infection are more likely to complain of dysuria than women with cervical chlamydial infection alone (Paavonen,

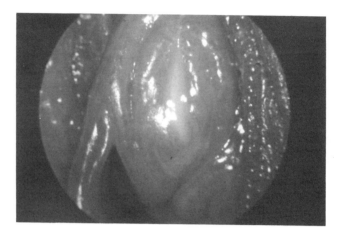

FIGURE 45. Acute urethral syndrome with pus expressed from the urethra.

1979). Thus *C. trachomatis* is a proven cause of acute urethral syndrome in young, sexually active women.

Although urethral symptoms in women with chlamydial infection are not uncommon, the majority of female STD clinic patients with chlamydial infection do not have dysuria or frequency (Bradley et al., 1985). Even in women with chlamydial urethritis, such signs of urethral inflammation as urethral discharge (Fig. 45), meatal redness, or urethral tenderness are infrequent. The presence of clinical signs suggestive of mucopurulent cervicitis, i.e., yellow endocervical exudate, edematous ectopy, and induced mucosal bleeding, strongly suggests chlamydial infection in a patient with urethral symptoms. Other predictors of chlamydial urethral syndrome are history of a new sex partner within the last one or two months, duration of dysuria for at least 7–10 days, lack of suprapubic tenderness, lack of hematuria, and use of birth control pills (Stamm et al., 1980; Stamm and Holmes, 1984).

Diagnosis

A urethral Gram stain showing an increased number of polymorphonuclear (PMN) leukocytes per oil immersion field in women with abacterial urethritis supports the diagnosis of chlamydial infection (Wallin et al., 1981). In order to establish a possible role of *C. trachomatis* in patients with acute urethral syndrome, a urethral (and cervical) chlamydial culture should be made. Screening studies in STD clinics suggest that up to half of all women with chlamydial infection are culture-positive both cervically and urethrally, and 25% are culture positive from either site alone (Ripa et al., 1978b; Paavonen and Vesterinen, 1982; Stamm and Holmes, 1984).

A possible concomitant gonorrhea should always be ruled out. Figure 46 shows a simple algorithm for the evaluation and management of women with urinary symptoms. This approach is recommended as it takes into account all known potential causes of acute urethral syndrome.

Therapy

Women with acute urethral syndrome and *C. trachomatis* infection should be treated with tetracyclines. Stamm and co-workers (1980) found that women with chlamydial urethritis given placebo remained culture-positive and symptomatic whereas those given doxycycline responded.

VAGINITIS/VAGINOSIS

An etiological role of *C. trachomatis* in vaginitis in adult women was not suggested until recently, when a causal relationship was proposed in women who had had hysterectomy (Barton et al., 1985). In prepubertal girls, *C. trachomatis* was isolated from the vagina and was thought to be the cause of vaginitis (Bump, 1985).

Bacterial vaginosis (also called nonspecific vaginitis) is the most common cause of abnormal vaginal discharge (Holst et al., 1987); it is characterized by decreased concentrations of lactobacilli and an increased concentration of anaerobic bacteria and mycoplasmas in the vaginal flora (Spiegel et al., 1980; Holmes, 1984). Diagnostic criteria include the presence of homogenous vaginal fluid, increased vaginal pH, positive KOH test, and "clue" cells on vaginal wet mount (Amsel et al., 1983).

Recently, bacterial vaginosis was diagnosed in up to one-third of women with vaginal discharge attending a primary health care facility (Holst et al., 1987). In women with bacterial vaginosis seen in a gynecological outpatient clinic, the recovery rate of *C. trachomatis* was significantly lower than would have been expected for the general age-matched female population in the same hospital catchment region (Holst et al., 1984a). This was also true for other STD agents, e.g., *N. gonorrhoeae*. Thus gonococci and chlamydiae were not recovered from any of 34 women harboring *Mobiluncus mulieris* (see below) who had attended because of increased vaginal discharge. In women with vaginal discharge seen in STD clinics, bacterial vaginosis was seen approximately as often in those with as in those without proven STD.

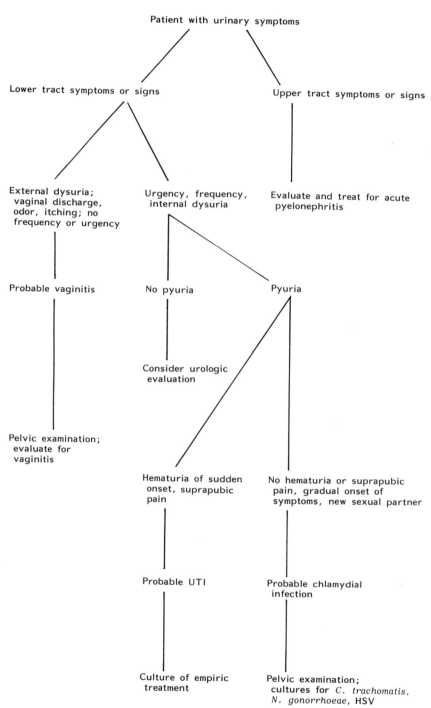

FIGURE 46. Suggested approach for evaluation of women with urinary symptoms.

Women with multiple STDs are at increased risk for chlamydial infection. Wølner-Hanssen and co-workers (1988b) studied the interrelationship between the occurrences of microorganisms among 700 randomly sampled STD clinic women. Isolation of *Trichomonas vaginalis* was significantly associated with the isolation of *Mycoplasma hominis, U. urealyticum, Gardnerella vaginalis, N. gonorrhoeae,* and with the clinical diagnosis of bacterial vaginosis. Surprisingly, *C. trachomatis* was recovered equally often from women with (15%) and without (13%) *T. vaginalis.* Vulvovaginal itching was associated with *T. vaginalis* in the presence of bacterial vaginosis, and lower abdominal pain was associated with *T. vaginalis* in the presence of *C. trachomatis* infection.

A large proportion of patients with PID (pelvic inflammatory disease) and chlamydial PID also has bacterial vaginosis. Laparoscopic studies have demonstrated that the nonchlamydial, nongonococcal organisms recovered from the upper tract are among those occurring in the vaginal flora of patients with bacterial vaginosis. However, no study has systematically addressed the efficacy of concomitant treatment of coexistent bacterial vaginosis and chlamydial PID.

In women with evidence of bacterial vaginosis but no concomitant cervicitis (and lacking signs of chlamydial infection), a vaginal wet mount generally does not show an increased number of polymorphonuclear leukocytes (Fig. 47), whereas women with concomitant chlamydial infection usually have increased number of leukocytes (Fig. 48).

Studies of male sexual consorts of women with bacterial vaginosis do not suggest that the condition is sexually transmitted (Holst et al., 1984b). On the

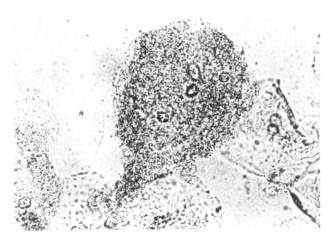

FIGURE 47. Wet mount of vaginal fluid from a case of bacterial vaginosis, showing clue cells (with no increase of leukocytes).

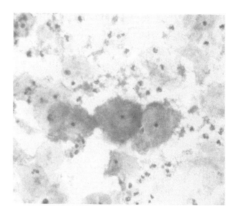

FIGURE 48. Wet mount of vaginal fluid from a woman with bacterial vaginosis and concomitant chlamydial cervicitis. (Courtesy of Dr. E. Purola.)

other hand, *M. hominis,* which so far has been regarded as an STD agent, is associated with *G. vaginalis, M. mulieris,* and *M. curtisii,* bacterial species that commonly occur vaginally in patients with bacterial vaginosis (Holst et al., 1984a). *Chlamydia trachomatis* was found in 21 female consorts of men with NGU, whereas *Mobiluncus* spp. have been found more than twice as often as *C. trachomatis* in such women (Pattman, 1984). An association between the occurrence of *Mobiluncus* spp. and that of *C. trachomatis,* but not *N. gonorrhoeae,* was found, although no explanation for this discrepancy has been given.

MUCOPURULENT CERVICITIS

Epidemiology

Both nongonococcal urethritis (NGU) in men and its counterpart mucopurulent cervicitis (MPC) in women are major public health problems (Holmes, 1981). Because MPC is frequently asymptomatic but sometimes leads to severe complications, a widespread application of specific diagnostic tests should be undertaken in high-risk populations and individuals (Handsfield et al., 1985; Stamm and Holmes, 1986). The prevalence of MPC in women approximates the prevalence of NGU plus gonorrhea in men. In a recent study, the prevalence of MPC was 29% in randomly selected women at an STD clinic and 8% in women attending a student health clinic for an annual examination (Paavonen et al., 1986). The major recognized infectious causes of cervicitis are *C. trachomatis, N. gonorrhoeae,* and HSV (Brunham et al., 1984; Holmes, 1984; Paavonen et al., 1988a).

The cervix is the reservoir for sexual and perinatal transmission of chlamydial infection. The columnar epithelium of the cervical canal is the primary target of *C. trachomatis* (Swanson et al., 1975).

An association between TRIC agent (*C. trachomatis*) and female genital infection (i.e., cervicitis) was first described by Dunlop and co-workers in 1964 in patients with concomitant eye infection and cervicitis from whom the agent could be recovered from both sites. Mordhorst (1964) studied neonatal blennorrhea and cervicitis as *Chlamydia*-related conditions.

In both gynecologic outpatient clinics and STD clinics one- to three-fourths of all cases of cervicitis are caused by *C. trachomatis* (Hilton et al., 1974; Burns et al., 1975; Rees et al., 1977a; Oriel et al., 1978; Ripa et al., 1978b; Thelin et al., 1980; Svensson et al., 1981; Osser and Persson, 1982, Paavonen and Vesterinen, 1982). In a study of women with MPC, *C. trachomatis* was isolated from 39% of women attending a university student health clinic and 48–67% of women attending an STD clinic (Paavonen et al., 1986) (Table 24). Although *T. vaginalis* and *U. urealyticum* were initially associated with MPC, both associations disappeared after adjustment was made for the presence or absence of *C. trachomatis*. Herpes simplex virus was associated with ulcerative lesions of the cervix. An unexpected finding was that *N. gonorrhoeae* did not correlate with MPC. This latter finding, however, should be interpreted with caution. It may be that women with gonorrhea develop symptoms of upper genital tract infection leading them to seek care in other clinical settings, such as gynecological and emergency clinics.

Diagnosis of Cervicitis

The clinical diagnosis of MPC is difficult to establish because of the lack of reproducible objective criteria. This is illustrated by the confusing nomenclature used for cervicitis, including such terms as acute or chronic cervicitis, cervical erosion, cervical discontinuity, papillary cervicitis, follicular cervicitis, and hypertrophic cervicitis. In a recent study conducted in an STD clinic population, simple objective criteria for the clinical diagnosis of cervicitis were established (Brunham et al., 1984). Cervical infection with the principal recognized infectious causes of MPC (*C. trachomatis, N. gonorrhoeae,* HSV) correlated best with the presence of mucopurulent endocervical discharge and the presence of 10 or more PMN leukocytes per ×100 microscopic (oil immersion) field in satisfactory Gram-stained endocervical smears.

TABLE 24. Associations of Cervical Microorganisms, Clinical Diagnoses, and Antichlamydial Antibodies with Mucopurulent Cervicitis by the Mantel–Haenzel Test, among 271 STD Clinic Women and 96 Student Health Clinic Women[a]

	Summary odds ratio	P value
C. trachomatis		
Cevical culture	16.39	<0.001
Serum antibody	4.24	<0.001
Cervical secretory IgA antibody	2.35	NS[b]
N. gonorrhoeae	1.66	NS
Herpes simplex virus	0.58	NS
T. vaginalis	3.17	<0.05
M. hominis	1.32	NS
U. urealyticum	2.70	<0.01
Group B streptococcus	1.14	NS
G. vaginalis	2.39	<0.05
Yeast	0.36	<0.05
Bacterial vaginosis	1.94	0.052
Oral contraceptive use	3.44	<0.001
Spermicide use	0,.42	<0.05

[a]From Paavonen et al. (1986).
[b]NS, no statistical difference.

Mucopurulent endocervical discharge is best confirmed by visualization of yellow endocervical mucopus on a white cotton swab (positive swab test). The yellow color of cervical mucopus (Fig. 49) can be more easily visualized against the white background of the swab than against the cervix (Brunham et al., 1984) (Fig. 50a and b). Other signs of MPC, i.e., edema and erythema in an area of ectopy and in the transformation zone, and induced mucosal bleeding (Fig. 51), are also more common in infected than in uninfected women (Paavonen et al., 1986). Handsfield and associates (1986) found strong independent associations between the isolation of C. trachomatis and the presence of mucopurulent endocervical exudate and induced mucosal bleeding. Colposcopic studies suggest that C. trachomatis produces severe erythema and edema of the area of ectopy and the transformation zone (hypertrophic cervicitis) (Paavonen et al., 1979, 1988a).

For quantitation of PMN leukocytes in endocervical secretions, the swab is withdrawn from the cervix and then rolled once onto a microscopic slide, air-dried, and Gram-stained. The slide is scanned at a magnification of 100 to identify the presence of inflammatory cells. The number of PMNs per oil immersion field in five nonadjacent fields is then established in the area of the cervical mucus, at a magnification of 1000×. The presence of a large number of squam-

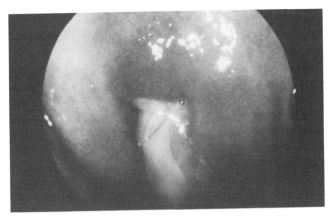

FIGURE 49. The cervical os of a woman with chlamydial cervicitis showing endocervical mucopus. A color version of this figure appears following p. xvi.

ous cells (vaginal epithelial cells) or of vaginal bacteria mixed with inflammatory cells suggests that the specimen includes ectocervical material and that the inflammatory cells might have vaginal rather than endocervical origins. Such specimens are unsatisfactory for the diagnosis of MPC. Both the swab test and PMN leukocyte quantitation are invalid during menstruation.

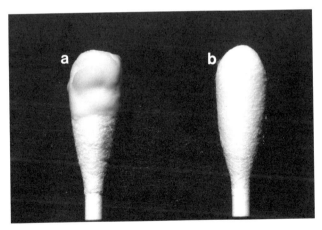

FIGURE 50. Swab test in a case of mucopurulent cervicitis (a) and control (b). A color version of this figure appears following p. xvi.

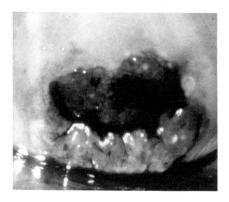

FIGURE 51. Edema, erythema, and induced bleeding in a patient with chlamydial cervicitis. A color version of this figure appears following p. xvi.

It is interesting that the criteria for the diagnosis of MPC are quite similar to those commonly used to make a presumptive diagnosis of nongonococcal urethritis in men, i.e., the demonstration of an urethral discharge and four or more PMN leukocytes per oil immersion field in a urethral smear.

Histopathology

The histopathological alterations of cervicitis have been little studied. Characteristic findings include severe inflammation involving both the epithelium and the subepithelial tissue. The inflammation is characterized by heavy PMN leukocyte and mononuclear cell infiltrations, microabscesses, and sometimes epithelial necrosis and ulceration. The presence of lymphoid germinal centers comprising transformed lymphocytes in cervical stroma is pathognomonic of chlamydial cervicitis (Paavonen et al., 1979; Kunimoto and Brunham, 1985; Kiviat et al., 1986a) (Fig. 14). (See also Chapter 3.)

Diagnosis of Chlamydial Cervicitis

The etiological diagnosis of chlamydial cervicitis should be based on either isolation of the agent or direct detection of chlamydial antigen in cervical samples. Some workers have found culture studies somewhat more efficient than antigen-detecting ELISA tests for the diagnosis of chlamydial cervicitis, whereas others have found these methods to be equally efficient (see also Chapter 6). Culture has been found more effective, than staining with fluorescent monoclonal antibodies (Taylor-Robinson et al., 1987). In cases of assumed chlamydial cervicitis, cultures should be made not only from the cervix but also from the urethra, a procedure which increases the overall recovery rate of chlamydiae (see also Chapter 6).

Serology plays a very limited role in the diagnosis of chlamydial cervicitis. High seroprevalence in the population restricts the use of serology in the diagnosis of chlamydial cervicitis. Similarly, differentiation of an acute ongoing cervical infection from past infection by serology alone is difficult.

Therapy

Proper recognition and treatment of MPC is essential to the control of chlamydial infections and the prevention of their complications.

Standard treatment of chlamydial cervicitis in *nonpregnant* women is a tetracycline analog, e.g., 2.0 g tetracycline HCl per day for 10 days, or 200 mg doxycycline for 10 days, or 300 mg lymecycline twice a day for the same period of time. The failure rates in therapeutic MPC studies vary from 0% to 34%. These rates are generally lower after tetracycline than after erythromycin or sulfonamide therapy. Currently, the treatment of choice for women with mucopurulent cervicitis, particularly when etiological studies cannot be performed, is a tetracycline in combination with an agent effective against *N. gonorrhoeae.*

Chlamydia trachomatis infection in *pregnant* women is a major concern. The prevalence of chlamydial infection of the cervix in pregnant women nationwide in the United States is approximately 5% (Hardy et al., 1984; Schachter et al., 1986a). It is well documented that infants delivered through an infected birth canal are likely to become infected. The newborn is a sensitive marker of chlamydial infection in the mother. The risk for conjunctivitis in U.S. studies ranges from 18% to 50% and that for pneumonia from 11% to 18% (Schachter et al., 1986; Alexander and Harrison, 1983). Lower risk figures appear in European studies (Mårdh et al., 1980b).

A cost–benefit analysis indicated that in situations in which the maternal infection rate exceeds 6%, screening of pregnant women for *C. trachomatis* is cost-effective (Schachter, 1986a). The treatment of those found to be infected prevents perinatal morbidity in infants (Schachter and Grossman, 1981; Schachter et al., 1986). Moreover, if *C. trachomatis* proves to be associated with preterm delivery and puerperal maternal infections, then the cost–benefit ratio further decreases.

Erythromycin is generally considered the drug of choice for treatment of chlamydial infections during pregnancy. Schachter and co-workers (1986a) reported that in a setting with a high prevalence of *C. trachomatis* infection (12%), a routine program of screening pregnant women followed by treatment with erythromycin ethylsuccinate 400 mg four times daily for 7 days was cost-effective and significantly reduced infant morbidity. They offered treatment with erythromycin at 36 weeks of pregnancy to 184 pregnant women with cervical infections by *C. trachomatis*. Thirty-two women refused the treatment; 24 of their infants were followed and served as controls. Chlamydial infection developed in 4 (7%) of 59 infants of the treated mothers, as compared with 12 (59%) of 24 infants of the untreated mothers ($p < 0.001$). The success rate for treatment of maternal infection was 92% with a relatively low intolerance rate (3%). Thus it is reasonable to recommend erythromycin for treating *C. trachomatis* infection during pregnancy.

Since both NGU and MPC are caused by *C. trachomatis* in the majority of cases, women should be screened for *C. trachomatis* in STD clinics, family-planning clinics, adolescent clinics, and similar high-risk settings.

Female partners of men with NGU or gonorrhea should be empirically treated for chlamydial MPC.

ENDOMETRITIS

Epidemiology

Pelvic inflammatory disease is usually a canalicularly ascending infection. The causative organisms can spread from the lower genital tract over the surface of the epithelium of the endometrium and the fallopian tubes. Experimental infections in grivet monkeys support the view of such a canalicular spread of *C. trachomatis* (Møller and Mårdh, 1980). Several factors may influence the spread of chlamydiae from the lower to the upper female genital tract (see Chapters 4 and 5).

Chlamydial endometritis was first described in 1981 by Mårdh and co-workers and by Gump and associates. Subsequent studies confirmed the causal role of *C. trachomatis* in plasma cell endometritis (Ingerslev et al., 1982; Wølner-Hansen et al., 1982b; Gump et al., 1983; Paavonen et al., 1985a; Sweet et al., 1983). Some believe that acute as well as chronic cases of endometritis might be associated with chlamydial infection (Ingerslev et al., 1982).

Mårdh and co-workers (1981a) found *C. trachomatis* in endometrial aspirates of 12 (46%) of 26 women with laparoscopic evidence of acute salpingitis. In three of the 26 patients, endometrial (but not cervical) cultures were positive for *C. trachomatis*. Plasma cell endometritis was found in 6 (75%) of 8 biopsies from patients who had had *C. trachomatis* isolated from the upper genital tract and in 2 (22%) of 9 biopsies from patients in whom *C. trachomatis* had not been recovered from such samples ($p < 0.05$). Sweet (1983) isolated *C. trachomatis* from the endometrium of 25% of patients hospitalized for PID. Wasserheit and co-workers (1986) studied 63 women with suspected PID by laparoscopy and endometrial biopsy. Endometrial or tubal *C. trachomatis* infection was detected in 8 (57%) of 14 patients with proven salpingitis and endometritis, but in none of 13 patients with neither of these conditions ($p < 0.001$). Paavonen and co-workers (1987) obtained endometrial biopsies from 45 women with suspected PID, 31 (69%) of whom had plasma cell endometritis; *Chlamydia trachomatis* was isolated from the endometrial specimens of 13 (42%) patients with plasma cell endometritis, but from none of those without endometritis ($p < 0.001$). Kiviat and associates (1986b) studied 55 women with suspected PID; *C. trachomatis* was detected by culture or immunofluorescence staining (using labeled monoclonal antibodies) of endometrial specimens from 12 (57%) of 21 patients who were positive for *C. trachomatis* at any sampling site.

Histopathology

The presence of plasma cells in the endometrial stroma is generally accepted as a histopathological definition of endometritis. Plasma cells can best be demonstrated in formalin-fixed, methyl green-pyronin-stained tissue sections (Ahlqvist and Andersson, 1972). The presence of PMN leukocytes or lymphocytes is not included in the histopathological definition of endometritis because these can also be found during certain phases of the normal menstrual cycle (Brudenell, 1955). Histopathological changes of the endometrium associated with PID are also described in Chapter 14.

Chlamydial Endometritis

The histopathological characteristics of chlamydial endometritis (Figs. 15 to 17) differ from those of nonchlamydial or gonococcal endometritis. Patients with *C. trachomatis* isolated from the endometrium show higher concentrations of plasma cells in the endometrial stroma and germinal centers comprising transformed lymphocytes (Paavonen et al., 1985a) (Fig. 17). Another histopathological feature of *C. trachomatis* is the presence of intraepithelial and intraluminal PMN leukocytes in the endometrial glands. Thus several histopathological endometrial findings are strongly associated with upper genital tract infection with *C. trachomatis*.

Correlation between Endometritis and Salpingitis

Recent studies from Finland and the United States showed a good correlation between the presence of plasma cell endometritis and laparoscopically proven salpingitis among patients hospitalized for acute PID (Paavonen et al., 1985a, 1987; Wasserheit et al., 1986). Plasma cell endometritis was found in approximately 80% of women with acute salpingitis, in 20–30% of women with suspected PID but no visible signs of salpingitis at laparoscopy, and never in controls. These results suggest that the finding of plasma cell endometritis has a high sensitivity and a high positive predictive value in the diagnosis of acute PID. Plasma cells do not persist in the endometrium after treatment of PID. Repeat endometrial biopsies were taken from 20 patients who underwent second laparoscopies 3–6 months after the acute episode. None had plasma cells in the endometrium (Teisala et al., 1987).

Diagnosis

Endometrial specimens can be collected transcervically with a Vabra suction curette equipped with a metallic tip (Mårdh et al., 1981c; Paavonen et al., 1985b) (Fig. 52). The procedure can be performed easily in the office and no anesthesia is needed. Such aspirated specimens can be used for histological and microbiological studies. The institution of antibiotic therapy after sampling is recommended.

Etiological diagnosis of chlamydial endometritis in routine health care should be based on urethral and cervical cultures. Preferably an endometrial aspirate should also be studied. A vaginal ''wet mount'' is advisable as well, since an increased number of leukocytes is generally associated with chlamydial endometritis. Serological studies (see below) complete the diagnostic battery.

As in chlamydial salpingitis, there may be cases that are cervically culture-negative but culture-positive upon endometrial aspiration (Kiviat et al., 1986b). This was found to be a comparatively common event in San Francisco (Schachter, personal communication), but less common in Seattle (Holmes, personal communication).

Immunoflourescence staining appears more sensitive than culture for the detection of *C. trachomatis* in the endometrium (Kiviat et al., 1986b). Such staining in patients with clinical evidence of PID has confirmed that *C. trachomatis* is actually present in the endometrial tissue and not simply introduced into the endometrial cavity by swabs and curettes contaminated with infected cervical chlamydiae. The use of monoclonal antibodies in studies of endometrial tissue with identification of the organism in endometrial glandular epithelium, inflammatory cells in the tissue, or underlying stromal cells allows one to distinguish true endometrial infection from contamination.

Kiviat and associates (1986b) found that staining of paraffin-embedded endometrial tissue with monoclonal antibody to *C. trachomatis* detected all infections demonstrated by culture and several others that had not been identified by this means. Thus endometrial biopsies for conventional histopathological

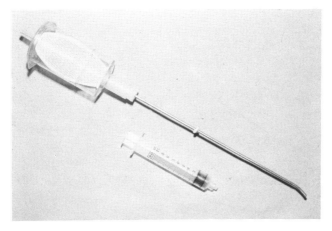

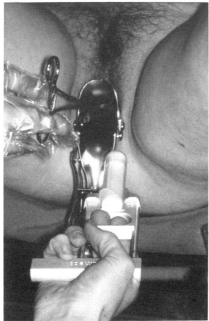

FIGURE 52. Vabra aspiration curette (upper) and transcervical endometrial sampling (lower).

studies and for immunofluorescent staining are useful for establishing the diagnosis of chlamydial endometritis.

Serological studies might add information that will increase diagnostic accuracy in chlamydial endometritis. High titers of antichlamydial micro-IF antibodies favor the diagnosis, whereas the lack of such antibodies does not. Furthermore, a significant change in the antibody titer strengthens the diagnosis of an ongoing, current chlamydial infection. However, such a titer change is likely to be found only in a proportion of all cases of chlamydial endometritis because by the time the patient seeks medical care, the acute phase of the chlamydial infection—from an immunological point of view—has often passed. Thus many patients have had chlamydial cervicitis for some time before they develop endometritis.

Therapy

Therapy for chlamydial endometritis should be the same as that for chlamydial salpingitis (see below). Investigation and treatment of sexual consorts of women with chlamydial endometritis is mandatory for a successful outcome, as with any STD.

SALPINGITIS

Epidemiology

Pelvic inflammatory disease (PID) is the most serious complication of bacterial and chlamydial lower genital tract infection and is a major public health problem that has risen to alarming proportions. The term PID refers to the presence of endometritis, salpingitis, or both, which seems justified by the usual concurrence of both conditions. Of all the known causes of infertility, PID is the most preventable. Every year in the United States up to 1 million women have an episode of frank PID and 300,000 are hospitalized for this condition. At least 25% of these women suffer long-term complications, including one or more of tubal infertility, tubal pregnancy, and chronic pelvic pain. The exact prevalence of salpingitis in most communities, however, has still not been established. The difficulty of establishing the diagnosis of acute salpingitis without visual inspection of the tubes contributes to this uncertainty (Jacobson and Weström, 1969; Falk, 1965; Wølner-Hanssen et al., 1983; Brihmer et al., 1987). In most countries in the last decade, the annual number of reported cases of acute salpingitis has increased steadily as might be expected in light of the prevailing STD pandemic (Weström and Mårdh, 1983a,b, 1984). In southern Sweden, the incidence of PID has been declining for several years. (See also Chapter 32.)

Since the first direct isolations of *C. trachomatis* from the fallopian tubes of patients with laparoscopically proven acute salpingitis in the 1970s (Hamark et al., 1976; Mårdh et al., 1977a,b), a growing number of laparoscopic studies has consistently demonstrated that *C. trachomatis* is the major cause of salpingitis. Selected studies showing the isolation rates of *C. trachomatis* from the upper genital tract are summarized in Table 25. Studies employing laparoscopy and endometrial biopsy have consistently demonstrated the high prevalence of *C. trachomatis* or *N. gonorrhoeae* in upper genital tract infection in proven PID. In recent studies, up to three-fourths of patients with confirmed endometritis and salpingitis had proven infection with either or both of these organisms (cf. Mårdh, 1980; cf. Mårdh and Svensson, 1982). A large number of seroepidemiological studies further support the etiological role of *C. trachomatis* in acute PID (cf. Mårdh et al., 1981c; cf. Paavonen and Mäkelä, 1984; cf. Eschenbach, 1986; cf. Mårdh, 1986). In a serological study of PID patients, antibody activity against *C. trachomatis, M. hominis,* and *N. gonorrhoeae* was found in approximately 80, 40, and 10%, respectively (Mårdh et al., 1981b). A significant titer change was detected with the three agents in approximately 40, 20, and 7%, respectively.

The relative importance of chlamydiae and gonococci as etiological agents of acute salpingitis has changed in many areas during the last decades; generally,

TABLE 25. *C. trachomatis* Infection among Women with PID

Study	Number of patients	Number of cervix/LGT		Present in UGT	
		C. trachomatis[a]			
Eschenbach et al., 1975	100	20	(20%)	1/54	(2%)
Eilard et al., 1976	22	6	(27%)	2	(9%)
Mårdh et al., 1977a	63	19/53	(36%)	6/20	(30%)
Thompson et al., 1980	30	3	(10%)	3/30	(10%)
Sweet et al., 1981	39	2	(5%)	0/35	
Henry-Suchet et al., 1982	16	6	(38%)	4/17	(24%)
Gjønnaess et al., 1982b	65	26/56	(46%)	5/31	(16%)
Bollerup et al., 1982	56	0/56	(—)		
Wölner-Hanssen et al., 1985	54			12/26	(46%)
Wasserheit et al., 1986	36	14/23	(61%)	10/23	(44%)
Kiviat et al., 1986b	55	21	(38%)	24/36	(67%)
Paavonen et al., 1987	45	16/31	(52%)	12/31	(39%)
Brihmer et al., 1987	187	50/187	(27%)	32/187	(12%)

[a]LGT, lower genital tract; UGT, upper genital tract.

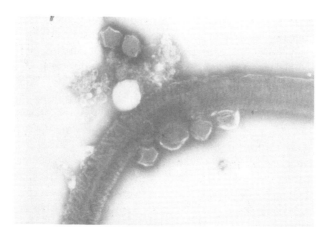

FIGURE 53. Spermatozoa with adherent chlamydiae, experimental study.

the proportion of cases caused by chlamydiae (nongonococcal salpingitis) has increased, whereas that associated with gonorrhea has decreased (Persson, 1986). In northern Europe, *C. trachomatis* is now the predominant cause of salpingitis (Mårdh et al., 1981b; Osser and Persson, 1982; Paavonen et al., 1987), whereas 25 years ago *N. gonorrhoeae* was probably the more common etiological agent of PID. The same trend has been registered in the United States, although less pronounced than that in Scandinavian countries. In many developing countries gonococcal infection is still thought to be the main cause of PID. However, recent African studies (Meheus et al., 1986) found gonococci and chlamydiae to be equally common in PID.

The general medical community has been remarkably slow to accept the importance of *C. trachomatis* in PID. Data from a national survey of office-based private physicians in the United States showed that from 1966 to 1983 most women with suspected PID were treated on an outpatient basis and most received a single antibiotic drug. Less than one-third received a tetracycline drug (Grimes et al., 1986; Wølner-Hanssen et al., 1986b). The proportion of patients hospitalized for PID who received a tetracycline actually declined from more than 30% in 1966 to less than 20% in 1980 through 1983. It is also alarming that cephalosporins and aminopenicillins were the drugs most commonly given to patients hospitalized for PID. As mentioned previously, cephalosporins usually have no clinical activity against *C. trachomatis,* which persists in the endometrium of PID patients treated with such antibiotics (Sweet et al., 1983). Treatment of PID is still one of the most neglected areas of medicine.

C. trachomatis has been found to adhere to spermatozoa in experimental studies (Fig. 53). Spermatozoa with adhered chlamydiae can pass through columns of egg yolk (Wølner-Hanssen and Mårdh, 1984). It has been postulated that chlamydiae or other PID pathogens attached to spermatozoa can "hitchhike" to the upper genital tract. More recently (Friberg et al., 1985), it was demonstrated that spermatozoa with adhered chlamydiae can be recovered from the peritoneal cavity, although a secondary attachment occurring first in the peritoneal cavity has not been ruled out. This spreading mechanism of chlamydiae might be hindered by the use of oral contraceptives that alter the composition of the cervical plug.

Diagnosis of Salpingitis

According to Jacobson and Weström's (1969) criteria, a laparoscopic diagnosis of acute salpingitis is made if tubal erythema, edema, and exudate are present (Fig. 54). Criteria for grading salpingitis by laparoscopic examination have been formulated by Hager and co-workers (1983). In mild salpingitis (grade I), the tubes are freely movable. Erythema and edema are seen. The tubes may require manipulation to produce purulent exudate. In moderately severe salpingitis (grade II), gross purulent material is evident, erythema and edema are more marked, and the tubes may not be freely movable. In severe salpingitis (grade III), an abscess, pyosalpinx, or inflammatory complex is seen.

Møller and co-workers (1979) were the first to report on the tubal histopathology in chlamydial salpingitis (Fig. 18). In histological sections the entire

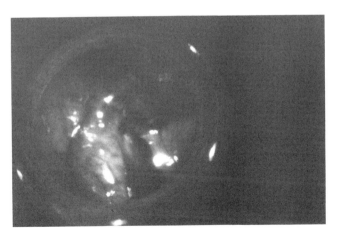

FIGURE 54. Fallopian tube of a woman with chlamydial salpingitis. Laparoscopic picture showing a swollen tube.

tubal mucosa may be destroyed and any intact ciliary cells difficult to find. The tubal lumen is filled by an inflammatory exudate. The tubal wall is infiltrated by inflammatory cells, mainly monocytic cells, through all layers. Tubal alterations similar to those in women with PID were found in experimentally infected grivet monkeys (Møller et al., 1980).

Laparoscopically, in cases of chlamydial salpingitis the tubes may show a full range of inflammatory changes, i.e., from mild to severe (grades I–III). Abscess formation can be seen. Hydro- and sactosalpinx may develop during the course of chlamydial salpingitis (cf. Mårdh et al., 1981b).

Wølner-Hanssen and associates (1987) derived a tubal abnormality score to quantitate the severity of tubal inflammation. This scoring system was based on the presence of periadnexal adhesions, tubal diameter, and the status of the fimbriated ends of the tubes. These authors, as well as others, demonstrated no correlation between the tubal abnormality score and the traditional clinical criteria for PID (i.e., erythrocyte sedimentation rate (ESR), white blood cell (WBC) count, fever, tenderness score, and duration of pain). Similarly, there was no correlation between the tubal abnormality score and the isolation of *C. trachomatis, N. gonorrhoeae,* or both, from the upper genital tract.

Patients with ultrasonic confirmation of a tubo-ovarian inflammatory complex had significantly more *C. trachomatis* infection than those with anaerobic infections (Kirshon et al., 1988).

Clinical Findings

Svensson and co-workers (1980) demonstrated a relationship between certain clinical signs and symptoms and the etiological agent of acute salpingitis. Chlamydial salpingitis patients often have irregular bleeding as a sign of endometritis and increased vaginal discharge as a sign of mucopurulent cervicitis. The body temperature is often normal or the patient may be subfebrile. The WBC count is either normal or only slightly elevated. Acute salpingitis caused by *C. trachomatis* is usually associated with less severe clinical findings (less pain, less frequent fever) than that caused by *N. gonorrhoeae.* Patients with chlamydial salpingitis have a higher ESR, and more severe tubal inflammatory findings as revealed by laparoscopy. Therefore the sensitivity of the clinical diagnosis of chlamydial salpingitis is probably even lower than that of nongonococcal, nonchlamydial salpingitis. Wølner-Hanssen and co-workers (1985) analyzed 104 consecutive *C. trachomatis* culture-positive women who underwent laparoscopy because of clinical signs and symptoms suggestive of acute salpingitis. *Chlamydia*-positive women with salpingitis were compared to those without. Clinical signs, symptoms, and laboratory findings were analyzed. Patients with chlamydial salpingitis had a longer history of pain, more frequent irregular bleeding, and more elevated ESRs. In fact, the presence of an elevated ESR and a history of irregular bleeding had the highest predictive values for chlamydial salpingitis. As yet, laparoscopy is the only diagnostic method that provides reliable information on the degree of tubal inflammation as well as an opportunity to obtain samples for microbiologic studies from the tubes of patients with salpingitis.

Further studies might include tubal minibiopsies, endotubal cytological smears, as well as endometrial biopsies to define the true sensitivity and specificity of laparoscopy for the diagnosis of all manifestations of PID. It is possible that the sensitivity of laparoscopy is less than 100% in the diagnosis of mild early endosalpingitis that is not visible as exosalpingitis.

Diagnosis of Chlamydial Salpingitis

The etiological diagnosis of chlamydial salpingitis is difficult to establish (Svensson et al., 1980, 1981a; Wølner-Hanssen et al., 1983). The most appropriate way to establish the diagnosis is to demonstrate the presence of the agent in the tubes by culture or antigen detection studies, a possibility only when laparoscopy or laparotomy is performed. If the abdominal ostia are closed, the tube can be punctured and the contents aspirated. If the tubal ostia are open, a baby-feeding catheter or swab can be introduced into the tubal lumina to obtain secretions. However, in routine health care, sampling from the tubes may be difficult and is not generally recommended. Fluid from the cul-de-sac has proved to have restricted value for chlamydial salpingitis culture studies (Mårdh et al., 1981c).

Urethral and cervical cultures for chlamydiae should also be taken. If possible, endometrial aspirates should be cultured since, as mentioned previously, such samples can be positive when cervical cultures are negative (see also Chapter 14) (Wølner-Hanssen et al., 1982a). If such an aspirate is made, antibiotic treatment should be instituted.

Experience has been limited regarding the use of ELISA tests and labeled monoclonal antibodies to *C. trachomatis* for the detection of chlamydial antigen or chlamydiae organisms in clinical samples from salpingitis patients. However, in some studies tubal samples of culture-negative patients were positive by immunofluorescence tests (Kiviat et al., 1986b).

The use of serological tests in the diagnosis of chlamydial salpingitis has limited value because antibodies are extremely common in the group of women who acquire chlamydial salpingitis (Treharne et al., 1979; Mårdh et al., 1981c; Gjønnaess et al., 1982b; Osser and Persson, 1982; cf. Paavonen and Mäkelä, 1984). The antichlamydial IgG antibody titers are often stationary. IgM antichlamydial antibodies occur in only a small portion of cases. A significant titer change during the course of the disease is seen in only up to 25% of chlamydial salpingitis patients. However, the micro-IF antibody titers are often high, ranging from 16–32 to 4096–8192.

Therapy

It is generally believed that PID has a polymicrobial etiology. Therefore the current CDC guidelines (see Appendix) recommend antimicrobial drugs that cover a broad spectrum of potential pathogens implicated in the etiology of PID. It should be noted, however, that the optimal treatment of PID is unknown. Furthermore, recent advances in the elucidation of the microbial etiology of PID do not seem to have been matched by improved treatment results.

As outlined by Svensson and Mårdh (1982) and by Brunham (1984), comprehensive assessment of the efficacy of antimicrobial treatment of PID should include evaluation of the short-term as well as the long-term clinical response. Evaluation of the long-term response should include relapse and recurrence rates, and rates of other sequelae such as tubal pregnancy, tubal infertility, and chronic pain. Very few studies have prospectively evaluated all these sequelae. Furthermore, few treatment studies have included uniform diagnostic criteria, comprehensive evaluation of the etiology of both lower and upper genital tract infections, grading of the severity of the tubal infection, and any systematic criteria for clinical cure or failure. Short-term clinical cure may not take into account or rule out persistent or subclinical tubal infection that sometimes results from inappropriate treatment. For instance, cephalosporins and aminopenicillins have been reported to result in clinical cure without eradicating *C. trachomatis* from the upper genital tract (Sweet et al., 1983).

The CDC recommendations for the outpatient and inpatient treatment of PID are outlined in the Appendix. Treatment of salpingitis cases should extend for (at least) 2 weeks. In severe cases, particularly those involving high body temperature and pelvic abscess formation, some clinicians institute a parenteral treatment with the combination of clindamycin and an aminoglycoside in order to eradicate pyrogenic bacteria, including anaerobes, or a combination of doxycycline and a β-lactam antibiotic (Wølner-Hanssen et al., 1986b) (see Appendix). Others give penicillin as a single-dose treatment, in case gonorrhea is present, followed the next day by a 14-day course of tetracycline. To cover anaerobes, a nitroimidazole, e.g., metronidazole, has been used in combination with tetracyclines or penicillins (Heinonen, 1986).

Brunham (1984) outlined several important issues regarding the antibiotic treatment of PID remain to be clarified: (1) choice of antimicrobial, (2) influence of disease severity, (3) the need for inpatient treatment, and (4) the effect of antimicrobial therapy on long-term tubal function (Brunham, 1984). The definitive treatment trial should be prospective, with patients enrolled after laparoscopic or endometrial biopsy verification of the diagnosis. Careful microbiological studies of the lower and upper genital tract are required. Patients enrolled in such studies should be randomized to therapy, and outcome should be evaluated using uniform clinical criteria. Long-term evaluation should determine recurrence rates and tubal function in order to define the optimal antimicrobial therapy of PID.

Peritoneal adhesion formation impairs the outcome of antimicrobial therapy of PID and has an impact on the fertility prognosis. Second laparoscopy studies have demonstrated unilateral or bilateral adhesion formation in 38–45% of patients treated for acute PID (Wølner-Hanssen et al., 1983; Teisala et al., 1987). Nonsteroidal anti-inflammatory drugs in PID are thought to act by decreasing the initial inflammatory tubal tissue response and by inhibiting significant adhesion formation.

Whether or not inpatient treatment for all cases of acute PID is required has not yet been adequately addressed. Currently in the United States, only 15–20% of all PID patients is hospitalized (Washington et al., 1984, 1986), whereas in the Scandinavian countries a larger proportion of patients is hospitalized. The CDC criteria for hospitalization of patients with PID are shown in the Appendix. More liberal hospitalization criteria for young patients with PID might lead to an improved outcome, although this has yet to be proven.

While therapy is in progress, bed rest and avoidance of intercourse are recommended. Intercourse should be avoided until all signs and symptoms have resolved and until the sex partners have been examined and treated. Separate studies have confirmed that a large proportion of male sex partners of women with PID has gonococcal or chlamydial infection (Osser and Persson, 1982; Danielsson et al., 1987). Frequently these men are asymptomatic and continue to be sexually active without being examined and treated. Treatment of sexual partners of chlamydial salpingitis patients is essential to avoid recurrent infections. In a group of salpingitis patients in which such measures were not undertaken (and contact tracing not performed), half of the patients once again became culture-positive for *C. trachomatis* within 6 months after having had been culture-negative (after finishing a 14-day course of tetracycline).

It is important that women who have had salpingitis not acquire additional tubal infections, since the risk of infertility increases markedly with each infection. This risk can be decreased by avoiding exposure to STD agents. Therefore barrier contraception should be recommended.

Several studies (Senanayake and Kramer, 1980) confirmed that up to 50% of women with PID have an intrauterine contraceptive device (IUD), and that having an IUD is an important risk factor for PID (Weström et al., 1976). Removal of an IUD in PID cases seems reasonable; the IUD should be removed soon after treatment is initiated. Contraceptive counseling should be given to all patients at the end of treatment.

Sequelae

Improper or suboptimal treatment of women with acute PID may result in serious complications. Recent estimates indicate that approximately 15% of women with acute PID fail to respond to initial treatment and that approximately 20% of women with acute PID will have at least one recurrence (Sanders et al., 1986). Fifteen percent become infertile (see also below) after one episode of salpingitis, 35% after two episodes, and 75% after three or more episodes (Weström, 1975). Among those who become pregnant, 8% have tubal pregnancy (Weström et al., 1981). It was recently reported that as many as 25% of all pregnancies following inpatient treatment of PID were tubal (ectopic) (Puolakkainen et al., 1986) (see Chapter 20). The risk of tubal pregnancy increases sevenfold after tubal infection (Weström et al., 1981). A large body of data is confirming the important causative role of *C. trachomatis* infection in PID and its sequelae (see also Chapters 15 and 20).

CHRONIC OR SUBCLINICAL PELVIC INFLAMMATORY DISEASE

Most studies of PID have focused on patients with acute symptoms, many of whom developed pelvic peritonitis. However, these cases may represent only the tip of the iceberg of all endometrial and tubal infections.

Chlamydial infections may produce chronic subclinical infection in the uterine cavity, analogous to ocular trachoma. Many women with tubal infertility and antibody to *C. trachomatis* has no history of past PID. Subclinical uterine or tubal infection may cause symptoms different from those in patients with acute PID.

The recent interest in chronic or subclinical PID is based on several observations (Table 26). Many investigators demonstrated that a large proportion (50% or more) of patients with tubal infertility had no history of clinical PID (Punnonen et al., 1979; Moore et al., 1982; Rosenfeld et al., 1983; Jones et al., 1982b). Furthermore, during the past few years, reports from several centers have documented a consistent association between the demonstration of antichlamydial antibodies to *C. trachomatis* and tubal factor infertility. Women with serological evidence of previous chlamydial infection have approximately two- to threefold increased risk of tubal abnormalities over infertile women with no

TABLE 26. Evidence of Chronic or Subclinical PID

1. Women with tubal infertility often have no history of PID.
2. Strong correlation of serum antibodies to *C. trachomatis* with tubal infertility and tubal pregnancy.
3. High prevalence of plasma cell endometritis among women with mucopurulent cervicitis.
4. Reports of chronic or subclinical chlamydial endometritis among asymptomatic high-risk STD clinic women.
5. Presence of plasma cell salpingitis in patients with tubal pregnancy.
6. Correlation of endometrial lymphoid aggregates with the presence of periadnexal adhesions.
7. Poor results of in vitro fertilization programs in women with antichlamydial antibodies.

antichlamydial antibodies. Similarly, infertile women with tubal disease are two to four times more likely to have elevated titers of *C. trachomatis* antibody than either infertile women with normal tubes or pregnant women (Cates, 1984).

There is a growing number of reports on subclinical or minimally symptomatic endometritis among women with mucopurulent cervicitis. Of 35 consecutive women referred for suspected cervicitis but without suspected PID who underwent endometrial biopsy, plasma cell endometritis was detected in 14 (40%) (Paavonen et al., 1985c). Plasma cell endometritis correlates with the isolation of *C. trachomatis* (Mårdh et al., 1981) and *N. gonorrhoeae* in women with a history of intermenstrual bleeding and uterine tenderness on pelvic examination.

Ingerslev and co-workers (1982) reported evidence of *C. trachomatis* as an etiological agent of chronic endometritis. Henry-Suchet and co-workers (1981) described chronic tubal inflammatory changes in women undergoing infertility evaluation that were supposed to be characteristic of chronic chlamydial infection. They reported isolation of *C. trachomatis* from the tubes or pelvic peritoneum of many such patients.

In a recent study (Henry-Suchet et al., 1987), 161 women undergoing laparoscopy for tubal infertility were analyzed. *Chlamydia trachomatis* infection did not correlate with a past history of salpingitis or pelvic pain, but current *C. trachomatis* infection did correlate with gross and histological evidence of chronic tubal inflammation. By contrast, Patton and co-workers (1986b) failed to isolate *C. trachomatis* from the tubes of 70 women with tubal infertility. Cleary and Jones (1985) isolated *C. trachomatis* from the cervix or the endometrium of 6 (32%) out of 19 infertile women with serum antichlamydial antibodies, usually in association with chronic salpingitis. *Chlamydia trachomatis* was isolated from the endometrium in five (26%) of the 19 cases. This finding indicates that a significant proportion of infertile women with serum antichlamydial antibodies may have active upper genital tract infection with *C. trachomatis* at the time of presentation. Jones and co-workers (1986b) obtained endometrial, endocervical, and urethral cultures for *C. trachomatis* from 60 women seen at an STD clinic who were at risk for chlamydial infection but did not have evidence of endometritis or salpingitis on pelvic examination. *Chlamydia trachomatis* was isolated from the lower tract in 26 (43%) and from the endometrium in 12 (20%) of the 60 women studied. Thus 12 of 29 (41%) women infected with *C. trachomatis* had endometrial infections. Two-thirds of the *Chlamydia*-positive endometrial specimens were positive only after blind passage to fresh monolayers. These studies support the view that a large proportion of chlamydial infections spreads to the upper genital tract in asymptomatic women.

Sweet and associates (1983) demonstrated (as discussed in the section "Endometritis") the persistence of upper genital tract infection with *C. trachomatis* in the face of apparent clinical cure of acute PID. Posttreatment cultures from the endometrial cavity yielded *C. trachomatis* in 12 of 13 patients treated solely with second or third generation cephalosporins as single-agent therapy. Their study suggests that women who apparently have been clinically cured may have a persistent chronic infection that can result in chronic tubal obstruction. Of further interest is the possibility that chronic chlamydial endometritis per se, or residual endometrial changes following chlamydial endometritis, can cause subfertility. This was supported in a report by Rowland and co-workers (1985), who demonstrated that in vitro fertilization was less successful in women with than without

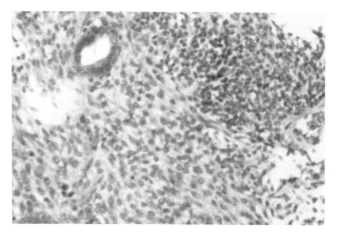

FIGURE 55. Endometrial biopsy showing a lymphoid aggregate in a patient treated for chlamydial PID. (Courtesy of Dr. R. Aine.)

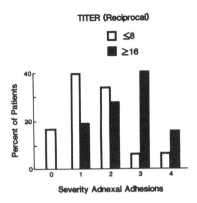

FIGURE 56. Association between antibodies to *Chlamydia trachomatis* and the severity of periadnexal adhesions. (From Gump et al., 1983.)

serum antibody to *C. trachomatis*. Burke and associates (1985) made the interesting observation of the occurrence of subacute focal inflammation and lymphoid aggregates in the endometrium of infertile women. They correlated the pelvic findings of 262 consecutive patients laparoscoped because of infertility with the histopathological diagnosis of endometrial biopsy of specimens that had been obtained as a part of the infertility evaluation. Pelvic adhesions were observed in 87% of women with lymphoid aggregates but in only 11% of women with no lymphoid aggregates. Lymphoid aggregates may represent so-called burned-out follicles characteristic of chlamydial endometritis (Fig. 55). Thus the development of pelvic adhesions may represent another manifestation of subclinical chlamydial PID. This is further supported by Gump and co-workers (1983b), who demonstrated a significant correlation between the prevalence of serum antibodies to *C. trachomatis* and the severity of periadnexal adhesions (Fig. 56).

Tubal pregnancy, like tubal factor infertility, is often associated with previous PID (Bone et al., 1961). Furthermore, Brunham and associates (1986) reported subepithelial lymphocytic and plasma cell infiltration of the tubes, suggesting ongoing salpingitis in 28% of women with tubal pregnancy (see below).

There is some evidence that abnormal menstrual bleeding or menometrorrhagia is associated with chronic endometritis. In studies of women with abnormal or dysfunctional menstrual bleeding, the prevalence of plasma cell endometritis (defined by varying criteria) ranged from 1% to 28% (Schröder, 1921;

Fluhmann, 1929; Keene and Payne, 1934; Dumoulin and Hughesdon, 1951; Rotterdam, 1978; Brudenell, 1955; Greenwood and Moran, 1981; von Bogaert, 1979; Vasudeva, 1972; Kiviat et al., unpublished data; Aine et al., unpublished data). The true prevalence of chronic PID in women with menometrorrhagia, tubal pregnancy, chronic pelvic pain, and infertility remains to be studied.

Infertility

EPIDEMIOLOGY

Pelvic inflammatory disease is often followed by permanent tubal dysfunction and consequent infertility. Swedish studies have shown that women with PID have a four- to sevenfold increased risk of infertility (Weström, 1975). Data from the U.S. National Survey of Family Growth show that 25% of American women with fertility problems had a self-reported history of PID (Aral et al., 1987). Each episode of PID approximately doubles the resulting rate of infertility. Permanent tubal oclusion depends greatly on the degree of acute tubal damage. The rate of permanent tubal damage is much lower after mild PID than after severe PID (3% versus 29%). Falk (1965) showed that tubal occlusion was more common after nongonococcal PID than after gonococcal PID. Postinflammatory tubal occlusion and peritubal adhesions are among the most common causes of infertility in industrialized countries, ranging from 14% to 38% (Hull et al., 1985; Cates et al., 1985). Most infertility in these countries is primary infertility, whereas in Africa and other developing countries most infertility is secondary infertility, and up to 85% is caused by tubal factors (Cates et al., 1985).

There is some evidence that the rate of infertility in the United States has increased over the last decade. Data from the National Diagnostic and Therapeutic Index (NDTI) show that the proportion of visits for infertility has increased steadily from 1968 to 1980 (Aral and Cates, 1983). According to these authors, at least four factors might be contributing to the increase in the demand for infertility services. First, there are more infertile women in the population. Second, a higher proportion of infertile couples is seeking infertility services. Third, more physicians have an interest in, and offer service for, infertility problems. Fourth, contemporary society now regards infertility as glamorous gynecology and a major health problem. Other factors that have contributed to more couples needing infertility services might include the following: the baby-boom generation has aged; infections and environmental exposures have increased age-specific rates; there is now a trend to delay childbearing into later reproductive years thus increasing the age-related biological risks of infertility; and, finally, in this same connection, the attempt to conceive is sometimes condensed into a relatively short time interval. These factors have cumulatively increased the number of couples with fertility problems (Aral and Cates, 1983).

PATHOGENETIC MECHANISMS

Women with PID often have damaged fallopian tubes at the time the diagnosis of PID is suspected, and there is no evidence that antimicrobial therapy can reverse existing tubal damage. It remains to be established if immunological reactions are responsible for tubal scarring in chlamydial salpingitis. Taylor et al. (1986) suggested that *C. trachomatis* possesses antigens that induce immunoprotective and immunopathological hypersensitivity reactions.

Several studies have shown that oral contraceptives (OCs) reduce the risk of PID and that users with clinical evidence of salpingitis develop visible tubal damage less often and manifest a less severe tubal infection when there are signs of salpingitis (Washington et al., 1985). The mechanism(s) of OC protection is(are) unknown. Animal models might help to determine how sex steroids are protective against salpingitis and if OCs modulate the immune response and thus modify the manifestations of chlamydial PID. The combined effects of sex steroids, antimicrobial drugs, and anti-inflammatory drugs on *C. trachomatis* infection should be investigated.

ROLE OF *CHLAMYDIA TRACHOMATIS* INFECTIONS

Cohort studies (Svensson et al., 1983; cf. Weström and Mårdh, 1983) have examined directly or indirectly the relationship between chlamydial infection and infertility. Data from the Swedish studies conducted between 1960 and 1974 suggested that women with nongonococcal salpingitis had a four- to sixfold higher rate of infertility then women with gonococcal salpingitis. More recent Swedish studies indicate that the rates of involuntary infertility among women who had had chlamydial salpingitis were threefold higher than among those without previous salpingitis. By contrast, women with clinically verified PID (but not laparoscopically verified, as in the Swedish studies), of whom 25% had serological or microbiological evidence of chlamydial infection, were no more likely to become infertile than controls, as suggested by a short (21 months) follow-up study (Adler et al., 1982). However, it is generally agreed that a follow-up period of 5–10 years is necessary for a true evaluation of the long-term impact of PID on fertility.

Several retrospective, seroepidemiological case control studies have complemented the cohort studies described. The studies demonstrated a consistent association between elevated titers of *C. trachomatis* antibody and tubal factor infertility. These studies, carried out by at least 13 centers (Table 27), showed that infertile women with serological evidence of past *C. trachomatis* infection have an increased risk of tubal abnormality compared to infertile women without such antibodies. Women with tubal factor infertility are more likely to have high titers of chlamydial antibodies than infertile women with normal tubes. In a study from Finland, Punnonen and associates (1979) showed that the prevalence and level of serum antibody to *C. trachomatis* was higher in women with abnormal hysterosalpingograms (HSGs) than in women with normal HSGs. In France, Henry-Suchet and co-workers (1981) found that infertile women with tubal obstruction and peritubal adhesions had a three times higher occurrence of antichlamydial antibodies than controls. Moore and associates (1982) studied 186 infertile women who underwent HSG or laparoscopy. Serum micro-IF antibodies at a titer of ≥ 32 were present in 73% of women with distal tubal obstruction as compared to none of women with normal tubes. Of women with peritubal adhesions, 21% had antichlamydial antibody. The demonstration of chlamydial antibodies with micro-IF was as accurate as HSG in predicting the presence of tubal disease. Chlamydial serology classified 72%, HSG 76%, and both factors 84%

TABLE 27. Presence of Serum Antibodies to *C. trachomatis* among Infertile Women with and without Tubal Abnormality

Study	Method to determine tubal abnormality	Number with antibodies/ total (%)		p value	Country
		Women with tubal abnormality	Women without tubal abnormality		
Punnonen et al., 1979	HSG	21/23 (91)	52/105 (49)	< 0.001	Finland
Henry-Suchet et al., 1981	L	32/64 (50)	8/40 (20)	< 0.01	France
Cevenini et al., 1982	HSG	36/40 (90)	8/30 (27)	< 0.001	Italy
Moore et al., 1982	L	24/33 (73)	0/35 (0)	< 0.001	USA
Jones et al., 1982b	HSG/L	46/77 (60)	13/77 (17)	< 0.001	USA
Gump et al., 1983b	HSG/L	34/53 (64)	38/134 (28)	< 0.001	USA
Conway et al., 1984	HSG/L	36/48 (75)	23/75 (31)	< 0.001	England
Gibson et al., 1984	HSG/L	33/58			USA
Kane et al., 1984b	L	25/70 (35)	6/52 (12)	< 0.01	England
Tjiam et al., 1985	HSG/L	7/33 (21)	0/20 (0)	< 0.01	Netherlands
Robertson et al., 1987	HSG/L	35/48 (73)	26/77 (34)	< 0.001	England
Ånestad et al., 1987	L	59/67 (88)	21/38 (55)	< 0.01	Norway
Sellors et al., 1988	L	34/43 (79)	29/77 (37)	< 0.001	Canada

of the patients correctly. Although none of the women with normal tubes had antichlamydial antibodies, tubal disease was also seen in 41% of women without serum antibodies to *C. trachomatis*. Interestingly, other infertility factors, including the cervical factor, abnormal sperms, abnormal sperm penetration assay, or endometriosis, were not associated with the occurrence of *C. trachomatis* antibody.

Jones and co-workers (1982b) in Indianapolis studied 172 women undergoing infertility evaluation. Tubal factor infertility was present in 75% of women with serum antibody to *C. trachomatis* compared with 28% of those who had no such antibody. Similarly, there was no correlation between serum antichlamydial antibodies and any other known infertility factor. Gump and co-workers (1983) studied 204 women attending an infertility clinic in Vermont. They found a significant correlation between the prevalence of serum antibody to *C. trachomatis* and adnexal postinflammatory adhesions detected by laparoscopy (64% versus 28%). The more severe the adhesions, the higher was the prevalence of serum antibody to *C. trachomatis*. Cevenini and associates (1982) in Italy also found the proportion of serum antichlamydial antibodies to be higher among women with abnormal HSGs than among infertile women with normal HSGs (90% versus 27%). No differences in the rates of serum antibodies to herpes simplex virus (HSV) or cytomegalovirus (CMV) were found between the groups.

In England, Conway and co-workers (1984) detected serum antichlamydial antibodies in 75% of women with hydrosalpinx or peritubal adhesions versus 21–46% in various control groups. The difference between the groups was even more marked when only high (>1024) antibody titers were considered. Brunham and associates (1985b) studied the role of *C. trachomatis* in tubal infertility by comparing the prevalence of antibody to *C. trachomatis* among 88 women undergoing evaluation for infertility and 49 women attending an antenatal clinic. Infertility patients with tubal infertility began sexual activity sooner, had more sex partners, and in more cases had a history of STDs, supporting the contention that tubal infertility is a sequelae of sexually transmitted infection. Independently of sexual behavior, tubal infertility correlated with the presence of serum antibody to *C. trachomatis*. Women with tubal infertility had a higher prevalence of *C. trachomatis* antibody (13 of 18) than women with nontubal infertility (6 of 70, $p < 0.0001$) or pregnant women (11 of 49, $p < 0.001$). In the population studied with a 20% prevalence of tubal factor infertility, a positive serological test had a predictive value of 68% for tubal infertility, whereas a negative test had a predictive value of 68% for tubal disease. A negative test had a predictive value of 92% for nontubal infertility. More recent seroepidemiological studies (Tjiam et al., 1985; Robertson et al., 1987; Ånestad et al., 1987; Sellors et al., 1988) basically confirmed the results of the previous investigations.

Serological tests for chlamydial antibodies should be part of routine infertility investigations since women with positive serological tests are most likely to have tubal disease and hence are candidates for laparoscopic evaluation. The liberal use of early laparoscopy in patients with antichlamydial antibody seems a reasonable approach. Only 20–50% of women with tubal occlusion and serum antibody to *C. trachomatis* have a history of a clinically recognized episode of PID. In such cases, bypassing HSG makes sense, since it is a procedure that may involve a risk of infection in women who have had PID and should be avoided until other measures have been tried (Stumpf and March al., 1980; Pittaway et al., 1983).

The importance of *C. trachomatis* in tubal infertility as compared to other microorganisms associated with PID, e.g., *N. gonorrhoeae,* has not been thoroughly established, partly because serological tests for gonococci or other microorganisms are less reliable than those for *C. trachomatis.*

More effective treatment for PID will probably not eliminate all cases of tubal infertility. Weström and associates (1975, 1979) observed that subsequent tubal occlusion rates were similar in women treated with various antibiotic regimens, some of which did and some of which did not inhibit *C. trachomatis* in vitro. This may suggest that much of the permanent tubal damage in salpingitis occurred before antibiotic therapy was instituted. Although early diagnosis and treatment of salpingitis might reduce the rate of total tubal occlusion, it might, on the other hand, increase the number of cases of only minor tubal damage, leading to increased risk for tubal (ectopic) pregnancy.

Periappendicitis

EPIDEMIOLOGY

Periappendicitis is defined as a serosal inflammation of the appendix with no involvement of the intestinal mucosa. The prevalence of periappendicitis among patients with histopathologically proven appendicitis varies from 4% to 6% (O'Neill and Moore, 1977; Butler, 1981). In 1912 Moritz detected periappendicitis in 12 of 27 patients with gonococcal salpingitis.

Mårdh and Wølner-Hanssen (1985) reported on periappendicitis as a novel manifestation of genital chlamydial infection. They described seven women with acute salpingitis and histologically proven periappendicitis. *Chlamydia trachomatis* was isolated in all seven cases. Three women showed a significant change in antichlamydial IgG antibody titer. None of the women had IgM antibodies. None had gonorrhea. In all cases the appendix was adherent to the right fallopian tube. In all but one case, the tubal inflammatory changes were more severe on the right side than on the left. They were unable to demonstrate the presence of chlamydial antigen in the appendix by immunofluorescence studies by using monoclonal antibodies to *C. trachomatis*.

In two other studies, periappendicitis was associated with high antichlamydial antibody titers (Lannigan et al., 1980; Poynard et al., 1982).

CLINICAL FINDINGS

Patients with chlamydial periappendicitis generally present with lower abdominal pain and vaginal discharge. They often have irregular bleeding and other signs suggesting (chlamydial) PID. The patients generally do not have fever. They may, however, be subfebrile. The WBC count is only slightly or moderately increased. The ESR is usually high, often 30–60 mm Hg/hr.

DIAGNOSIS

The diagnosis of periappendicitis must be based on visual inspection of the appendix. There are signs of inflammation at inspection, i.e., the peritoneal surface is inflamed, whereas the mucosa is generally normal. In other words, in cases of assumed chlamydial periappendicitis, the inflamed appendix should be removed and the intestinal mucosa inspected.

Also in cases of assumed chlamydial periappendicitis, cultures for chlamydiae and for gonococci should be made from the urethra, the cervix, the peritoneal surface of the appendix, and, if possible, from the fallopian tubes and aspirates from the endometrium (see Chapter 14).

Serological tests for antichlamydial antibodies might add to the diagnostic battery but have the same limited value as in chlamydial salpingitis.

THERAPY

Treatment of chlamydial periappendicitis should be the same as that for chlamydial PID (see Chapter 14). The surgeon should be aware of the possibility of a concomitant salpingitis when removing an inflamed appendix, and if periappendicitis is diagnosed an appropriate antibiotic treatment should be instituted. Contact tracing is important.

Peritonitis and Perihepatitis

EPIDEMIOLOGY

Perihepatitis, or Fitz-Hugh–Curtis syndrome, is a localized fibrinous inflammation affecting the anterior surface of the liver and the adjacent parietal peritoneum. Perihepatitis, first described by Stajano in 1920, is almost always associated with acute salpingitis. Curtis (1930) described the typical "violin string" adhesions between the liver and the abdominal wall in patients with previous salpingitis.

The prevalence of perihepatitis among patients with acute PID has varied considerably in different studies, i.e., from 4% (Wang et al., 1980; Paavonen et al., 1981) to 28% (Gjønnaess et al., 1982b). This difference might be explained by differences in the study populations or in the diagnostic criteria or tests employed.

Early studies related perihepatitis to gonococcal infection (Curtis, 1930; Fitz-Hugh, 1934). Since Fitz-Hugh's report, perihepatitis was thought to be a specific reaction to a gonococcal infection (Amman et al., 1971; Semchyschyn, 1979; von Knorring et al., 1979; Sundal and Stalder, 1980). Litt and Cohen (1978) were the first to consider other etiological agents in this syndrome. They reported 37 patients with signs and symptoms of perihepatitis. They found that two-thirds of their perihepatitis patients did *not* have gonorrhea. *Chlamydia trachomatis* was first suggested as a possible cause of perihepatitis by Müller-Schoop and co-workers (1978) when they found serological evidence of a recent chlamydial infection in patients with peritonitis and perihepatitis. Wølner-Hanssen and associates (1980) were the first to describe perihepatitis in patients with chlamydial salpingitis. Subsequent studies further strengthened the association between *C. trachomatis* and perihepatitis (Wang et al., 1980; Paavonen and Valtonen, 1980; Paavonen et al., 1981; Darougar et al., 1981; Dalaker et al., 1981; cf. Eschenbach, 1984). In 1982, for the first time, *C. trachomatis* was isolated directly from the liver capsule of a patient with perihepatitis (Wølner-Hanssen et al., 1982a).

Soon after Wølner-Hanssen and co-workers (1980) had reported on three cases of perihepatitis associated with chlamydial infection, they (1982a) described 17 (5%) cases of perihepatitis among 339 women with laparoscopically proven salpingitis who had been seen during the period 1978–1983. All but two of the patients presented with right upper quadrant abdominal pain. The serum levels of the liver and pancreatic enzymes were within normal limits in all but one patient. Subsequently, patients with salpingitis and perihepatitis were compared to such patients with no signs of perihepatitis (Wølner-Hansson, 1986). Patients with perihepatitis had high ESRs and high serum IgG antichlamydial antibody titers in micro-IF tests significantly more often. The geometric mean titer of antibodies to *C. trachomatis* was 1217 in women with and 67 in women without perihepatitis ($p < 0.0001$).

Chlamydial infection can also cause peritonitis without signs of perihepatitis. Pericolitis and perisplenitis are also seen in some patients affected by *C. trachomatis*.

IMMUNOPATHOLOGY

Isolation of *C. trachomatis* from the liver capsule suggests a canalicular spread of the microorganism from the lower genital tract to the upper abdomen, although the possibility of a hematogenous or lymphatic spread cannot be excluded. Interestingly, Kimball and Knee (1970) reported on a male patient with gonococcal urethritis who apparently developed perihepatitis and had *N. gonorrhoeae* isolated from a liver biopsy. Møller and Mårdh (1980a) inoculated *C. trachomatis* into the uterine cavity of grivet monkeys following ligature of the tubal isthmus. One of the monkeys died 14 days later and had peritonitis and perihepatitis at autopsy, which might suggest a lymphatic or hematogenous spread. However, clinical studies support a canalicular spread of the organism as the common mode of spread in humans.

Wang and co-workers (1980) suggested that chlamydial perihepatitis might be the result of an immunological reaction induced by a reinfection with a heterologous serotype of *C. trachomatis*. They found that the serotype specificity of IgM antibodies differed from that of the IgG antibodies in 7 of 11 patient with chlamydial perihepatitis.

In an experimental animal model, Patton and associates (1985) found that the primary infection produced salpingitis but reinoculation of the tubes with another serotype of *C. trachomatis* produced perihepatitis. In a study of cell-mediated immunity to *C. trachomatis* among women with perihepatitis and salpingitis, lymphocytes from patients with perihepatitis tended to maintain a higher level of responsiveness at follow-up than those from patients with salpingitis alone (Hallberg et al., 1985). These data also suggest that the perihepatitis might be the result of a hyperimmune reaction to chlamydial reinfection.

DIAGNOSIS

Perihepatitis is usually diagnosed by the finding of a severe, acute right upper abdominal pain that is accentuated by deep inspiration, coughing, laughing, and twisting of the upper body. Some patients experience only minor subcostal discomfort. The pain can be similar to that found in cholecystitis. Cholecystography may give evidence of pathology since the chlamydial peritonitis found in perihepatitis patients can interfere with gallbladder motility. There can be referred pain to the right shoulder. Young women who are seen in the emergency room with symptoms suggestive of acute cholecystitis should always be evaluated for salpingitis and perihepatitis. The recognition of Fitz-Hugh–Curtis syndrome is important to avoid unnecessary laboratory and radiological examinations and even laparotomy. If not properly recognized and treated, tubal dysfunction is likely to follow. Pelvic examination usually reveals pelvic pathology suggesting PID, although the findings may be minimal.

Chlamydial perihepatitis is characterized by a fibrin deposit on the liver surface (Fig. 57), adhesions between the liver surface and the anterior abdominal

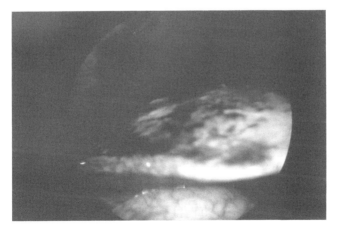

FIGURE 57. Chlamydial perihepatitis (Fitz-Hugh–Curtis syndrome) showing a liver surface with fibrin deposits. (Courtesy of Dr. F. Nordenskiöld.)

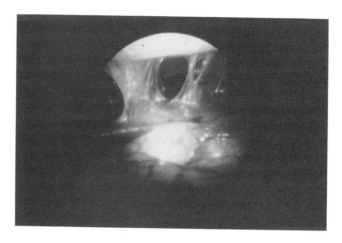

FIGURE 58. Violin string adhesions in a case of chlamydial perihepatitis. (Courtesy of Dr. F. Nordenskiöld.)

wall, so-called violin-string adhesions that can be seen at laparoscopy (Fig. 58). There may also be signs of peritonitis.

Liver biopsies will generally reveal only minor inflammatory cell infiltration in the liver capsule. There might also be a slight congestion in the capsule (Fig. 59). The liver parenchyma is usually normal.

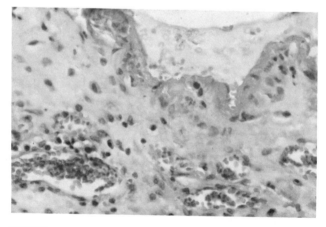

FIGURE 59. Histology of the liver capsule in a case of perihepatitis.

Liver enzyme (i.e., ASAT, ALAT, and pancreatic amylase) levels are usually within the normal range. The ESR is usually high. The white blood cell count may be normal or high. The etiological diagnosis in chlamydial perihepatitis should be based on isolation of *C. trachomatis* from the urethra, the cervix, and, if possible, from the tubes and liver capsule.

Serum antibodies to *C. trachomatis* should be determined when a woman of fertile age presents with acute upper abdominal pain and also when a young woman presents with pain suggestive of acute cholecystitis. Patients with chlamydial perihepatitis usually have exceptionally high serum antichlamydial antibody titers compared to patients with PID who lack signs of perihepatitis, or to controls (Wang et al., 1980; Puolakkainen et al., 1984). The antibody response to perihepatitis involves antibodies to both major antigenic components of *C. trachomatis*, the lipopolysaccharide antigen and the major outer membrane protein, MOMP. With a finding of a high-IgG ELISA antibody titer in MOMP EIA or in EIA using crude chlamydial antigen, a presumptive diagnosis of perihepatitis was obtained in 88–96% of patients (Puolakkainen et al., 1984). Although seroconversion was found in 11% to 44% of the patients for IgG and in 28–36% for IgM antichlamydial antibodies, a high-IgG titer was the best predictive test for chlamydial perihepatitis.

THERAPY

Patients with acute right upper abdominal pain suggestive of perihepatitis should be hospitalized and treated with antimicrobials active against *C. trachomatis* and *N. gonorrhoeae*. If laparoscopy is performed, liver adhesions should probably be released. A second laparoscopy to accomplish further release of adhesions should be considered in cases of chronic postinflammatory right upper abdominal pain. This can lead to a dramatic resolution of pain in such cases (Reichert and Valle, 1976).

Patients with chlamydial perihepatitis should be treated with antibiotics, and the therapy should be the same as that described for patients with chlamydial salpingitis.

As in other types of genital chlamydial infections, contact tracing is essential in cases of chlamydial perihepatitis. Experience indicates that this measure is often neglected.

Adverse Pregnancy Outcome

Chlamydia trachomatis is a common infectious agent in pregnant women. Depending on the population studied, 2% to 37% of pregnant women have been *C. trachomatis* culture-positive. The infection is clinically more difficult to recognize in pregnant than in nonpregnant women. Pregnant women usually have increased vaginal discharge, their endocervical mucus frequently has a cloudy appearance, and their Gram-stained endocervical smears often show an increased number of PMN leukocytes.

Infection by several microorganisms has been associated with adverse pregnancy outcome, i.e., abortion, stillbirth, premature labor, or premature rupture of membranes (PROM). These microorganisms include β-hemolytic streptococci Group B (Regan et al., 1981; Thomsen et al., 1987), *Ureaplasma urealyticum* (Braun et al., 1971; Kass et al., 1981; Minkoff et al., 1984; Cassell et al., 1983; Shurin et al., 1975; Gibbs et al., 1983; Waites et al., 1988), *Mycoplasma hominis* (Harwick et al., 1970; Christensen et al., 1982; Thompson et al., 1982; Harrison et al., 1983a; Waites et al., 1988), and *Trichomonas vaginalis* (Minkoff et al., 1984; Hardy et al., 1984). The clinical condition known as bacterial vaginosis is also associated with adverse pregnancy outcome (Gravett et al., 1986a, 1986b).

Chlamydia trachomatis has also been associated with PROM and prematurity (Martin et al., 1982; Harrison et al., 1983b; Gravett et al., 1986a). Because *C. trachomatis* can infect primary cultures of human amniotic cells (Harrison et al., 1979b), it is plausible that *C. trachomatis* can infect the amniotic membranes, causing inflammation of the membranes, release of prostaglandin precursors, and PROM (McDonald et al., 1978; Minkoff, 1983). Studies have shown that women at high risk for placental and amniotic fluid infection are women recently exposed to *C. trachomatis*. Martin and others (1982), in a small study, first demonstrated an association between *C. trachomatis* and adverse pregnancy outcome. Later studies found adverse pregnancy outcome related to recent chlamydial infection as demonstrated by the presence of antichlamydial IgM antibody (Harrison et al., 1983b; Sweet et al., 1987). Other studies indicated no correlation between *C. trachomatis* and adverse pregnancy outcome (Thompson et al., 1982; Hardy et al., 1984).

The early prospective studies of *C. trachomatis* infection during pregnancy did not find any correlation between prematurity and the presence of *C. trachomatis* (Chandler et al., 1977; Schachter et al., 1979b; Frommel et al., 1979; Hammerschlag et al., 1979; Mårdh et al., 1980b). This might be due to the fact that the women studied had usually entered into the studies during the last trimester of pregnancy. Martin and co-workers (1982) enrolled patients before the 18th week of pregnancy and found that stillbirth, premature delivery, and perinatal death were all associated with *C. trachomatis* infection. Six of 18 women with and only 3% of 238 women without *C. trachomatis* had an adverse pregnancy outcome.

Gravett and associates (1986a), in a case control study, found that *C. trachomatis* was independently associated with premature birth (Table 28). In a larger prospective study of more than 1300 women, Harrison and others (1983b) found no overall increase in the rate of adverse pregnancy outcome in those harboring *C. trachomatis*. However, women with *C. trachomatis* and antichlamydial IgM antibody were more likely to have premature delivery and low birth weight infants than antichlamydial IgM-negative culture-positive or culture-negative women. Other confounding variables did not explain the association.

Although a few studies have shown a link between cervical chlamydial infection and adverse pregnancy outcome, not all studies have confirmed such an association. In a recent prospective study, Sweet and co-workers (1987) com-

TABLE 28. Multiple Logistic Analysis of the Association of *Chlamydia Trachomatis* with Adverse Pregnancy Outcome[a,b]

| | *C. trachomatis* | | | Confidence |
	Present (%)	Absent (%)	Odds ratio	interval (95%)
Preterm labor				
< 34 weeks	23	9	4.0	(1.7–9.2)[c]
< 37 weeks	36	12	4.3	(2.1–8.8)[c]
Preterm PROM < 37 weeks	23	11	2.4	(1.1–5.4)[d]
Birth weight < 2500 g	32	15	2.7	(1.3–5.7)[c]

[a]From Gravett et al. (1986).
[b]Adjusted for 11 variables (age, race, parity, marital status, welfare status, smoking, prior abortion, prior preterm delivery, anemia, third trimester bleeding, and urinary tract infection with the current pregnancy).
[c]$p < 0.01$.
[d]$p < 0.05$.

pared 270 pregnant women with cervical chlamydial infection to matched controls. No significant differences were noted between cases and controls for PROM, preterm delivery, amnionitis, intrapartum fever, small for gestational age, postpartum endometritis, and neonatal sepsis. However, in the subset of cases with IgM antibody against *C. trachomatis,* preterm delivery occurred in 13 of 67 IgM-positive versus 8 of 99 IgM-negative cases ($p < 0.03$). The presence of serum IgM antibody to *C. trachomatis* might imply a recently acquired or a more invasive infection. It is probable that a large proportion of young, pregnant women with *C. trachomatis* has antichlamydial IgG antibody. These women may not be at risk for an adverse pregnancy outcome, since the presence of IgG antibody may be protective. Contrary to this, women with recent *C. trachomatis* infection who have antichlamydial IgM antibodies may be at risk.

Nevertheless, the inconsistency between different studies raises uncertainty as to whether or not *C. trachomatis* is related to adverse pregnancy outcome. In addition, the importance of *C. trachomatis* relative to other microorganisms must be more thoroughly studied before definite conclusions can be drawn. Many pregnancy outcome studies focused on a limited number of organisms known to be associated with adverse pregnancy outcome, and the numbers of cases studied were generally small. Much larger investigations will be necessary to reach any definitive conclusions. In such investigations all microorganisms known to be associated with adverse pregnancy outcome should be considered in the same study. Both qualitative and quantitative cultures should be performed, and adjustment for demographic, socioeconomic, and other confounding factors is important. At the present time, studies seem to suggest an association between *C. trachomatis* and an adverse pregnancy outcome, the relative risk being in the range of 2–4%, and perhaps only among women with a recently acquired IgM-positive chlamydial infection.

Postpartum Endometritis

Early ophthalmological studies on chlamydial infections reported that mothers or infants with inclusion conjunctivitis had a high rate of postpartum fever (Thygeson and Mengert, 1936; Mordhorst and Dawson, 1971).

In a prospective study, Rees and others (1977b) confirmed that *C. trachomatis* is associated with postpartum endometritis, and that most of the infants born to mothers with postpartum endometritis developed inclusion conjunctivitis. Wager and co-workers (1980) reported that *C. trachomatis* was associated with late postpartum endometritis, i.e., endometritis that developed from 2 days to 6 weeks postpartum, but not with early postpartum endometritis that developed within 2 days postpartum. Late postpartum endometritis developed in 22% of patients with *C. trachomatis* versus 5% of those without *C. trachomatis*. Similarly, Watts and Eschenbach (1986) did not find *C. trachomatis* to be associated with early (<48 hr) onset postpartum endometritis, which they usually found to be caused by a pyrogenic bacterial infection. However, Harrison and co-workers (1983) reported only a weak association between postpartum endometritis and *C. trachomatis* (or *U. urealyticum*). They found a stronger association between antepartum presence of *M. hominis* and the risk of postpartum endometritis. There is also evidence from culture studies linking *C. trachomatis* with postpartum endometritis. In a recent study, *C. trachomatis* was isolated from the cervix or endometrium of 60% and from the endometrium of 23% of patients with postpartum endometritis who had delivered vaginally (Hoyme et al., 1986).

The impact of *C. trachomatis*-associated late postpartum endometritis is not fully understood. Postpartum infections may cause a considerable proportion of secondary tubal infertility. Certainly in developing countries secondary infertility is a major problem and most of this infertility is tubal factor infertility. In the obstetrical wards of African hospitals, postpartum and postabortal endometritis are very common diagnoses.

In the Western industrialized countries, most infertility is primary infertility, whereas in developing countries most infertility is secondary infertility, suggesting that postpartum infections play an important role (Cates et al., 1985).

Chlamydia trachomatis is probably one of the leading causes of postabortal endometritis. Approximately 20% of women with *C. trachomatis* undergoing induced abortion develop postabortal PID (Møller et al., 1982; Westergaard et al., 1982; Qvigstad et al., 1983; Barbucci et al., 1986). Møller and co-workers (1982) studied 943 healthy, pregnant women from Denmark and Sweden in the first trimester of pregnancy who were all undergoing elective abortion. They found that the development of postabortion PID was significantly associated with the isolation of *C. trachomatis* before the intervention ($p < 0.04$). Westergaard and associates (1982) reported that 28% of 29 women with *C. trachomatis* and 10% of 241 women without *C. trachomatis* developed postabortal PID ($p < 0.025$). Barbucci and associates (1986) studied 505 women presenting for elective abortion. They found that 6 of 17 patients with postabortal endometritis were positive for *C. trachomatis,* with a significant correlation between chlamydial infection and development of postabortal endometritis.

Qvigstad and co-workers (1983) isolated *C. trachomatis* from the cervix of 70 of 557 (13%) patients admitted for therapeutic abortion. Twenty percent of the *C. trachomatis*-positive patients developed PID versus only 2% of the *C. trachomatis*-negative patients.

In summary, the results of these adverse pregnancy outcome studies are consistent with the hypothesis that patients with *C. trachomatis* infection at the time of pregnancy termination are at high risk for the development of postoperative PID.

20

Tubal (Ectopic) Pregnancy

In the early 1980s a woman with a history of documented PID had a sevenfold increased risk of tubal pregnancy over a woman with no history of PID (Weström et al., 1981; Persson, 1986). In 1983, 70,000 ectopic pregnancies were reported in the United States. During the surveillance period 1970–1983, the rate of ectopic pregnancy increased more than threefold from 4.5 per 1000 pregnancies in 1970 to 14.0 per 1000 pregnancies in 1983 (*MMWR*, 1986) (Fig. 60). Maternal mortality resulting from ectopic pregnancy has dropped dramatically since the early 1970s; however, ectopic pregnancy still has major long-term effects on the reproductive capacity of women. The infertility rate after an ectopic pregnancy is 50%, and 10–15% of patients develop recurrent ectopic pregnancy (Eschenbach and Daling, 1983).

Only 10% of women with ectopic pregnancy had a history of clinically recognized PID. Asymptomatic or subclinical tubal infections may contribute to tubal pathology resulting in ectopic pregnancy or tubal infertility.

Gump and others (1983) reported that the presence of antichlamydial serum antibody correlated with the subsequent risk of ectopic pregnancy. These data suggest that if *C. trachomatis* is involved in tubal infection leading to ectopic pregnancy, the infection is often subclinical.

Svensson and others (1985) studied 112 women with ectopic pregnancy and found that 75% had IgG antibodies to *C. trachomatis*, whereas only 21% of women with intrauterine pregnancy had such antibodies. There was a correlation between the presence of IgG antibodies to *C. trachomatis* and a history of PID. They concluded that chlamydial infection is etiologically related to ectopic pregnancy and that such a pregnancy is one sequelae of genital chlamydial infection.

Brunham and co-workers (1985b) reported that subepithelial lymphocytic and plasma cell tubal infiltration was suggestive of an ongoing salpingitis in 9 (28%) of 32 women with tubal pregnancy who lacked other known risk factors. They found antibody to *C. trachomatis* in all of 7 cases with plasma cell salpingitis, but in only 8 of 23 nonsalpingitic women ($p < 0.001$).

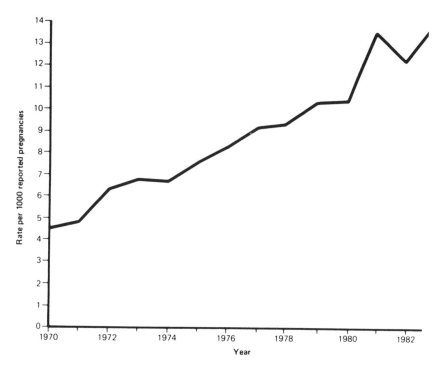

CHAPTER 20

FIGURE 60. Ectopic pregnancy rates for females aged 15–44 by year in United Sates 1970–1983. (From *MMWR*, 1986.)

Ectopic pregnancy, which can be a sequelae of both gonorrhea and chlamydial infection, seems to be an epidemiological marker of STDs in a community. However, it highlights the epidemic situation that prevailed years earlier in the community. Thus Persson (1986) found a mean age of 29 years for women with ectopic pregnancy, whereas that for women with acute salpingitis in the same hospital catchment region was only 24 years. Among the salpingitis patients, those with proven chlamydial infection were even younger (mean age 20 years).

Tubal pregnancy contributes significantly to the heavy economic consequences of STDs (Washington, 1985).

Contraceptive Use and Infection by *Chlamydia trachomatis*

There seems to be a consensus that chlamydial infection generally spreads canalicularly from the cervix to the tubes. In women in whom such a passage is impossible (such as pregnant women) or in whom the tubes have been ligated, primary salpingitis does not occur. In other women, where intraluminar passage of microbes may be facilitated (such as in women with intrauterine devices, or IUDs), salpingitis occurs more often than in controls (Weström et al., 1976). The use of contraceptives decreased the risk of salpingitis in women with chlamydial cervicitis and diminished the severity of tubal inflammatory alterations (Svensson et al., 1984).

Several studies have shown a significantly increased risk of *C. trachomatis* infection in oral contraceptive (OC) users. Of 14 studies reviewed by Washington and co-workers (1985) all but two showed a significantly increased relative risk (range 1.5–3.9) for *C. trachomatis* infection among OC users (Table 29). This increase could be the result of more sexual activity among women who use such contraceptives than among those who do not. It could also be due to the presence of OC-induced cervical ectopy (Jordan and Singer, 1976). Women with cervical ectopy not only had increased rates of *C. trachomatis* infection but increased concentrations of the organism as well (Hobson et al., 1980). *Chlamydia trachomatis* infects columnar endocervical cells. Cervical ectopy is therefore believed to increase the number of potential host cells available to *C. trachomatis* and also enables detection of chlamydial infection in OC users.

Oral contraceptives increase the viscosity and otherwise change the character of cervical mucus, thereby providing a more effective barrier to microorganisms and sperms, and probably decreasing the ascent of microorganisms from the lower genital tract to the upper genital tract. Oral contraceptive users

TABLE 29. Epidemiological Evidence for Association between Oral Contraceptive (OC) Use and Cervical *C. trachomatis* Infection[a]

Study	Proportion (number) of cases with *C. trachomatis* infection[b]		Relative risk (90% CI)[d]
	OC users	Non-OC users[c]	
Hilton et al., 1974	0.45 (92)	0.24 (187)	1.9 (1.3–2.6)
Oriel et al., 1974	0.26 (102)	0.12 (145)	2.1 (1.2–3.7)
Oriel et al., 1978	0.28 (121)	0.16 (138)	1.8 (1.1–2.8)
Ripa et al., 1978	0.41 (44)	0.15 (34)	2.8 (1.1–6.7)
Tait et al., 1980	0.46 (99)	0.22 (95)	2.1 (1.4–3.2)
Kinghorn and Waugh, 1981	0.27 (601)	0.15 (479)	1.8 (1.4–2.3)
Svensson et al., 1981	0.72 (204)	0.54 (282)	2.2 (1.5–3.3)
Arya et al., 1981	0.43 (191)	0.23 (121)	1.9 (1.3–2.7)
Schachter et al., 1983	0.13 (1.146)	0.05 (761)	2.5 (1.8–3.5)
Fraser et al., 1983	0.18 (34)	0.05 (89)	3.9 (1.2–13.1)
Shafer et al., 1984	0.24 (107)	0.11 (194)	2.1 (1.2–3.5)
Burns et al., 1975	0.13 (287)	0.13 (289)	1.0 (0.6–1.5)
Nayyar et al., 1976	0.24 (161)	0.16 (139)	1.5 (0.9–2.4)
Woolfitt and Watt, 1977	0.26 (66)	0.26 (88)	1.0 (0.6–1.7)

[a]From Washington et al. (1985).
[b]Patient sources were sexually transmitted disease clinics, gynecological clinics, family-planning clinics, and adolescent clinics.
[c]Generally includes no method of contraception and all contraceptive methods other than oral contraceptives.
[d]Relative risk of *C. trachomatis* infection among women using oral contraception vs. all other contraceptive methods plus no contraception; 95% confidence intervals (CI) were calculated from published data.

also generally have shorter duration of menstrual bleeding and therefore possibly a decreased risk of infection.

In tissue cell cultures, sex hormones enhance the growth of *C. trachomatis* (Mårdh, 1981; Wenman et al., 1982). Thus both estrogen and progesterone, when added to McCoy tissue cell cultures, influenced the rate of formation of *C. trachomatis* intracytoplasmic inclusions (Mårdh, 1981) (see also Chapter 5). In animal models (Rank et al., 1982; Pasley et al., 1985; Taylor-Robinson et al., 1982), the development and persistence of ascending *C. trachomatis* genital infection is influenced by sex hormones. Experimental chlamydial infection in estrogen- and progesterone-treated mice lasts longer than in untreated mice (Barron et al., 1981; Tuffrey and Taylor-Robinson, 1981).

The results of animal model studies suggest that oral contraceptive steroids may enhance chlamydial infection. However, extrapolating observations from such studies to humans is difficult (Washington et al., 1985). Nevertheless, present knowledge suggests that contraceptive steroids may stimulate genital chlamydial infections.

Use of OCs is less common in women with acute PID than in controls without PID. This unexpected finding has been convincingly demonstrated in many case-control and cross-sectional studies (Eschenbach et al., 1977; cf. Washington et al., 1985), although these studies were generally limited to women hospitalized for acute PID. Furthermore, the studies were designed to analyze the relationship between IUD usage and PID. Wølner-Hanssen and co-workers (1985) studied contraception among 738 women laparoscoped because of acute signs of salpingitis. The relative risk using no contraception was 0.24 ($p < 0.001$). The same relative risk was found for the group of women infected with *C. trachomatis*. Twice as many OC users as IUD users, and almost three times as many OC users as users of barrier methods or women using no contraception, had no laparoscopic evidence of salpingitis even though PID was clinically suspected. Possible differences between specific OCs were not analyzed.

If women using OCs have higher rates of cervical *C. trachomatis*, it is difficult to explain how OCs can protect against PID if the rate of ascending infection remains the same. Furthermore, one would expect OC users to have higher rates of chlamydial PID and long-term sequelae related to PID, such as tubal infertility and tubal pregnancy. No such data have been presented.

There is evidence that OC use modifies the manifestations of PID. Svensson and associates (1984) were the first to show that OC users had significantly milder tubal disease than nonusers. In a controlled study from Lund, Sweden (Wølner-Hanssen, 1986), among 94 women with salpingitis and 12 women with salpingitis and perihepatitis (all culture-positive for *C. trachomatis*), a negative association was found between OC use and the presence of perihepatitis ($p = 0.002$). A trend toward milder salpingitis was seen among OC users. The OC users also had a lower mean antichlamydial IgG antibody titer than the nonusers. Paavonen and co-workers (1987) laparoscoped 45 women with suspected PID, of whom 30 (67%) had salpingitis. *C. trachomatis, N. gonorrhoeae*, or both organisms were isolated from any sampling site in 24 (80%) and from the upper genital tract in 14 (47%) of the 30 women. It was notable that pill users were more likely to have mild salpingitis than IUD users or women using other or no contraceptive methods ($p = 0.0025$). In fact, all OC users had mild salpingitis.

Washington and co-workers (1985) concluded that current information does not permit the generalization that OCs protect against all forms of PID from mild subclinical to severe emergency. A vast majority (at least 75%) of PID episodes are actually less acute and are generally managed on an outpatient basis. Clinicians should suspect *C. trachomatis* when evaluating nonspecific complaints suggesting lower genital tract infection in women using OCs. Even mild clinical signs of PID should be assumed to possibly represent PID caused by *C. trachomatis*. Oral contraceptives obviously do not protect against all PID, and it is not known whether or not OC usage increases the rate of subclinical or chronic PID. The advisability of prescribing OCs to women after a first episode of PID in order to prevent recurrences remains to be established.

The mechanisms of the possible modifying effect of OCs on PID are not yet understood (Svensson et al., 1984). The OCs might modify PID by suppressing immune infection (Paavonen et al., 1981; Grossman, 1985). More studies are needed on possible interactions between chlamydial infection, sex steroid hormones, and the immune system.

Concomitant Infection with *Chlamydia trachomatis, Neisseria gonorrhoeae,* and Other Genital Pathogens, and Treatment of Mixed Infections

Genital chlamydial infection is common in patients with gonorrhea, although the reverse is no longer true in many Western industrialized countries. Some years ago up to 30–50% of both male and female chlamydial patients had gonorrhea (Oriel et al., 1972; Holmes et al., 1975; Ripa et al., 1978). Today this figure is much lower in many countries. However, in many developing countries gonorrhea is still quite common, and in fact should be interpreted as a marker of concomitant chlamydial infection.

In cases of concomitant chlamydial and gonococcal infection that have been treated with penicillins or cephalosporins, postgonococcal urethritis (PGU), postgonococcal cervicitis, postgonococcal PID, and postgonococcal conjunctivitis may be seen.

Approximately 15–30% of heterosexual men with gonococcal urethritis simultaneously have urethral infection by *C. trachomatis.* When these men receive penicillin, single-dose ampicillin, or spectinomycin for treatment of their gonorrhea, the chlamydial infection persists and causes PGU or asymptomatic urethral infection (Holmes et al., 1967a; Richmond et al., 1972; Oriel et al., 1976; Karney et al., 1977; Bowie, 1984). Some cases of PGU first become culture-positive for *C. trachomatis* after β-lactam antibiotic therapy has begun.

An even higher (25–50%) proportion of women with gonorrhea also has *C. trachomatis* infection of the cervix (Brunham et al., 1982b). Rees (1980) treated women who had uncomplicated gonococcal and chlamydial infections with either intramuscular penicillin G or oral tetracycline, and found that subsequent PID developed in 11 of 103 women given penicillin, but in only 1 of 105 given tetracycline. Brunham and co-workers (1982c) associated postgonococcal cervicitis in *C. trachomatis*-infected women with the use of gonorrhea treatment regimens that were ineffective for *C. trachomatis*.

Treatment of concomitant chlamydial and gonococcal infections may create problems if a single-drug alternative is looked for. In many areas a marked resistance to tetracycline has long been common in gonococcal strains.

Stamm and co-workers (1984) evaluated the effect of treatment for gonorrhea on simultaneous *C. trachomatis* infection by assigning 293 heterosexual men and 549 heterosexual women with gonorrhea to one of the following treatment regimens: (1) 4.8 million units of procaine penicillin plus 1 g of probenecid, (2) nine tablets of trimethoprim-sulfamethoxazole for 3 days, or (3) 500 mg of tetracycline four times a day for 5 days. Among the men, gonococcal infection was cured in 99% given penicillin plus probenecid, 96% given trimethoprim-sulfamethoxazole, and 98% given tetracycline. Among the women given tetracycline, only 90% were cured. This is in contrast to cure rates of 97% for those given penicillin plus probenecid and 99% for those given trimethoprim-sulfamethoxazole. The chlamydial infection, present in 15% of the men and 26% of the women, was cured in 30 of 32 patients given trimethoprim-sulfamethoxazole, in 27 of 29 given tetracycline, but in only 10 of 23 given penicillin plus probenecid. Among *C. trachomatis*-positive patients, postgonococcal urethritis in men and postgonoccal cervicitis in women occurred more often in patients given penicillin plus probenecid, but in only 1 of 26 given trimethoprim-sulfamethoxazole and in none of 24 given tetracycline.

For the above-mentioned and other reasons, an expert panel from the Centers for Disease Control recommended that heterosexual men and women treated with a single dose of ampicillin, amoxicillin, or penicillin also be given a 7-day course of tetracycline (cf. Appendix). In gonorrhea treatment, erythromycin should be reserved for pregnant, penicillin-allergic women. It should be remembered that erythromycin is not very effective against gonorrhea and many of the newer cephalosporins with a high activity against gonococci have a poor activity against chlamydiae (Stamm and Cole, 1986). This may be especially important in cases of uncertain etiology.

Fortunately, *C. trachomatis* has not yet developed resistance to tetracycline, although the increased use of tetracycline for genital as well as other infections regardless of microbial etiology is probably one factor responsible for the growing spread of tetracycline resistance among many genital pathogens, including *N. gonorrhoeae, M. hominis,* and *U. urealyticum* (Koutsky et al., 1983; Christiansson and Mårdh, 1983; Stamm and Holmes, 1986). The newly discovered, pronounced tetracycline resistance of *N. gonorrhoeae,* i.e., with an MIC

$\geqslant 4\mu g/ml$, may create further therapeutic problems, as resistant gonococcal strains are now spreading rapidly in some parts of the world.

Differences in the male and female reproductive tracts contribute to greater difficulty in the differential diagnosis of various urogenital tract infections in women and greater risk of complications of many STDs in women. The difficulty of diagnosing sexually transmitted urogenital infections in women often results in delay of proper therapy, which contributes to a higher risk of complications. In heterosexual men, gonococcal and chlamydial infections are limited to the anterior urethra in most cases, and symptoms and signs of urethral discharge are readily recognized by both the patient and the clinician. On the other hand, in women several STD pathogens including *N. gonorrhoeae, C. trachomatis,* HSV, *M. hominis, Trichomonas vaginalis, Gardnerella vaginalis,* and *Candida albicans* have a predilection for infection of the urethra, the introitus, the vagina, the cervix, and the rectum, simultaneously producing variable patterns of symptoms and signs. Mixed infections are also common.

Chlamydial cervicitis was found to be uncommon in gynecological outpatient clinic patients with bacterial vaginosis (BV), i.e., women with an increased vaginal discharge, a vaginal pH $\geqslant 4.7$, a positive amine test (fishy odor), and the presence of ''clue'' cells (Fig. 47) in wet mounts (Holst et al., 1984). However, in STD clinic patients, both conditions have been diagnosed with high frequency (Fig. 48). In women with bacterial vaginosis, a nitroimidazole compound, e.g., metronidazole or tinidazole, should be prescribed along with a tetracycline drug or a macrolide. These drugs have a therapeutic effect, although their in vitro activity against *G. vaginalis* and *Mobiluncus* spp., i.e., bacteria that are strongly associated with bacterial vaginosis, is limited. It is believed that metabolites formed in vivo are responsible for the in vivo effect. Erythromycin has a poor clinical effect on bacterial vaginosis. Combined therapy with tetracycline (or erythromycin) and a nitroimidazole should be instituted in known or possible cases of concomitant chlamydial infection and trichomoniasis.

A polymicrobial etiology of PID was implicated in previous U.S. studies (Eschenbach et al., 1975, 1977; Eschenbach, 1980; Sweet et al., 1980); therefore it is no longer appropriate to apply single-drug therapy to PID unless the drug is active in vitro against both *N. gonorrhoeae* and *C. trachomatis* as a minimum. *Chlamydia trachomatis* was cervically isolated from 5% to 56% (mean 29%) of women with clinically suspected PID, whereas *N. gonorrhoeae* was demonstrated in 5–80% (mean 26%) (Eschenbach, 1986). Double infections with these agents are relatively common in the cervix of PID patients, but not in the fallopian tubes.

In case of possible concomitant syphilis, treatment of a chlamydial infection should be chosen that does not mask the treponemal infection. Trimethoprim-sulfa has been recommended in such cases.

Reiter's Syndrome

EPIDEMIOLOGY

Of NGU cases, 1–3% are complicated by reactive arthritis (Keat et al., 1978; Kousa et al., 1978). Asymmetrical polyarthritis (especially in the lower extremities, sometimes occurring as sacroilitis) and tenosynovitis (in the achilles and other tendons of the feet) (Kousa, 1978; Keat et al., 1983) are the most common manifestations. Arthritis can occur in association with uveitis and urethritis, a triad that has been named Reiter's syndrome. However, all three manifestations are seldom present simultaneously. Reiter's syndrome can occur after intestinal infections (enteroarthritis) or after urogenital infections (uroarthritis). Uroarthritis is also called sexually acquired reactive arthritis (SARA) (Keat et al., 1983). Patients with HLA B27 antigen are a special risk group for reactive arthritis.

Sexually acquired reactive arthritis most often affects young, sexually active males. Thus it is more common in males than in females (20 : 1) (Leirisalo et al., 1982). The male preponderance might be partly due to difficulties in diagnosing SARA and Reiter's syndrome in women. The often asymptomatic character of the genital manifestation in women can result in a high degree of nondiagnosis or misdiagnosis of Reiter's syndrome among females.

A disease called rheumatic salpingitis has been proposed as a manifestation of reactive arthritis in females (Yli-Kerttula et al., 1984).

CHLAMYDIAL INFECTION

Since chlamydial infection has long been known as a comparatively common cause of polyarthritis in a variety of animals (Storz, 1961), there was early interest in a possible association of chlamydial infection with reactive arthritis in human beings.

The first report of the isolation of *C. trachomatis* (from the urethra) in a case of Reiter's syndrome appeared in 1962 (Siboulet and Galestin, 1962). Since then there has been a continuous attempt to establish a firm etiological relationship between this organism and SARA and Reiter's syndrome. However, a great number of partly controversial and/or contradictory data have been presented over the years (cf. Kousa, 1982; cf. Keat, 1983). The precise role of *C. trachomatis* in the pathogenesis of SARA and Reiter's syndrome is still unknown, although a large proportion of patients have recently been or still are infected by the organism.

A Scandinavian study (Bengtsson et al., 1983) of 25 cases of complete and incomplete Reiter's syndrome indicated that infections with *C. trachomatis, Yersinia enterocolitica,* and *Campylobacter jejuni,* serotype 3, were associated with the syndrome in 17, 4, and 1 case, respectively.

Chlamydia trachomatis has been recovered from the urethra of a large portion of acute Reiter or SARA cases with signs of genital infection (Siboulet and Galestin, 1962; Kousa et al., 1978; Keat et al., 1980; Martin et al., 1984).

Culture studies (including isolation on embryonated hen's egg) of synovial fluid and synovial biopsies have given contradictory results. Most chlamydial isolates have been made in eggs and very few in tissue cell cultures (Schachter et al., 1966; Dunlop et al., 1968; Gordon et al., 1973).

The geometric mean titer (GMT) of antichlamydial micro-IF antibodies is higher in SARA than in nongonoccocal urethritis (NGU), systemic lupus erythematosus (SLE), rheumatoid arthritis (RA), and ankylosing spondylitis (AS) (Keat et al., 1980). The latter authors also found the GMT to be greater in culture-positive than culture-negative cases. Kousa and colleagues (1978) found 79 (87%) of 91 men with Reiter's syndrome to have micro-IF IgG antibodies to *C. trachomatis* as compared to 24% of controls. The GMT of antichlamydial IgG antibodies was 47.5 (Keat et al., 1980) and 69 (Kousa et al., 1978) in the two study groups, respectively. The GMT was greater in those with a less-than-3-month history of disease than those with disease of longer duration. The GMT was 188 in those with positive chlamydial urethral culture as compared to 15.2 in those with positive culture but no signs of Reiter's syndrome (Keat et al., 1980). In men with ankylosing spondylitis, no humoral antichlamydial antibody response was detected (Keat et al., 1980).

Cellular immunity to *C. trachomatis* has been found in up to 75% of Reiter cases (Schachter and Dawson, 1978). When uncomplicated chlamydial urethritis cases were compared with Reiter's syndrome cases, no difference in cellular immune reactivity was found (Amor et al., 1972).

CLINICAL FINDINGS

Synovitis may develop up to 1 month prior to other symptoms. The Reiter patient may also present concomitantly with genitourinary or bowel symptoms.

The genital chlamydial infection is generally acquired approximately 1 month, often longer, before the start of SARA symptoms. The genital chlamydial infection may have been asymptomatic.

Arthritis symptoms usually emerge from peripheral joints. The knees (in 50% of cases) or the joints in the feet are most often engaged, but the mandibular, shoulder, elbow, wrist, and hand joints can also be involved. In addition, back pain may occur. The initial symptoms are often misinterpreted or ignored. The arthritis symptoms develop over a 2- to 3-week period. Monoarthritis (knee, ankle, or wrist) is rather uncommon (10%). Often several joints are engaged but characteristically not all the small joints in a group are affected, as is common in rheumatic disease.

Many of the mucosal membranes might be engaged and some patients might develop keratoderma blennorrhagicum, circinate balanitis (Fig. 61), or circinate vulvitis. Changes in the mouth and nails might also be seen in patients with SARA (Kousa, 1978).

Ophthalmological symptoms occur in one-third to one-half of all cases of Reiter's syndrome. Acute uveitis is seen comparatively seldom during the period of acute arthritis but may debut later. Conjunctivitis is common but often overlooked. Iritis occurs in approximately 10% of Reiter patients. Keratitis, retinitis, and hemorrhage are other, less common eye manifestations (Kousa, 1978).

Carditis and neurological disorders are other rare manifestations of Reiter's syndrome.

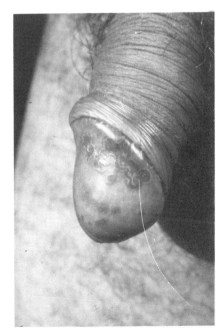

FIGURE 61. Circinate balanitis in a case of Reiter's syndrome infected by *C. trachomatis*. (Courtesy of Department of Dermato-Venereology, University of Lund.)

DIAGNOSIS

Synovial fluid in the acute phase of the disease is turbid and rich in polymorphonuclear leukocytes. Bacterial cultures and microscopy will exclude bacterial arthritis and crystal synovitis. Synovial biopsy is not diagnostic since it shows a nonspecific inflammatory cell infiltration.

Chlamydial cultures should be made from the urethra and, in women, from the cervix as well. Synovial fluid and biopsy specimens might be examined by labeled monoclonal antichlamydial antibodies (Keat et al., 1987) for detection of *C. trachomatis* elementary bodies.

Paired sera may be studied by micro-IF tests for IgM and IgG antichlamydial antibodies. IgM antibodies and/or a significant IgG antibody response to *C. trachomatis* is seen only in a minority of Reiter patients. One may also have stationary high titers of IgG antichlamydial antibodies. Thus serology plays mainly a supportive role in the diagnosis of current infections by *C. trachomatis* in Reiter's syndrome.

THERAPY

Antibiotic therapy is not believed to alter the course of SARA and Reiter's syndrome. If a current chlamydial infection is detected, treatment with tetracyclines should be given.

There is evidence that maybe half of all SARA cases are associated with infection by *C. trachomatis,* although in some cases the infection is not acute or is even healed when the patient presents. However, active treatment against *C. trachomatis* should be instituted in order to eradicate the organism and hinder further spread to other individuals. Sexual partners should also be treated, a fact that is too often forgotten. Anti-inflammatory drugs can be given as therapy against rheumatic symptoms. Antirheumatic drugs have little or no influence on the course of the disease. Uveitis symptoms may require topical steroids.

The majority of SARA cases heal within 2–6 months (Kousa, 1978). In approximately 15% of patients with Reiter's syndrome, any of the clinical symptoms may reappear annually (Csonka, 1960).

Lymphogranuloma Venereum

EPIDEMIOLOGY

Lymphogranuloma venereum (LGV) is caused by *C. trachomatis,* serotypes L_1–L_3. It is mainly a tropical and subtropical disease (Meheus et al., 1983), and therefore is endemic in eastern and western Africa, in India and Southeast Asia, as well as in some areas of South America and the Caribbean. Sporadic cases of LGV—often import cases from the endemic areas—are diagnosed each year in Australia, Europe, and the United States.

Patients with LGV disease carry many of the same stereotypes as persons who acquire STDs. Thus, in Western STD clinics, LGV is most often seen in prostitutes, sailors, soldiers, globe trotters, and other adventurers. In industrialized countries, homosexual men also constitute a risk group for LGV.

In endemic areas LGV is most often seen in the lower socioeconomic strata of the population and in promiscuous groups, e.g., soldiers, prostitutes, and male (immigrant) workers living separately from their families.

A male-to-female ratio of 5 : 1 for LGV has been reported in most countries. It is likely that there is an underdiagnosis of female cases, possibly caused by the lack of easily detectable genital ulcers and bubos (see below) that are apparent in males with LGV.

PATHOLOGY

An infection by L_1–L_3 engages not only superficial epithelial tissues, as is generally the case in infections with other *C. trachomatis* serotypes, but also underlying structures.

The LGV infection causes the initial stage genital ulcer(s) (Fig. 62) and

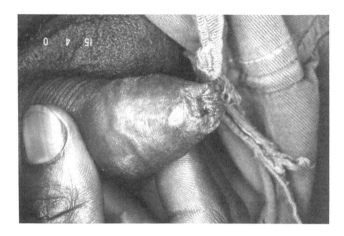

FIGURE 62. Genital ulcer caused by *C. trachomatis* of any serotypes L_1-L_3. (Courtesy of Dr. R. Ballard.)

lymphoadenopathia. In males the inguinal lymph nodes may be engaged (bubos) (Fig. 63). Still later in the course of the disease, involvement of the urogenital and gastrointestinal tracts can be seen, resulting in stricturing processes and lymphoedema (elephantiasis) (Schachter and Dawson, 1976; cf. Schachter and Dawson, 1978). The LGV infection can thus result in irreparable progressive tissue damage. Tissue damage may also occur secondarily to fibrosis and altered lymphatic drainage. The result may be fistulas, edema, ulcerations, strictures, and elephantiasis. The latter complications can be seen in approximately 5% of LGV cases.

Affected tissues generally show a heavy monocytic inflammatory cell response. In LGV cases rectal biopsies may histologically mimic Crohn's disease (Quinn et al., 1981).

CLINICAL FINDINGS

The incubation period of LGV varies from a few days to up to 3 weeks. The first stages of LGV may be clinically overlooked. In the *primary stage* of LGV there is a transient vesicle, papule, or ulceration in the genitalia that is painless. The lesion may mimic that of chancroid.

Men with LGV may also present with painful inguinal or femoral lymphadenopathy without penile ulcerations. In one-third of male LGV cases, the inguinal lymphadenopathy is bilateral. The inguinal lymph nodes are usually painful. Inguinal redness and erythema generally occur. In the San Francisco

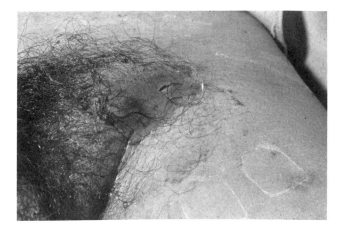

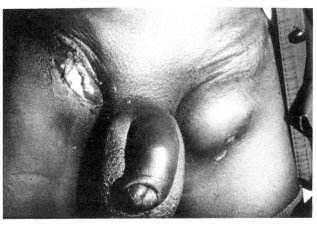

FIGURE 63. Bubo that has suppurated in a case (upper) of lymphogranuloma venereum (courtesy of Dr. D. Oriel) and in another case (lower) where the inguinal gland is suppurated only on the right side. (Courtesy of Dr. R. Ballard.)

area, LGV in homosexual men has manifested itself as proctitis rather than as the classical LGV disease (Quinn et al., 1981).

The ulcerative lesions in women are often overlooked. In women with vaginal lesions, the iliac rather than the inguinal lymph nodes become involved.

After 2–16 weeks, a *secondary stage* follows. In the secondary stage constitutional symptoms may occur, such as fever, chills, headache, myalgias, arthralgias, and anorexia. During this stage there might be hepatitis, arthritis, meningitis, and meningoencephalitis. However, none of these manifestations is common. Fistulas involving the rectum and the bladder may also occur in the secondary stage.

Reactive arthritis and Reiter's syndrome has been seen in some LGV cases (cf. Keat et al., 1983). Follicular conjunctivitis is an uncommon manifestation of LGV. In this type of conjunctivitis, lymphadenitis of the posterior auricular and maxillary lymph nodes is often seen. Autoinoculation of the eye by infected genital secretion is thought to be the mode of transmission. *Chlamydia trachomatis*, LGV serotypes, may cause Parinaud's oculoglandular syndrome with marginal corneal perforation (Burrs et al., 1988).

Chlamydia trachomatis, serotype L_2, caused pneumonia in a man preparing antigen for serological studies. The infection was thought to have been spread by aerosol formation. Using complement fixation tests, a seroconversion was seen with maximum titer of >4000. The patient became febrile after several weeks. X ray demonstrated pneumonia, which was cleared by treatment; X ray also showed pulmonary cancer, from which the patient later died (Cevenini, personal communication). Other cases of laboratory infection by L_2 resulting in pneumonia have been described (Paran et al., 1986).

Penoscrotal elephantiasis can appear a year after infection, but it can also occur after one or two decades. It can affect the preputium or the scrotum. In a few cases the scrotum may reach a monstrous size, pictures of which are often shown in pathology textbooks. A misdiagnosis of LGV is often made in cases of elephantiasis since other conditions, e.g., filariasis, can result in the same deformations.

DIAGNOSIS

The diagnosis of LGV in the acute phase can be based on both isolation studies and serological tests. Sampling for culture of *C. trachomatis*, serotypes L_1–L_3, should be made from pus from lymph nodes, from the urethra, the cervix, and from genital lesions. Chlamydial urethritis caused by serotypes D–K is not uncommon in men with LGV which should be remembered in the culture diagnosis of LGV. Thus strains urethrally isolated from assumed cases of LGV must be serotyped to obtain an (accurate) etiological diagnosis. In chronic LGV cases, isolation studies are less rewarding.

The methods for sampling, transporting samples, and culturing are the same as those indicated for the diagnosis of *C. trachomatis*, serotypes D–K (cf. Chapter 6).

The complement fixation test can generally be used to diagnose lymphogranuloma venereum. It must be noted that the L_1–L_3 antigens cross-react in this test with antibodies formed against all serotypes of *C. trachomatis*, *C. psittaci*, and TWAR chlamydiae.

The microimmunofluorescence (micro-IF) test is also useful for the diagnosis of LGV (Wang and Grayston, 1970). The risk of misinterpretations due to cross-reactions must be kept in mind when this test is used, particularly when three pools of antigen (A–C, D–K, and L_1–L_3) are employed (Treharne et al., 1977). Duncan and co-workers (1986) found that micro-IF IgG antichlamydial antibody titers of 256 were highly suggestive of lymphogranuloma venereum in South African mine workers with genital lesions. However, half of their LGV cases had titers of <256.

The so-called Frei skin test (Fig. 21) was recommended earlier as a diagnostic test for LGV. The test becomes positive 2 to 8 weeks after infection and is positive in the vast majority of LGV cases. The antigen is no longer commercially available (since the 1970s). In the test, an intradermal injection of heat-sterilized pus from unruptured bubos and later yolk sac antigen from embryonated eggs (also used in complement tests for detection of antibodies to *C. trachomatis*) was given. Frei's test was thought to demonstrate a delayed hypersensitivity reaction to the infectious agent. The cell-mediated immune response is induced by a genus-specific *C. trachomatis* antigen and can thus be caused by all serotypes of this species as well as by various strains of *C. psittaci*. Therefore it is understandable that Frei test results are often nonspecific.

THERAPY

The standard treatment of lymphogranuloma venereum is a course of tetracycline for at least 2 weeks, e.g., tetracycline hydrochloride 500 mg orally four times a day, doxycycline 100 mg orally twice a day, or lymecycline 250 mg orally also twice daily.

Trimethoprim-sulfamethoxazole (80 mg/40 mg) twice daily for 2 weeks has also been used but today would be considered a second alternative because of the potential side-effects of the sulfa component. One advantage of using sulfonamides to treat LGV is that such treatment will not mask a concomitantly acquired syphilis.

Among other drugs tested in the treatment of LGV, rifampicin has been reported effective (Menke et al., 1979). Chloramphenicol has a poor effect, like penicillin and streptomycin (Coutts, 1950). Antibiotic therapy is often effective in healing genital ulcers and stopping systemic symptoms during the primary and secondary stages of LGV. However, relapses after treatment often occur. Therefore repeated courses of antibiotics are sometimes needed. After the acute stage, the infection can enter a chronic phase. Late complications may need surgical correction, which should be preceded by antibiotic treatment.

Fluctuating bubos should be aspirated under antibiotic cover in order to prevent spontaneous drainage. The bubos may resolve slowly. Incision and drainage of the abscesses might be necessary.

Sexual contacts of LGV cases should be identified and treated. Also sexual contacts lacking clinical evidence of LGV should be given prophylactic treatment.

Neonatal Infections

INTRODUCTION

Currently, *C. trachomatis* is a major cause of perinatally acquired infections. Infants born to women with genital chlamydial infection have a high risk, i.e., 30–50%, of contracting *C. trachomatis* infection during vaginal delivery (Chandler et al., 1977; Schachter et al., 1979b; Alexander et al., 1982; Beem and Saxon, 1982; Grossman et al., 1988; Alexander and Harrison, 1983) (Table 30). The risk figures from Europe (Mårdh et al., 1980b; Persson et al., 1983; Persson, 1986) are lower than those from the United States. For example, Persson (1986) reported an attack rate of 17% in Swedish children born to *Chlamydia*-infected mothers.

In a most comprehensive study on perinatal chlamydial infections, Schachter and co-workers (1986) found 4–7% of 5531 pregnant women to be cervically culture-positive for *C. trachomatis*. Of the newborn infants in this population, 2.8% had serological evidence of perinatal chlamydial infection and 1.4% developed either conjunctivitis or pneumonia. Of the infants born to *Chlamydia*-infected mothers, 131 were followed prospectively. Culture-positive conjunctivitis was diagnosed in 18% and chlamydial pneumonia in 16%. Rectal and vaginal colonization occurred in 14% of the infants. Of the infants, 79 (60%) had serological evidence of chlamydial infection, whereas only 36% were culture-positive. Only 56 cases had clinical signs of infection. Thus in 18% there was serological evidence of infection alone.

Serological studies usually have limited diagnostic value during the first months of life due to newborn's poorly developed immune system. Moreover, serum IgG antibodies are mainly of maternal origin. Serum IgM antibodies, to the contrary, represent the infant's own seroresponse. However, a local anti-chlamydial antibody response (tear fluid IgA) can be seen in some infants with chlamydial conjunctivitis. In chlamydial pneumonia, which usually develops

TABLE 30. Transmission of *C. trachomatis* to Infants Born to Infected Mothers

Author	Number of infants followed	Number of infants with		Number of infants with		
		Culture + (%)	Serology + (%)	Conjunctivitis	Pneumonia	Other[a]
Chandler et al., 1977	18	3 (17)	12 (67)	3 (8)[b]	ND[c]	ND
Frommel et al., 1979	18	8 (44)	11 (61)	8	2	3 (rectum)
Hammerschlag et al., 1979	6	4 (67)	ND	2	1	ND
Schachter et al., 1979b	20	10 (50)	14 (70)	7	4	ND
Hammerschlag et al., 1980a	36 + 24[d]	ND	ND	12 + 0	3 + 1	ND
Mårdh et al., 1980b	23	5 (22)	ND	5	ND	ND
Heggie et al., 1981	95	27 (28)	ND	20	3	ND
Schachter et al., 1986b	131	47 (36)	79 (60)	23	21	18 (rectum/vagina)

[a]Other infection or colonization detected.
[b]Three infants had *C. trachomatis* isolated from the eye, although eight had clinical conjunctivitis.
[c]ND, not determined, or data not available.
[d]Of the exposed infants, 36 received ocular silver nitrate and 24 ocular erythromycin prophylaxis.

later than conjunctivitis—usually not before the age of 6 weeks—an anti-chlamydial antibody response can usually be demonstrated and an (often high) antichlamydial IgM antibody titer is pathognomonic.

Infants delivered by caesarean section have also been reported to have acquired *C. trachomatis* perinatal infections. However, Givner et al. (1981) considered this to be an uncommon event. On the other hand, Barry and co-workers (1986) found four children among 38 chlamydial neonatal conjunctivitis cases to have been delivered by caesarean section. The mode of transmission of infection to such infants has not been firmly established.

A risk of transmission of *C. trachomatis* to the mother by artificial insemination has been documented (Nagel et al., 1986), resulting in the possibility that a sperm donor may be the source of infection in a newborn.

A *Chlamydia*-infected baby is a marker of infected parents. The parents should be examined and treated adequately in order to hinder spread to new partners or to hinder the development of complications in the parents themselves. Reinfection of the baby could also occur if the parents remain carriers.

CONJUNCTIVITIS

Epidemiology

Conjunctival chlamydial infection, or inclusion conjunctivitis, is generally the earliest occurring marker of neonatal chlamydial infection. The conjunctivitis is usually observed between the fifth and fourteenth day of life, i.e., several days later than gonococcal ophthalmia, and often not until mother and baby have left the hospital after delivery.

In an English series of neonatal chlamydial conjunctivitis cases, the mean age at presentation was 12 days for ambulatory clinic patients but only 4 days for hospitalized patients (Barry et al., 1986). Of consecutive neonatal ophthalmia cases, 38% were culture-positive for *C. trachomatis*. The latter authors found no difference in gestation length, mode of vaginal delivery, sex, maternal age, or race between neonates with positive and negative eye cultures for *C. trachomatis*.

Neonatal *C. trachomatis* and *N. gonorrhoeae* may be demonstrated in the same eye, an event that seems uncommon in Western countries (Barry et al., 1986) but fairly common in certain developing countries.

Clinical Findings

The symptoms of neonatal conjunctivitis vary in severity. Subclinical cases seem to occur frequently. Symptomatic cases are characterized by swelling of the

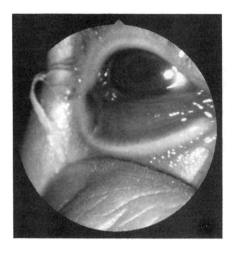

FIGURE 64. The conjunctiva of a new-born child with mild chlamydial ophthalmia neonatorum. A color version of this figure appears following p. xvi. (Courtesy of Dr. L. Salminen.)

eyelids, erythematous conjunctivae (Fig. 64), and mucopurulent discharge (Fig. 65). On rare occasions pseudomembrane formation and papillary hypertrophy may also be present (Allen, 1944; Freedman et al., 1966). The infection is often bilateral when the patient presents, having started on one side and spreading within a week.

Sandström (1987) used a scoring system whereby purulent discharge, edema and erythema of the lids, and edema and erythema of the palpebral conjunctivae were studied in cases of assumed chlamydial conjunctivitis.

Chlamydial infant conjunctivitis sometimes spreads from infected neonates to their siblings, parents, grandparents, and medical personnel (Lindner, 1911; Thygeson and Stone, 1942; Jones, 1964; Rees et al., 1977b).

Diagnosis

To establish the diagnosis of neonatal chlamydial conjunctivitis, a sample from the inferior palpebral conjunctival mucosa should be collected for culture and for other diagnostic tests (see below) (Table 31). Conjunctival secretion can also be stained with labeled monoclonal antichlamydial antibodies (Bell et al., 1984). Culture is the most sensitive diagnostic method in neonatal conjunctivitis. The sensitivity of other diagnostic methods relative to culture as the "golden standard" have varied by up to 100%. The quality of the culture procedure influences how favorably other methods turn out in comparative studies. The poorer the quality of the culture technique, the better will appear the sensitivity of the alternative method. Reliable clinical predictors of neonatal chlamydial conjunctivitis do not exist.

Scrapings from the conjunctivae can be collected for detection of intra-cytoplasmic inclusions in Giemsa-stained smears. In one series, such staining for

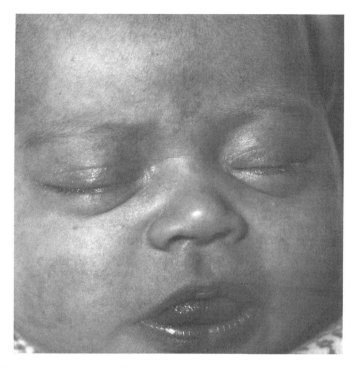

FIGURE 65. A newborn child with chlamydial conjunctivitic. (Courtesy of Dr. B. Møller.)

the demonstration of chlamydial inclusions in neonatal chlamydial conjunctivitis had a sensitivity of 42%, a specificity of 98%, a predictive value of a positive test (PVP) of 95%, and a predictive value of a negative test (PVN) of 69%, respectively (Rapoza et al., 1986).

Direct-specimen antigen detection test sensitivities of 75–100% have been

TABLE 31. Diagnosis of *C. trachomatis* Infections in Infants[a]

Manifestation	Clinical criteria	Laboratory criteria	
		Presumptive	Diagnostic
Conjunctivitis	Watery to purulent discharge, swollen lids usually unilateral	—	Positive culture or direct-antigen test (C)
Pneumonitis	Lower respiratory tract infection of variable severity, no fever, cough, tachypnea	Elevated CRP, bilateral interstitial infiltrates in chest X ray, eosinophilia	Positive culture or direct-antigen test (NP) High-titer IgM antibody to *C.t.*

[a]*C.t.*, *C. trachomatis;* C, conjunctiva; NP, nasopharynx.

reported in the diagnosis of neonatal chlamydial conjunctivitis. Mårdh and co-workers (1987) recently reported that culture is more favorable than both ELISA and IF, with the latter two showing sensitivity of only 74% ± 14.4 as compared to culture.

Rapoza and co-workers (1986) found the predictive values for positive and negative IF test results to be 94 and 100%, respectively. Hammerschlag and associates (1985) found the EIA (Abbott) test to have a sensitivity of 93% and a specificity of 98%. The predictive values for positive and negative EIA tests were 97.6% and 95%, respectively.

Prophylaxis

In 1980, the American Academy of Pediatrics and the CDC recommended that Credé prophylaxis could be replaced with ophthalmic ointments or solutions containing either 1% tetracycline or 0.5% erythromycin for the prevention of neonatal ophthalmia (CDC, 1985). Both drugs are provided in tubes containing 3.5 g ointment (Committee, 1980). One advantage of using antimicrobial ointment prophylaxis is that the chemical conjunctivitis that often results from the installation of silver nitrate can be avoided.

In a series of 46 neonatal chlamydial conjunctivitis cases, 19% had clinical and laboratory evidence of persistent chlamydial conjunctivitis despite the fact that erythromycin ointment had been applied after delivery (Rapoza et al., 1986). Other investigators reported failures in 5% to 14% of infants studied (Heggie et al., 1986; Rapoza et al., 1986). These and similar negative results have brought into question the value of prophylactic antibiotic therapy.

Although Credé prophylaxis has not been considered effective against chlamydial conjunctivitis, experimental infections and therapeutic trials in animals have contradicted this view (Sandström, 1987). The Credé prophylaxis probably prevents certain cases of bacterial conjunctivitis, e.g., infections by such respiratory tract pathogens as *Haemophilus influenzae* and pneumococci.

Colostrum applied locally has been indicated to reduce markedly the incidence of "sticky eyes" (Singh et al., 1982). Whether it also prevents neonatal *C. trachomatis* eye infections remains to be established. One objection to this approach has to do with the possibility of infected breast milk transmitting other agents to the infant's eyes, particularly when the colostrum has been donated by another mother.

Treatment

Systemic treatment with erythromycin, which is more effective than local therapy in the treatment of chlamydial conjunctivitis (cf. Patamasucon et al., 1982), should always be given since many of the infected infants also have nasopharyngeal chlamydiae. Treatment is 25 mg/kg twice daily for 2 weeks (Sandström, 1987). Lower doses have been found unsatisfactory. The absorption of erythromycin ethylsuccinate is increased when administered with milk; however, this is not the case for some other erythromycin analogs.

Systemic treatment with erythromycin can also fail (Barry et al., 1985), and therefore follow-up of treated neonatal chlamydial conjunctivitis cases is recommended. Topical sulfacetamide has proved noneffective in eradicating chlamydial conjunctivitis in infants (Heggie et al., 1985).

We have yet to see whether the markedly tetracycline-resistant gonococcal strains that have spread rapidly around the world during the last years, and *C. trachomatis* strains with reduced susceptibility to erythromycin will negatively influence the efficiency of antibiotic prophylaxis and treatment of neonatal ophthalmia.

Good lid hygiene is recommended for neonates with chlamydial conjunctivitis.

Sequelae

Left untreated, neonatal conjunctivitis is usually self-limiting (Allen, 1944), although permanent sequelae can occur. In a few cases, corneal pannus formation (neovascularization), conjunctival scarring, and subsequent visual impairment were reported (Mordhorst and Dawson, 1971; Chandler et al., 1977).

PNEUMONIA

Epidemiology

Most infants with chlamydial conjunctivitis also harbor the agent nasopharyngeally, where it can spread to the lower respiratory tract and cause pneumonitis (Schachter et al., 1975; Beem and Saxon, 1977; Hammerschlag et al., 1980a; Attenburrow and Baker, 1985) (Table 32).

In prospective U.S. studies, *C. trachomatis* accounted for 15–73% of afebrile pneumonia in early infancy (Beem and Saxon, 1977; Harrison et al., 1978; cf. Rettig, 1986a). Lower prevalence figures have been reported from Europe. Differences as to socioeconomic backgrounds have been proposed to explain the difference in the populations observed.

The pneumonitis generally begins at the age of 2–12 weeks. In a series of 21 cases of chlamydial pneumonia, the average age at onset was 62 + 19 days, with a range of 39–111 days (Schachter et al., 1986b).

TABLE 32. Respiratory Infections Due to *Chlamydia*

Factor	Infant pneumonitis	Adult respiratory infections due to *C. trachomatis*	Psittacosis pneumonia	Respiratory infections due to TWAR chlamydiae
Causative agent	*C. trachomatis*	*C. trachomatis*	*C. psittaci*	*C. sp. novum* (TWAR strains)
Epidemiology	Common cause of perinatal respiratory infections	Rarely found, diagnosis difficult to establish	Infrequent	Very common
Target population	Infants exposed to *C.t.* during birth	Immunocompromised	All ages, pet shop clientele, farmers	Military recruits, young adults, but probably all ages
Clinical characteristics	Gradual onset, no fever, cough, tachypnea	?	Pneumonia of variable severity, extrapulmonary manifestations occur	Respiratory infections of variable severity, usually mild pneumonia, pharyngitis
Diagnosis	Isolation of *C.t* or demonstration of *C.t.*-specific antigen in nasopharynx, IgM-antibodies in *C.t.*-specific test	Isolation of *C.t.* or demonstration of *C.t.*-specific antigen in lower respiratory tract	Serology: titer rise or high titer in CF test	Serology: IgG titer rise or IgM present in TWAR-specific micro-IF test
Therapy	Erythromycin 50 mg/kg per day for 21 days	Tetracycline 2 g/day for 7–10 days	Tetracycline 2 g/day for 7–10 days	Tetracycline 2 g/day for 7–10 days, or 1 g/day for 21 days, erythromycin (?)
Sequelae	Chronic obstructive lung disease, asthma?	?	?	?

Clinical Findings

Clinically, chlamydial infant pneumonitis is characterized by a mild pertussis-like cough (Beem and Saxon, 1977; Harrison et al., 1978; Tipple et al., 1979; Hallberg et al., 1979; Schaad and Rossi, 1982). The diseased infants are tachypneic and afebrile. They may have rhinitis. Cyanosis, vomiting, malaise, and poor weight gain may occur. Often the cough and the tachypnea are preceded by 1 to 2 weeks of rhinitis. The cough differs from that of pertussis in that it does not build up to a crescendo and does not cause emesis or a whoop. The chlamydial pneumonia is seldom clinically severe. On auscultation, near-normal breath sounds can often be heard. About 50% of chlamydial pneumonic infants have either active conjunctivitis or a history of chlamydial eye infection (Beem and Saxon, 1977).

Symptoms increase gradually over several weeks. Untreated children usually improve after approximately 1½ months.

Recently, Brayden and co-workers (1987) found that 6 of 23 infants with chlamydial pneumonia presented with apneic episodes. Zouari and co-workers (1986) also reported such a case. Infants with episodes of apnea should therefore be studied for the possible occurrence of chlamydial pneumonia.

It is likely that many chlamydial infant pneumonia cases remain undiagnosed.

Diagnosis

Chest X ray usually shows bilateral, diffuse, and symmetrical interstitial infiltrates, scattered areas of atelectasis, and hyperexpansion of the lungs (Tipple et al., 1979; Hallberg et al., 1979; Radkowski et al., 1981) (Fig. 66). Pleural effusion is rare. Histological examination of lung biopsies has shown pleural congestion as well as alveolar and bronchiolar consolidation with a mononuclear exudate containing some eosinophils. There have been no interstitial infiltrates.

As already mentioned, chlamydial conjunctivitis occurs in half of all cases of neonatal chlamydial pneumonitis. *Chlamydia trachomatis* can also be demonstrated nasopharyngeally in many such patients (Bell et al., 1984) (Table 30).

Chlamydia trachomatis can be isolated from lung biopsies in chlamydial pneumonitis (Frommell et al., 1977). Staining of respiratory tract secretion using labeled monoclonal antibodies has also been used in the diagnosis of infant chlamydial pneumonia. Nasopharyngeal colonization can, however, occur without evidence of developing pneumonitis (Hammerschlag et al., 1979). As indicated by isolation studies, Mårdh et al. (1987) found approximately 80% of neonates with conjunctivitis positive for *C. trachomatis* in eye samples to also have chlamydiae in the nasopharynx. Direct-specimen antigen detection tests were less sensitive than culture: IF was positive in only three-fourths of culture-

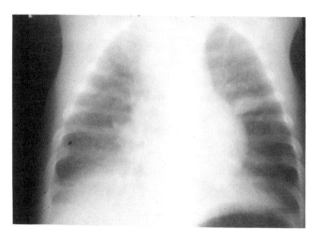

FIGURE 66. A chest X ray of an infant suffering from chlamydial pneumonitis showing bilateral interstitial pulmonary infiltrates. (Courtesy of Department of Pediatrics, Helsinki University.)

positive cases. ELISA was only somewhat more sensitive than IF. None of the children developed pneumonia, although the infection had in some cases been going on for several weeks before investigation and institution of antimicrobial chemotherapy.

Serology may be a useful diagnostic tool in perinatal chlamydial infections. According to Schachter and co-workers (1982b), the presence of antichlamydial IgM antibodies in systemic infant infections is a rule. They proposed that a high IgM titer ($\geqslant$64) in the micro-IF test is a marker of chlamydial pneumonia. In one study (Schachter et al., 1986b), all infected infants had marked elevated levels of serum IgM and IgG antichlamydial antibodies. The IgM titers ranged from 32 to 4.096 (mean titer 512). Only half of the infants studied (12 cases) were culture-positive when the condition was diagnosed. *Chlamydia trachomatis*-specific IgM antibodies can also be detected by an EIA with major outer membrane protein (MOMP) of *C. trachomatis* as antigen (Puolakkainen et al., 1984). Spurious IgM antibodies in a micro-IF test might also occur, although the titers of such antibodies are usually <64 (Person and Bröms, 1986).

Antichlamydial IgG antibodies are also nearly always present in high titers in chlamydial infant pneumonia (Schachter et al., 1982b), but the diagnostic value of their demonstration is questionable as they are partially of maternal origin.

In neonatal chlamydial pneumonia, the total white blood cell count is usually within the normal range. Fifty percent to 65% of infected infants have moderate eosinophilia. The total serum IgM level is generally elevated, and the total level of IgG might also be slightly elevated (cf. Rettig, 1986a).

Treatment

Erythromycin treatment should be given as 25 mg/kg twice daily for at least 3 weeks. In infants with chlamydial pneumonia given erythromycin or sulfonamides, clinical improvement occurred within 7 days as compared with 24–61 days in untreated cases (Beem et al., 1979).

Certain studies (Schachter et al., 1986a) indicate that surveillance of *C. trachomatis* in late pregnancy and treatment of infected mothers can effectively hinder vertical transmission to the offspring. Of 18 culture-positive women who had been given treatment during the 36th gestational week, 16 returned with their children 4 to 8 weeks postdelivery with no signs of chlamydial infection. All the children were culture-negative at follow-up.

Sequelae

Chronic chlamydial pneumonia or recurring infection has not yet been proved to occur. However, some studies have reported obstructive respiratory tract problems to occur later in life more often in neonatal *Chlamydia*-pneumonia cases than in controls (Harrison et al., 1982; Schaefer et al., 1985). This was the case at follow-up at 4 years of age (Harrison et al., 1982).

Pulmonary status was evaluated in 18 children 7–8 years after chlamydial pneumonia had been diagnosed in their infancy (Weiss et al., 1986). Significant limitations of expiratory air flow were found (FEV_1, FEV_1/FVC, PEF, and FEF). There were also signs of abnormally elevated volumes of trapped air (altered functional residual capacity and residual volume/total lung capacity ratio). The obstructive patterns were responsive to inhalation of isoproterenol. A significantly greater number of patients had bronchial asthma than did age-matched controls (Beem et al., 1986).

VARIOUS OTHER NEONATAL INFECTIONS

Multiple sites are often colonized in newborns infected by *C. trachomatis.* Schachter and co-workers (1979c, 1986b) found 47 (36%) of 131 infants to be culture-positive from any of the following sites: the eyes, the nasopharynx, the rectum, the vagina. From these sites, 17.5, 11.5, 13.5, and 13.9% (only 36 were cultured from the vagina) of the infants were positive, respectively. The 17 rectal culture-positive cases were believed to have subclinical gastrointestinal tract infection (enteritis) by chlamydiae. In several infants, the rectum was the only culture-positive site. The rectal shedding often had a late onset. The vaginal colonization did not produce any clinical disease.

Bell (1985) described a chlamydial condition in infancy characterized by chancrous nasal congestion without rhinorrhea lasting for weeks or months.

Pus can be found in the nasopharynx. Such infants rarely develop chlamydial pneumonia.

Otitis media has been diagnosed in infants infected with *C. trachomatis* (Tipple et al., 1979), but the possible pathogenic role of the organism in this condition is still controversial (Hammerschlag et al., 1980b; Chang et al., 1982). Tipple and co-workers (1979) noted that half of the infants with chlamydial pneumonia had abnormal tympanic membranes.

An etiological role of *C. trachomatis* in infant gastroenteritis has been considered (Schaefer et al., 1985), but no proof that the agent is capable of producing clinical gastroenteritis has been brought forward (cf. Rettig, 1986). Allergy to bovine milk is considered a differential diagnosis in chlamydial gastroenteritis.

Samples for the diagnosis of neonatal chlamydial infection should be collected from the nasopharynx and from the eyes if there are clinical signs of conjunctivitis. The oropharynx should also be sampled in assumed cases of infant chlamydial infection. Vaginal or rectal swabs might also be useful in diagnosing such infections.

Infections in Childhood

SEROEPIDEMIOLOGY

As suggested by seroepidemiological studies, chlamydial infections also occur during childhood. Antibodies to *C. trachomatis* can be detected in sera from healthy children (Black et al., 1981; Grayston et al., 1982; San Joaquin et al., 1982; Gray et al., 1986) (Fig. 67). In some studies, antichlamydial antibodies were found more often in girls than boys, whereas in other series such antibodies were found equally often in both sexes. Frequently, after the disappearance of maternal antibodies, a slow age-related increase in the seropositivity rate, i.e., up to 7–12%, throughout childhood up to puberty has been found Gray and co-workers (1986) found antibodies in boys to occur most often at the age of 7–8 years, whereas in girls the peak incidence occurred at puberty. The prevalence of antibody to *C. trachomatis* was similar in healthy children and children with respiratory complaints.

Currently, there is no explanation for the occurrence and distribution of antichlamydial antibodies in children. The prevalence of antibody varies with the method of analysis and the criteria for antibody positivity (Fig. 67). Chlamydial infection following sexual abuse (Bump et al., 1985; Hammerschlag et al., 1984; Fuster and Neinstein, 1987) has been suggested to explain only a few seropositive cases (Chapter 28).

The presence of infectious agents other than chlamydiae that cause an unspecific polyclonal B-lymphocyte stimulation resulting in the formation of antibodies that react with chlamydial antigen might explain the occurrence of positive chlamydial serology in some children (Banck and Forsgren, 1978; Persson, 1986; Gray et al., 1986). Many respiratory tract pathogens are mitogenic for B lymphocytes.

Antichlamydial IgM antibodies found to react with *C. trachomatis* in hospitalized children with lower respiratory tract infections were thought to be spu-

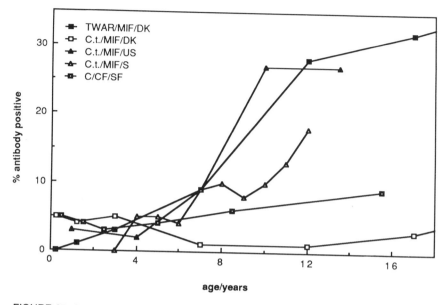

FIGURE 67. Antibodies to *Chlamydia* in children. Abbreviations: TWAR, TWAR strains of *Chlamydia*; MIF, micro-immunofluorescence test; DK, Denmark; C.t., *C. trachomatis*; US, United States; S, Sweden; C, *Chlamydia;* CF, complement fixation; SF, Finland.

rious, and their formation was considered to represent a nonspecific B-lymphocyte stimulation. *Chlamydia trachomatis* was not isolated from any of 254 children studied (Persson and Bröms, 1986).

One of the most plausible explanations of the serum antibody activity to *C. trachomatis* found in many children is the existence of antibodies against TWAR chlamydiae that cross-react with the former agent in genus-specific tests. TWAR antibodies occur in some children. This means that much of the data from previous seroepidemiological studies of *C. trachomatis* in children (and other age groups) must be reevaluated. However, careful interpretation of micro-IF tests allows distinction of antibodies to *C. trachomatis, C. psittaci,* and TWAR chlamydiae. Antichlamydial serum antibodies are only infrequently found in complement fixation tests because of the insensitivity of the test and the poor immunogenicity of lipopolysaccharides during childhood (Puolakkainen et al., 1984; Puolakkainen, 1987).

CLINICAL FINDINGS

Although the role of *C. trachomatis* in neonatal pneumonia is well documented (Beem and Saxon, 1977), reports concerning *C.trachomatis* pneumonia in childhood are based on serological studies only (Komaroff et al., 1981) and the data are not convincing for an etiological relationship. Pharyngeal colonization occurs in infants without clinical signs of pneumonia (Schachter et al., 1979b; Hammerschlag et al., 1980a). *Chlamydia trachomatis* has also been demonstrated in the pharynx of a child with atypical croup (Miller et al., 1982) and in children with trachoma (Malaty et al., 1981). However, according to more recent studies, *C. trachomatis* appears not to be an important cause of upper respiratory infections in children aged 6 months to 15 years (San Joaquin and Rettig, 1987), including acute pharyngitis in children and young adults (aged 2 to 24 years) with fever, pharyngeal infection, headache, and cervical lymphadenitis (Gerber et al., 1987). Otitis media sometimes accompanies chlamydial pneumonia in infants (Tipple et al., 1979). In subsequent studies, attempts to isolate *C. trachomatis* from middle ear fluid of older children undergoing tympanocentesis or myringotomy were unsuccessful (cf. Myhre and Mårdh, 1982a). Hammerschlag and co-workers (1980a) could not isolate the organism in any of 68 children with chronic effusion. Chang and associates (1982), however, reported the recovery of *C. trachomatis* from the middle ear fluid of two of 12 children with acute otitis media, and from one of 14 children with persistent otitis media with effusion. *Chlamydia trachomatis* might thus occasionally be associated with otitis media in children older than 6 months, but its possible role in this and other respiratory tract infections requires further studies.

Chlamydial eye infections offer another explanation for the observed antichlamydial antibody prevalence in children. Trachoma is a rarity in western Europe and the United States. Purulent conjunctivitis in children is often caused by *S. aureus, Streptococcus pneumoniae,* or *H. influenzae* (Baum, 1978), and only infrequently by *C. trachomatis.* Persistence of *C. trachomatis* in the eye for years after perinatal transmission seems possible. Recently, a persistent chlamydial eye infection, most probably originating from a neonatally acquired infection, was described in a 6-year-old girl (Stenberg and Mårdh, 1986). Persistence of chlamydiae at other sites is also a possibility. Intrafamiliar nonsexual transfer might also occur. However, it is not yet known how frequently such chlamydial spreads take place.

C. trachomatis has been believed to be the etiological agent in a case of vaginitis in a prepubertal girl (Bump, 1985).

27

Chlamydial Infections in Adolescence

EPIDEMIOLOGY

The influence of youth on the epidemiology, pathophysiology, and manifestations of STDs has only recently been appreciated. Although the clinical manifestations of STDs are essentially the same in adolescents and adults, the maturing female reproductive system is often more susceptible to STD organisms than during later life. In some instances chlamydial infections in adolescents lead to more severe manifestations as well as to more severe complications and late sequelae. For instance, the immature metaplastic epithelial cells in the squamocolumnar junction of the cervix are less well differentiated than cells from other areas of the cervix. Therefore adolescent women have increased susceptibility to selected STD organisms and increased vulnerability to the action of oncogenic agents (Briggs and Paavonen, 1984). Cervical ectopy with endocervical columnar cells extending well out on the ectocervix may increase this susceptibility to *C. trachomatis*.

Sexually active adolescents constitute a risk group for chlamydial and gonococcal infections. Studies from Sweden and the United States revealed an unexpectedly high prevalence of genital *C. trachomatis* infections in adolescent males and females, i.e., in up to 35–37% (Shafer et al., 1982, 1984; Weström et al., 1982; Bell et al., 1984; Fraser et al., 1983, 1984; Chacko and Lovchik, 1984; Golden et al., 1984; Hardy et al., 1984). Asymptomatic disease, many sexual partners, and oral contraceptive use are evidently factors contributing to the high prevalence of genital chlamydial infection in adolescents.

Mulcahy and Lacey (1987) screened 210 adolescent girls in England for several STDs. The prevalence figures for *N. gonorrhoeae*, *C. trachomatis*, and *T. vaginalis* were 14, 16, and 16%, respectively. A surprisingly high prevalence of *C. trachomatis* infections was found in an Alaskan Eskimo population (39% of teenagers and 47% among pregnant teens) (Toomey et al., 1987). Of particular concern are the reports of an extremely high prevalence of *C. trachomatis* among young women seen in antenatal clinics (Brunham et al., 1984; Martin et al., 1986; Ismail et al., 1985; Nugent et al., 1986; Toomey et al., 1987).

Chlamydial infections occurring in pregnancy increase the risk of adverse pregnancy outcome, including perinatal and puerperal infections (see Chapter 18). Pelvic inflammatory disease (PID) is the most common serious complication of genital chlamydial infection in adolescents. The incidence of PID in sexually active 15-year-old women is approximately 10 times higher than in 24-year-old women (Weström, 1980). In the United States, the incidence of hospitalization for PID was highest in very young women (Bell and Hein, 1984). As a result of the increase in sexual activity and sexually transmitted diseases, PID has become an important cause of morbidity in the adolescent female population (Shafer et al., 1982; Bell, 1983; Bell and Hein, 1984; Toomey et al., 1987; Mulcahy and Lacey, 1987).

DIAGNOSIS

For the diagnosis of symptomatic and asymptomatic chlamydial infections in sexually active adolescent males and females, the same diagnostic procedures as described for adults should be undertaken. Recently, a urine leukocyte esterase dipstick test was introduced and evaluated for the detection of pyuria and for the screening of venereal diseases in adolescent males (Shafer et al., 1987). It was found to be a rather efficient, noninvasive, painless screening method for asymptomatic urethral infection due to *C. trachomatis* and *N. gonorrhoeae*.

Female adolescents at risk (i.e., sexually active girls, including those who are asymptomatic) should be screened for sexually transmitted diseases when they are seen in family-planning clinics for contraceptive counseling. Asymptomatic *Chlamydia*-infected males are more difficult to reach.

PROPHYLAXIS

Asymptomatic infection is an effective reservoir for STDs among adolescents. To preserve the fertility of teenagers, diagnosis and adequate treatment of genital chlamydial infections are important prophylactic measures. Treatment should be given as recommended for adults with genital chlamydial infection. In college girls, *C. trachomatis* can persist for years in the genital tract after an initially positive culture (McCormack et al., 1979). Spontaneous cure of the infection is less common, at least during the initial months.

The general medical health care of sexually active adolescents should include screening for *C. trachomatis*. Cost–benefit analyses have convincingly shown that screening of young women not only in STD clinics but also in adolescent clinics, antenatal clinics, and family-planning clinics is cost-effective. The cost-effectiveness increases rapidly if the prevalence of *C. trachomatis* is higher than 5% (Schachter et al., 1986a).

In the context discussed, it should be remembered that early sexual intercourse in girls imports a great risk of infectious complications. A Swedish study showed that a girl who is sexually active at the age of 15 has a $1:4$ risk of acquiring an acute (most commonly chlamydial) salpingitits before age 16.

It is important to discuss safe-sex practices and contraceptive use with adolescent boys and girls. The impact of contraceptives on the pathogenesis of genital chlamydial infection should be stressed (see also Chapter 21).

Sexual Abuse of Children

Child abuse is heavily underreported. Recommendations for management of children with suspected abuse have been given by the CDC (see Appendix) (Kramer and Jason, 1982).

Chlamydia trachomatis can be transmitted to children via sexual abuse (Hammerschlag et al., 1984; Ingram et al., 1984). Chlamydial infection in abused children can occur without vaginal intercourse. However, chlamydial infection was found more frequently in children with a history of rectal and vaginal penetration than in otherwise sexually abused children (Fuster and Neinstein, 1987).

The finding of *C. trachomatis* in a child's rectum or vagina does not necessarily indicate sexual abuse, but rather can represent a persistence of chlamydial organisms in this area following perinatal colonization (Schachter et al., 1979c). Past sexual abuse can also be an explanation (Hammerschlag et al., 1984). The possible persistence of chlamydial infections acquired at birth, even up to school age, has been discussed (Stenberg and Mårdh, 1987). Chlamydial infection should always be considered in abused children as well as in children with gonorrhea, since double infections with *C. trachomatis* do occur (Ingram et al., 1984).

In one study, *C. trachomatis* was demonstrated equally often in abused adolescent girls and age-matched controls (Hammerschlag et al., 1984), which should be remembered in medicolegal situations. Vaginal chlamydial infection in abused girls can be asymptomatic, which should also be considered in legal situations. Likewise, the infection can produce symptoms, e.g., vaginal discharge (Fuster and Neinstein, 1987).

In the adult female genital tract, *C. trachomatis* shows a marked predilection for the columnar epithelium of the endocervix. The estrogen-stimulated vaginal epithelium is rather resistant to infection. In prepubertal girls the vaginal cuboidal epithelium has been found to be susceptible to chlamydial infection

(Bump et al., 1985), which forms the basis for a chlamydial vaginitis rather than cervicitis in young girls. Rectal colonization, when present, is often asymptomatic, although symptoms and signs of proctitis should be demonstrable.

In a case of suspected sexual abuse, the clinical examination should be completed with vaginal and rectal specimens for isolation of C. *trachomatis*. In abused boys, urethral meatal and rectal cultures should be investigated. Serology by micro-IF should be done and interpreted with caution (see also Chapter 26).

Treatment of chlamydial infections in abused children should consist of erythromycin given in doses of 25 mg/kg body weight twice daily for 3 weeks.

So far no studies have been published regarding the possible sequelae of chlamydial infections in abused children.

Ocular Nontrachoma Infections in Adults

EPIDEMIOLOGY

In addition to trachoma and perinatal conjunctivitis, *C. trachomatis* can cause inclusion conjunctivitis in adults, which is also known as paratrachoma (Jones, 1961, 1966). The disease is often overlooked or misdiagnosed, with many patients receiving their diagnosis weeks or months after the manifestation of symptoms. Most affected individuals belong to the age group 15–45 years (Viswalingam et al., 1983; Rönnerstam et al., 1985). It is estimated that chlamydial conjunctivitis in adults is seen in 0.3–1.0% of cases with genital *C. trachomatis* infection. Chlamydial conjunctivitis does not seem to occur more often in deep-sited chlamydial infections (e.g., in salpingitis cases) than in uncomplicated nongonococcal infections.

Transmission of adult inclusion conjunctivitis usually occurs by auto-inoculation with infective genital or ocular discharge. Genital infection with *C. trachomatis* is a concomitant finding in up to 80–90% of females and 50% of males with chlamydial conjunctivitis (Jones, 1964; Dawson and Schachter, 1967; Darougar et al., 1971a; Grayston and Wang, 1975). Eye-to-eye transmission of chlamydiae has been shown to occur rarely (Jones, 1964).

CLINICAL FINDINGS

The incubation time for adult chlamydial conjunctivitis varies from 2 days to 3 weeks (Dawson et al., 1966). As is often the case in chlamydial urethritis, a chlamydial eye infection can present clinically after a gonococcal eye infection

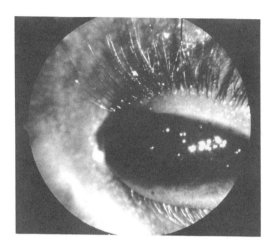

FIGURE 68. Chlamydial conjunctivitis in an adult patient with edematous congested mucosa that bleeds easily. A color version of this figure appears following p. xvi. (Courtesy of Dr. L. Salminen.)

has been cured by antibiotic therapy. Such a postgonococcal chlamydial conjunctivitis was recently described in an adolescent female (Scott and Fortenberry, 1986).

Swollen lids, mucopurulent discharge, papillary hypertrophy (Fig. 68) due to congestion and neovascularization, and follicular hypertrophy (Fig. 69) due to stimulation of lymphoid tissue are typical clinical features of chlamydial adult conjunctivitis. The disease is generally regarded as benign and self-limiting. However, the healing may take months. Upper respiratory tract symptoms may accompany chlamydial conjunctivitis (Jones et al., 1966). The nasopharynx may be colonized, but symptoms of nasopharyngitis are generally absent.

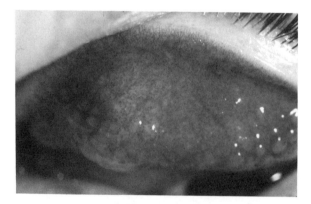

FIGURE 69. Follicles on the upper tarsal conjunctiva in a case of chlamydial conjunctivitis (paratrachoma). A color version of this figure appears following p. xvi. (Courtesy of Dr. J. Treharne.)

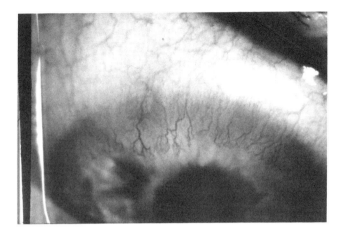

FIGURE 70. The rare event of pannus formation in a case of chlamydial conjunctivitis (paratrachoma). (Courtesy of Dr. J. Treharne.)

In a few chlamydial conjunctivitis cases, corneal lesions (keratitis punctata), pannus formation (Fig. 70), and scarring were noted (Jones et al., 1966). Iritis is a rare complication of adult inclusion conjunctivitis (Dawson et al., 1967, 1970).

The course of the infection is influenced by the patient's immunological status. Previously infected individuals seem to develop more severe disease, likely due to cell-mediated immune reactions (hypersensitivity) (Darougar et al., 1978); this is a counterpart to the pathogenetic process of trachoma (Brewerton et al., 1973).

DIAGNOSIS

The diagnosis of chlamydial conjunctivitis in adults can be established by studies of Giemsa-stained conjunctival scrapings, isolation studies, and direct-specimen antigen detection tests. A comparison of culture (using cycloheximide-treated McCoy cells) on the one hand, and two immunofluorescence tests and ELISA on the other, showed culture to detect a chlamydial infection in approximately 25% more cases than any of the other diagnostic methods. The direct-specimen antigen detection tests were equally effective (Mårdh et al., 1987). Culturing the clinically unaffected eye in cases of unilateral conjunctivitis did not add to the diagnostic sensitivity, nor did culturing the nasopharynx.

Seroconversions are seldom noted in adult chlamydial conjunctivitis because often a concomitant long-standing genital infection has preceded the diagnosis of chlamydial conjunctivitis. This limits the value of serology in the diagnosis of current chlamydial eye infection.

The presence by micro-IF of antichlamydial IgA and IgG antibodies in tears as well as high serum titers of IgM and IgG antibodies have been shown to correlate with the presence and severity of ocular chlamydial infection. Antichlamydial IgG and IgA antibodies were found in tears of 95% and 65% of patients with isolation-positive chlamydial conjunctivitis, respectively. Antichlamydial serum IgM antibodies were detected in 30% of such patients. Most patients had high levels of antichlamydial IgG antibodies (Darougar et al., 1978).

TREATMENT

Oral treatment with tetracycline or erythromycin for 2–3 weeks is recommended in adult chlamydial conjunctivitis. Standard dosages, as recommended for C. trachomatis genital infections should be used. Chlamydiae in the respiratory or genital tract will thus be treated as well. Topical treatment might abolish ocular symptoms but does not eradicate chlamydiae from extraocular sites, or even from the eyes in most cases. If general treatment is not given, recurrences will occur. In fact, local treatment of chlamydial conjunctivitis is not even needed. The only rationale for local treatment is the avoidance of bacterial superinfection in the eyes, which is uncommon in adults.

To keep the eye free from pus, washing the eye at least three times a day, or when pus is present, is recommended. Since adult chlamydial (inclusion) conjunctivitis is generally believed to be transmitted sexually, sexual consorts should also be examined. This is a frequently forgotten step in ophthalmological as well as in many other clinical settings.

SEQUELAE

Sequelae of chlamydial conjunctivitis in adults are not common. However, micropannus formation has been described in nontreated paratrachoma cases. Conjunctival scarring can also develop (Jones et al., 1966; Darougar and Jones, 1983). Pseudoptosis has been noted in some cases as a sequelae of upper eyelid alterations caused by infection. Impairment of vision is rare.

Chlamydia trachomatis Respiratory Tract Infections in Adults

According to seroepidemiological data, serum antibodies against *C. trachomatis* occur in the general adult population more frequently than can be accounted for by diseases known to be caused by this organism (Grayston et al., 1982). For the time being, unrecognized *C. trachomatis* infections, possibly in the respiratory tract, are thought to explain the observed antibody prevalence. Culture studies, however, have not supported this assumption. Respiratory tract infections caused by TWAR chlamydiae and by other *C. psittaci* strains—probably often subclinical—may partially explain the common occurrence of antichlamydial antibodies in adults. Whether or not cross-reactions with other microbes can explain the demonstration of an antichlamydial antibody response in healthy individuals, e.g., with *Legionella, Coxiella,* and *Acinetobacter,* should also be evaluated. In acute respiratory tract infections, a polyclonal B-lymphocyte stimulation could explain the presence of antibodies. Group A streptococci, *H. influenzae, S. pneumoniae, Staphylococcus aureus,* and *Mycoplasma pneumoniae,* i.e., the majority of respiratory tract pathogens, are also known B-cells stimulators, another factor that could partly account for the discrepancy discussed (cf. Gray et al., 1986).

Serological studies suggest, however, that *C. trachomatis* might be a potential pathogen in the nasopharynx. One such study detected antichlamydial serum antibodies in 21% of patients with a sore throat (Komaroff et al., 1983). Later studies did not confirm these findings unanimously. In two studies (Gerber et al., 1984; Huss et al., 1985), none of the individuals with symptomatic pharyngitis studied were positive in isolation studies or in direct-specimen antigen detection tests using monoclonal antibodies to *C. trachomatis.* Jones and associates (1985) reported a pharyngeal isolation frequency for *C. trachomatis* of 3.7% among heterosexual men and 3.2% among heterosexual women without any pharyngeal symptoms.

Bowie and co-workers (1977b) could not demonstrate *C. trachomatis* in the pharynx of women practicing fellatio with isolation-positive men. In the study by Jones and co-workers (1985), a positive pharyngeal culture in women, but not in men, was associated with the performance of oral–genital sex. In a series of 100 teenagers, 42% of whom had a history of sexual intercourse and 11.5% of whom had had oral–genital sex, only one was culture-positive for *C. trachomatis* (Neinstein and Inderlied, 1986).

Chlamydia trachomatis is an uncommon isolate from the pharynx of homosexual men (Sulaiman et al., 1987). However, antichlamydial antibodies occur in half of all such men (McMillan et al., 1981; Persson, 1986). It is possible that difficulties in recovering *C. trachomatis* can explain the discrepancy.

As in gonococcal infections, the role of the oro- and nasopharynx as a reservoir for the transmission of *C. trachomatis* to other persons or for the spread to other sites within the infected individual is poorly understood.

An association between *C. trachomatis* and adult pneumonia is still uncertain, although the etiological role of chlamydiae in infant pneumonitis is well established (Beem and Saxon, 1977). *Chlamydia trachomatis* has been isolated from the lower respiratory tract of immunocompromised adults with signs of pneumonia (Tack et al., 1980). Serological tests seem to implicate *C. trachomatis* as an etiological agent in community-acquired pneumonia in nonimmunocompromised adults (Komaroff et al., 1981).

Pneumonitis was reported in a laboratory worker exposed to *C. trachomatis* (Bernstein et al., 1984). Two other laboratory workers were reported to have developed pneumonia after exposing themselves in the laboratory to a strain (434 bu) of serotype L_2 of *C. trachomatis*. Both developed a marked antibody response to the agent. No characteristic clinical and radiological pulmonary X-ray pattern was found and the findings did not resemble those seen in primary atypical pneumonia (Paran et al., 1987). Pneumonia also developed in yet another laboratory worker who was preparing L_2 antigen. The patient seroconverted in complement fixation tests and developed extremely high titers (>4000) in a micro-IF test (Cevenini, personal communication).

The prevalence of *C. trachomatis* in lung infection in AIDS patients was evaluated by studying brush biopsies and lung lavages in 658 hospitalization episodes, with the conclusion that this organism is not an important respiratory tract pathogen in AIDS patients (Moncada et al., 1986).

Disseminated Infections with *Chlamydia trachomatis*

Disseminated infections seem to be more common with *C. psittaci* than with *C. trachomatis* (see Chapter 33). Apparently, *C. trachomatis* is killed rapidly in the bloodstream (Yong et al., 1982), and reports of disseminated infections caused by this agent are rare.

Endocarditis can be one manifestation of disseminated infection by *C. psittaci* in humans (Levison et al., 1971; Dick et al., 1977; Regan et al., 1978). There have also been single reports of endocarditis caused by *C. trachomatis* (Van der Bel-Kahn et al., 1978). The authors describe a 25-year-old, 30-week-pregnant woman who developed a fulminating endocarditis with heart failure and cerebral infarction. She died within 2 weeks of admission. Finger-shaped vegetations were found on the aortic valves. Electron microscopy of the vegetations revealed chlamydial inclusions. Serum IgM antibodies to *C. trachomatis* serotype F were demonstrated.

Cardiac involvement can occur as a complication in lymphogranuloma venereum, i.e., in a *C. trachomatis* infection (serotypes L_1–L_3) (Sheldon et al., 1948). There have also been reports of meningitis and meningoencephalitis occurring in cases of *C. trachomatis* infection. In these cases chlamydiae were not recovered from cerebrospinal fluid. However, a chlamydial genital tract infection was diagnosed by culture. A significant antichlamydial antibody response was detected in all cases using micro-IF tests (Myhre and Mårdh, 1982a). Whether these cases represent an invasion of the central nervous system by chlamydiae or an adverse immunological response to the cross-reaction of *C. trachomatis* antigen with an unknown agent is not known.

Prevention and Control of Genital Chlamydial Infections

MAGNITUDE OF THE PROBLEM

As in all epidemiological situations, recognition of the extent of the problem is important. Generally speaking, the prevalence of *C. trachomatis* infections has been greatly underestimated in most countries. However, wherever chlamydial infections have been registered, they have been recognized as one of the most common infections in the community studied. For example, in Sweden it has been estimated that up to one-third of the entire population of young people will have had one or more genital chlamydial infections during their lifetime, i.e., if the present epidemic situation does not change markedly during the years to come. Projections from the United States are more optimistic (Judson, 1985), although prevalence figures from the two countries are very similar.

Relatively few countries practice large-scale screening for chlamydial infections and very few countries require reporting of chlamydial cases. Sweden was one of the first countries to implement the reporting of chlamydial infections on a national basis, i.e., reports on positive laboratory diagnoses have been made on a voluntary basis since the late 1970s. For some countries, e.g., Finland and Sweden, physicians are now required by law to report cases with genital chlamydial infection.

In 1984, there were approximately 8000 reported cases of gonorrhea and 36,000 cases of chlamydial infection in Sweden. The population of Sweden is approximately 8.5 million. The present estimate is that there are more than 100,000 new cases of *C. trachomatis* infection per year. England is one of the few countries in which nongonococcal urethritis (NGU) in males has been reported (by clinics for genitourinary medicine) in the last three decades (Catterall, 1975) (Fig. 40). These reports show that the occurrence of NGU has increased steadily during the past decades, whereas the number of cases of gonococcal urethritis during the same period of time first increased, then leveled off, and during recent years decreased.

In certain regions of some countries, e.g., Seattle and Malmö (see above)— there has been a leveling-off of chlamydial infections in recent years. In certain parts of Sweden, where culture service for *C. trachomatis* has generally been available since the late 1970s, i.e., in the county of Malmöhus and the city of Malmö, the annual number of cases of chlamydial infections had already started to decrease since 1982 (Persson, 1986), whereas the number of cases of gonorrhea in the same area had already started to decrease in the early 1970s. The prevalence of chlamydial infections in many other areas of Sweden does not seem to have been affected in the same way. In Finland in 1987, *C. trachomatis* infections were reported three times more often than gonococcal infections (Puolakkainen and Saikku, 1988).

Registration not only of diagnosed chlamydial cases but also of cases of cervicitis, salpingitis, and epididymitis (in younger men) might improve the monitoring of alterations in the local epidemic situation regarding genital chlamydial infections, since these conditions are known to be caused by *C. trachomatis* in many instances. In areas where gonococcal infections are less common, infection by *C. trachomatis* accounts for the vast majority of cases of exogenous genital bacterial infections. Sequelae of genital chlamydial infections, i.e., ectopic pregnancy and infertility (cf. Mårdh, 1986), would also be relevant to such a program, although those conditions would reflect the epidemic situation 5–10 years earlier.

The trends in chlamydial epidemiology in eastern Europe and in the developing world are still uncertain. However, data available from Poland (Zdrodowska-Stefanow, 1988) and Russia (Shatkin, 1988) suggest a situation very similar to that in most Western industrialized countries. In terms of severe sequelae of chlamydial infections, e.g., salpingitis, the situation in the industrialized and developing countries also seems to be quite similar (Mabey et al., 1985; Meheus et al., 1986; Frost et al., 1987). The relative proportion of gonococcal vs. chlamydial PID cases in the developing world is similar to that seen in many industrialized countries 10 or more years ago. Presently there seems to be a decrease in gonococcal infections and an increase in chlamydial infections in most countries.

COSTS

It has been estimated that chlamydial infections in the United States are now costing Americans over $1.4 billion per year in direct and indirect costs (Table 33). Women were estimated to account for 79%, and men and infants for the

TABLE 33. Annual Cost of *C. trachomatis* Infections in Men,
Women, and Infants in the United States[a]

Infection	Annual cost (millions of $)		
	Direct costs	Indirect costs	Total
Men			
Urethritis	73.50	115.44	188.94
Epididymitis			
Outpatient treatment	7.94	28.79	36.73
Hospitalization	13.13	4.87	18.00
All infections	94.57	149.10	243.67
Women			
Uncomplicated illness	80.50	108.35	188.85
(MPC and ure-			
thritis)			
PID (and sequelae)			
Outpatient treatment	60.33	174.52	234.85
Hospitalization	365.70	132.45	498.15
Ectopic pregnancy	58.87	23.00	81.87
Infertility	20.13	7.49	27.62
Deaths	—	84.44	84.44
All infections	585.53	530.25	1115.78
Infants			
Conjunctivitis	3.32	4.93	8.25
Pneumonia	0.33	0.25	0.58
Outpatient treatment	0.33	0.25	0.58
Hospitalization	42.91	2.23	45.14
All infections	46.56	7.71	53.97

[a]From Washington et al. (1987).

rest, of these costs. Three-quarters of the cost has been estimated to relate to sequelae of untreated, uncomplicated infections. It is believed that if the current rate of genital chlamydial infection persists, the annual cost for these infections in 1990 will exceed $2.8 billion (Washington et al., 1987).

EPIDEMIOLOGICAL MARKERS

A large number of data now support an etiological association of chlamydial infection with both tubal (ectopic) pregnancy and infertility resulting from damage to the fallopian tubes. Since chlamydial infections seem to be an important cause of tubal pregnancy, the latter condition might be one epidemiological marker of chlamydial infection in areas lacking etiological diagnostic capabilities. Involuntary childlessness might also be such a marker in countries where *C. trachomatis* is the main cause of salpingitis, although the diagnosis of tubal factor infertility is much less easily recognized than an actual tubal pregnancy. At present both tubal pregnancy and infertility in women are steadily increasing in many countries because of the chlamydial epidemic that prevailed over the last decades.

In Western countries there is a mean lag time of 5–10 years between the diagnosis of an acute episode of primary acute salpingitis, and the diagnosis of ectopic pregnancy or the evaluation for involuntary childlessness (Persson, 1986). Consequently, during the coming years we can expect an increase in both the number of women attending emergency rooms because of extrauterine pregnancy and those seeking intervention for suspected infertility. In many countries such a marked increase has already been registered. It is possible that the modulating effect of oral contraceptives on upper genital tract infections has contributed to an increase in the number of subclinical tubal chlamydial infections resulting in an increase of the type of conditions discussed (see also below). Chlamydial eye infection might also be an easily recognized marker of genital chlamydial infections.

CONTRACEPTIVES INFLUENCING CHLAMYDIAL EPIDEMIOLOGY

The influence of contraceptives, i.e., oral contraceptives (OCs), intrauterine devices (IUDs), and barrier methods such as condoms and pessaries, on the course of genital chlamydial infections must be considered when discussing the prevention and control of such infections. The prescription of contraceptives to a woman means that she—without risk of pregnancy—can expose herself to STDs, chlamydial infections being no exception. Several studies have shown a higher prevalence of genital chlamydial infection as well as a higher carrier rate in users than in nonusers of oral contraceptives.

Intrauterine device usage increases the risk of ascending chlamydial infections in women with cervicitis (Weström et al., 1976). Because of this risk, an IUD should not be inserted in a nullipara. In women using the pill, a decreased risk of ascending genital infection, including chlamydial infection, has been reported (Svensson et al., 1984). In OC users with proven upper genital chlamydial tract infection, the tubal inflammatory reactions were generally less severe than those of nonusers. Women with chlamydial salpingitis who were on the pill when the tubal infection was acquired had a significantly better chance of retaining their fertility than nonusers (Svensson et al., 1984). However, other studies (Cramer, 1985) involving somewhat older women hospitalized for severe PID in whom infertility was not only associated with the tubal factor did not show such a benefit of contraceptive use. All the above-mentioned studies were, however, conducted before the introduction of low-dose estrogen pills and the new gestagen pills. Thus the influence of the most recently introduced OCs on the natural course of genital infections, e.g., chlamydial infections, remains to be established.

In one study (Worm and Petersen, 1987), condom use was the only contraceptive technique that lowered the risk of transmitting chlamydial infections, although it should be stressed that the risk of transferring such infections was still far from abolished.

In summary, contraceptive use might have an important impact on the epidemiology of genital *C. trachomatis* infections in women, which must be kept in mind when recommending contraceptive techniques, particularly to younger individuals.

CONTACT TRACING AND PARTNER TREATMENT

As in other STDs, contact tracing is important in genital chlamydial infections. In fact, it is generally a highly rewarding method in combatting the chlamydial epidemic. Thus in VD clinic patients, the agent was recovered from more than every second consort (in both sexes). In one series, when the index case was a woman and a man, respectively, the incidence of culture positivity in heterosexual consorts was 66 and 52%, respectively (Thelin et al., 1980; Thelin and Mårdh, 1982). The same sex difference, i.e., a lower isolation rate in male than in female consorts, was reported in a more recent study (Worm and Petersen, 1987) in which 62% of male and 42% of female partners to a heterosexual index case were *Chlamydia*-positive.

One reason it is important to perform contact tracing is that the consort, if a carrier, may develop complications. Pelvic inflammatory disease is likely to develop in approximately 10% of infected young females. Of course, another important reason for performing contact tracing is that treatment of infected partner(s) stops the spread of infection to new partners as well as preventing reinfection of the index case. Finally, the finding of *Chlamydia*-positive partners opens up the possibility of extending the contact tracing to new partners, thereby detecting and treating even more cases of chlamydial infection.

Experience indicates that contact tracing is particularly neglected in cases of SARA and Reiter's syndrome, chlamydial eye infections in adults, and intraperitoneal chlamydial infections, e.g., in cases of peritonitis, periappendicitis, and perihepatitis, and in cases of proctitis seen in surgical departments. Thus reinfection occurs frequently in such cases.

SCREENING PROGRAMS

Genital chlamydial infections are often asymptomatic or minimally symptomatic. Therefore, screening is mandatory in order to successfully combat the present *Chlamydia* epidemic. The search for chlamydial infections in high-risk groups is very rewarding, particularly in family-planning clinics and antenatal clinics. Other groups considered as candidates for chlamydial screening programs are young women undergoing elective abortion and young men recruited to military service as well as men in active service; all these groups have proved to have a high prevalence of chlamydial infections.

Some investigators in the United States (Schachter et al., 1986a) have found the rate of genital chlamydial infection in pregnant women so high that they recommend the initiation of national programs to prevent perinatal transmission of *C. trachomatis*. Treatment of culture-positive pregnant women (and their sexual partners) with a 2-week course of erythromycin will prevent infection of the neonate (Schachter et al., 1986a).

Postabortal genital infections have been found more often in *Chlamydia*-positive than *Chlamydia*-negative women. In one study (Shiótz and Csángo, 1985), such an infection occurred in 7.4 and 2.0% of cases, respectively. Screening for *C. trachomatis* in abortion patients and institution of antibiotic treatment for infected patients has been found to reduce the rate of postoperative pelvic inflammatory disease (Møller et al., 1982; Shiótz and Csángo, 1985).

In some family-planning clinics, screening for *C. trachomatis* is performed regularly in women requesting an IUD. Screening should also be done in women from whom an IUD has been removed, since the removal procedure is also likely to increase the risk of ascending chlamydial infection in asymptomatic carriers. In *C. trachomatis* culture-positive women, treatment should be given before the insertion or in conjunction with the removal of an IUD.

EFFICIENCY OF LABORATORY TESTS

In order to effectively prevent chlamydial infections, not only the implementation of screening for *C. trachomatis* (Table 34) but also the development of new, more sensitive and specific diagnostic methods is required. Today one-fourth to one-half of all *C. trachomatis* cases may be missed, even when optimum laboratory techniques are used. Many of the direct-specimen antigen detection techniques have been evaluated with culture as the standard, but the culture techniques used have not been optimal in many of the studies. Thus the direct-specimen antigen tests, i.e., immunofluorescence and ELISA, appear to have better sensitivities than is actually the case. These tests perform better in high- than in low-prevalence groups, which restricts their use, for example, in

TABLE 34. Measures for Combating the Current Pandemic
of *C. trachomatis* Genital Infections

Establishing nationwide laboratory diagnostic facilities for the diagnosis of *C. trachomatis* infections.

Implementing liberal sampling for *C. trachomatis* in patients with signs of genital infection and in their partners, including cases in which other STDs have been diagnosed.

Establishing national surveillance programs.

Screening high-risk groups.

Using antibiotics active against *C. trachomatis* in the treatment of syndromes frequently caused by the agent, regardless of results of etiological studies.

Implementing contact tracing and treatment of infected partners; partners in ongoing relations should be treated regardless of symptoms.

Educating professionals.

Informing teenagers and other high-risk groups about chlamydial infections.

Providing opportunities for young people to consult with integrity and without bureaucracy, at low or no cost.

---

many screening situations and in follow-up studies after antibiotic treatment. Sensitivities of 40 to 70% of IF and ELISA tests have been obtained, not only in low-prevalence groups (Stamm et al., 1984; Taylor-Tobinson et al., 1987) but, recently, in high-prevalence groups as well (e.g., in men and women with acute urethritis and cervicitis).

More basic and applied research is needed to increase the sensitivity of the so-called direct-specimen antigen detection tests, e.g., methods for amplifying the signal in ELISA tests (cf. Mabey et al., 1987).

Optimized methods for the sampling and transport of specimens (taking into account local conditions) as well as reference methods for the laboratory diagnosis of *C. trachomatis* should be worked out. Means for quality control in the performance of laboratory tests for the diagnosis of chlamydial infections should be established on a state- or nationwide basis. In 1987, such measures were undertaken in Sweden, and helped many laboratories achieve better service.

The limited sensitivity of diagnostic tests for genital chlamydial infections implies that antibiotic treatment should be liberally instituted in cases presenting with syndromes commonly caused by *C. trachomatis* (see also below).

PREVENTIVE MEASURES

Despite evidence that genital chlamydial infections poses a significant health problem, very few countries have undertaken any large-scale preventive measures (cf. Mårdh, 1988). The present AIDS situation seems in many countries to have partially drained personal initiatives and economic resources from and to have detracted activities concerning other STDs, including genital chlamydial infections.

One of the most important medical measures would be to prevent further spread of HIV infections in the community. As already mentioned, reducing the pool of persons with genital infections would likely reduce the risk of HIV being transmitted. In this context, chlamydial infections are of particular interest since they are so common. In women with chlamydial infection of the endometrium causing bleeding from the uterine cavity, an efficient mode for spreading blood-borne infections, such as HIV, is established. The mere inflammation of genital tissue with transudation of serum as seen in cervicitis may also represent an increased risk of transferring HIV from carriers. Likewise, a person with a chlamydial infection seems to be more susceptible to HIV infections than noninfected individuals; mucosal lesions might be a port of entrance for the virus.

It seems important to establish risk factors for aquiring genital infections by *C. trachomatis* (Martin et al., 1986), as for any other STD.

National policy guidelines for the prevention and control of genital chlamydial infections are urgently needed (Table 33). So far, few countries, e.g., United States and Sweden, have such guidelines (*MMWR*, 1985; Socialstyrelsens Allmänna Råd och Anvisningar angående *Chlamydia trachomatis* infektioner, 1987).

In the United States, a prevention program was started in 1985. *Morbidity and Mortality Weekly Report* (*MMWR*) has disseminated information on diagnostic and therapeutic measures for chlamydial infections for years (*MMWR*, 1985).

In Sweden, since April 1988, genital chlamydial infections have been legally declared a venereal disease. That is, the disease is reportable, contact tracing is required, patients and partners must allow investigation and therapy (both of which are free of charge at certain clinics), and legal action can be taken if needed.

In most countries, information on chlamydial infection has spread only through drug companies, since the official health authorities have generally not bothered probably due to lack of knowledge and insight, or both.

The local epidemiological status of STDs and the way the health care system is organized influence how preventive measures against chlamydial infections can be undertaken. Screening for chlamydial infections in young women attending maternal health and birth control clinics seems to be a key preventive approach. It is also important to provide for young persons seeking attention for symptoms of genital tract infection with little or no bureaucracy, with short or no waiting time, and at little or no cost. Control programs should include recommendations about the groups that should be screened for chlamydial infections. Table 35 lists a number of situations in which the patient [and partner(s)] should be investigated for *Chlamydia*.

TABLE 35. Populations to Be Considered
for Chlamydial Infection

Women with increased vaginal discharge, particularly of recent manifestation
Women with signs of cervicitis or urethritis
Young, sexually active women with irregular bleeding
Women with the assumed diagnosis of PID (acute salpingitis)
Young, sexually active women, particularly with newly acquired partner, with
    signs of appendicitis, cholecystitis/pleuritis, and diffuse peritonitis where
    surgical diseases have been excluded
Males with signs of urethritis or with urethral discomfort
Young men with epididymitis
Young men with prostatitis symptoms, particularly after having changed
    partners
Men with proctitis and in some cases with hemorrhoidal disorders
Young persons with reactive arthritis (Reiter's syndrome)
Sexually active persons with one-sided conjunctivitis
Sexually active persons who have developed genital symptoms
Partners of patients with genital or other *C. trachomatis* infections
Persons with nonchlamydial STD
Newborns with bilateral conjunctivitis
Newborns with afebrile, nonproductive cough or signs of pneumonia

---

Control programs should spread information on the spectrum of syndromes and sequelae associated with *C. trachomatis*. Knowledge of the various manifestations of infection with *C. trachomatis* is still not well established in the medical community. Control programs should also make an effort to disseminate information to groups and individuals whose behavior puts them at risk for acquiring chlamydial infection (or any STD). Educational material should be available, e.g., pamphlets, video tapes, television programs. Guidelines for antibiotic therapy of *C. trachomatis* infection should be given and the need for contract tracing and partner treatment stressed.

Recommendations for the treatment of *C. trachomatis* infections were first established by the Centers for Disease Control (CDC) in 1982. These recommendations were revised in 1985 (*MMWR*, 1985) (see Appendix). Most antimicrobial agents effective against chlamydial infections were initially evaluated in men. Although one might expect regimens proved effective in men to be similarly effective in women, this is not necessarily the case. Differences in drug efficiency are often noted. There may be variations in the bioavailability of antimicrobial agents in men and women. Thus differences may exist in the ability of an antimicrobial agent to penetrate cervical mucosal and male urethral cells, or in the relative burden of epithelial cells infected by *C. trachomatis* in women and men (Sanders et al., 1986). Furthermore, the effectiveness of different regimens in pregnant women may be different from that in nonpregnant women. In fact, very little is known about the optimal treatment of *C. trachomatis* infection in pregnant women. Particularly important to clarify is the optimal regimen for PID, a condition in which *C. trachomatis* is known to play a major etiological role. Obviously, prevention and early treatment of lower genital tract chlamydial infections before they ascend to the upper genital tract remains the most cost-effective way to reduce PID-associated morbidity.

Because a laboratory diagnosis of *C. trachomatis* infection cannot be obtained in many places or, as discussed, is often missed due to the low sensitivity of existing diagnostic techniques, recommendations for treatment of cervicitis, acute salpingitits (PID), NGU, and epididymitis in younger men should include drugs that are active against *C. trachomatis*. Perinatal infections affecting the eyes and the lungs should also be included in such treatment recommendations.

Education should be given to medical and paramedical staff, school-children, military personnel, women attending family-planning clinics and antenatal clinics, as well as to groups of individuals known to be at high risk for nonchlamydial STD agents. Such persons should be considered appropriate candidates for information, whether oral or written, on chlamydial infections (Table 34).

IV

Chlamydia psittaci Infections

Chlamydia psittaci Infections in Humans

PSITTACOSIS/ORNITHOSIS

Introduction

During the late 1920s, there was a great deal of interest in *C. psittaci* infections related to the ongoing pandemic of "parrot fever," i.e., of psittacosis, caused by transmission of avian chlamydiae to humans. Small outbreaks of psittacosis/ornithosis occur constantly, particularly among shopkeepers selling caged birds, among visitors of such shops, and among persons working in the poultry industry.

Recent decades have shown a neglect of the study of human infections by *C. psittaci*, despite the well-documented importance of this species in avian and lower mammalian infections (Storz, 1971). In the last few years, however, there has been a renewed interest in chlamydial, nontrachomatis infections (Grayston et al., 1984) because of the fact that TWAR chlamydiae are known to be a very common cause of pneumonia (Grayston et al., 1985b; Saikku et al., 1985) (see below). There has probably been an overdiagnosis of nonepidemic ornithosis cases due to false serological diagnoses based on cross-reactions of TWAR antibodies and *C. psittaci* antigen in CF tests (see Chapter 36).

The spectrum of known clinical syndromes caused by *C. psittaci* infection in humans has recently expanded. The newer studies indicate *C. psittaci* to be associated with abortion in women involved in sheep farming (Johnson et al., 1985).

Epidemiology

The disease has been called psittacosis if acquired from psittacine birds, e.g., parrots and parakeets, and ornithosis if acquired from other birds, e.g., ducks, turkeys, pigeons, and chickens. Psittacosis/ornithosis is primarily a respiratory tract infection, although it can cause a variety of manifestations involving many other organ systems. It should also be remembered that respiratory tract infections due to TWAR are acquired from humans (see Chapter 36).

The incubation time of psittacosis/ornithosis in humans is generally 7–15 days but can be as long as 5–6 weeks. Psittacosis seems to be rare in children less than 10 years of age.

Humans are generally infected by inhaling contaminated particles from birds with serous conjunctivitis or purulent rhinitis. Dried excrement of infected birds occurring in the environment or on contaminated feathers are a further source of infection. Clinically healthy birds can spread the disease as well. Bird bites are a less common mode of transmission. Sea gulls are a source of ornithosis, and pickers of their eggs can be infected. Workers in the poultry industry, particularly those engaged in plucking and eviscerating birds (e.g., turkeys and ducks), belong to a high-risk group for infection (Schachter, 1978; Isaacs, 1984; Nagington, 1984; Maffei et al., 1987). Sporadic cases of psittacosis/ornithosis are seen in persons in contact with birds at home or at work. Laboratory infections in veterinary and medical clinical laboratory workers are reported comparatively frequently. Human-to-human transmission of classical psittacosis has been discussed (Dalgaard, 1957; Broholm et al., 1977; Pether et al., 1984), but this mode of spread is unimportant (Maffei et al., 1984). Many reported instances of a human-to-human transfer have to be reconsidered in light of the present knowledge on TWAR infections (Saikku et al., 1985) (see also Chapter 36).

Clinical Findings

Psittacosis/ornithosis in humans is a feverish respiratory infection of variable severity (MacFarlane and Macrae, 1983) (Table 31). In a series of 46 psittacosis cases, headache occurred in 96%, chills in 93%, fever in 89%, nonproductive cough in 65%, while rales or rhonchi were detected in 6 of the 33 cases examined by pulmonary auscultation (Kuritsky, 1984). Yong and Grayson (1988) recently reviewed 129 cases of psittacosis. Respiratory symptoms were absent in 18% of the patients. Most patients had a normal leukocyte count. Diarrhea and sore throat were occasional complaints.

Psittacosis/ornithosis is occasionally accompanied by diverse extrapulmonary manifestations. Abdominal symptoms, especially vague abdominal pain and vomiting, and severe headache are often found whereas a few cases present with fever (Maclachlan et al., 1953; Jansson, 1960; cf. Myhre and Mårdh, 1982b; Puolakkainen et al., 1987a). Hepatic involvement in psittacosis/ornithosis is comparatively common. In one study (Ragnaud et al., 1986) of 32 patients with psittacosis, 14 had moderately increased hepatic transaminases and alkaline phosphatases. Endocarditis can also occur in psittacosis (Birkhead and Apostolov, 1974; editorial, 1980).

Reiter's syndrome (Bhopal and Thomas, 1982) and other types of reactive arthritis (Langham and Doyle, 1984) may also be seen in psittacosis. Erythema nodosum is seen in cases with *C. psittaci* infection (Sarner and Wilson, 1965).

Differential diagnoses to psittacosis/ornithosis include, e.g., TWAR infection and *M. pneumoniae,* tularemia, tuberculosis, histoplasmosis, and coccidioidomycosis.

Diagnosis

Isolation of *C. psittaci* is potentially hazardous, with the exception of TWAR chlamydiae. Because safe laboratory facilities are rarely available, serology remains the diagnostic method of choice for *C. psittaci.*

Antibodies to *C. psittaci* can be detected by CF and micro-IF tests. Serum CF antibodies at titers of >32 and/or a fourfold or greater change in the IgG titer in both CF and micro-IF tests are considered indicative of an acute, ongoing infection (Potter et al., 1983). In some ornithosis cases, no CF antichlamydial antibodies can be detected, although micro-IF tests may reveal the diagnosis (Myhre and Mårdh, 1982b).

Sera of 22 patients with the diagnosis of psittacosis/ornithosis were used in micro-IF test for the study of IgG, IgM, and IgA antichlamydial antibodies (Myhre and Mårdh, 1982b). Twenty of the patients were positive in CF tests. By the micro-IF test, no antichlamydial antibodies were detected on day 5 after onset of symptoms, whereas all sera were positive on day 22. Seroconversion was found in 21 of the 22 patients studied. In 10 cases the seroconversion was restricted to IgG, whereas in the remaining cases two or more of the three Ig classes converted. The noted micro-IF IgG titers ranged from 16 to 1024, while the IgM and IgA titers varied between 16 and 128. The patient who had a stable micro-IF titer had a fourfold rise in CF antibodies. The two patients lacking CF antibodies had an eightfold titer change of micro-IF antibodies. Conversion with regard to IgG, IgM, and IgA antibodies was seen in 20, 7, and 6 patients, respectively.

Groups of psittacosis cases with and without hepatic involvement did not differ serologically (Ragnaud et al., 1986).

Cross-reactions with antibodies formed against other chlamydiae, e.g., TWAR chlamydiae, constitute a differential diagnostic problem when the genus-specific CF test is used (Mordhorst et al., 1986). Thus, as mentioned, it seems plausible that many cases diagnosed as ornithosis/psittacosis with the aid of CF test might in fact have been TWAR infections. The use of CF tests may result not only in overdiagnosis of ornithosis cases but also in missed cases of chlamydial pneumonia, as indicated by the study cited (Myhre and Mårdh, 1982b).

Wreghitt and Taylor (1988) have noted a correlation between the number of serologically (with CF tests) diagnosed human chlamydial respiratory tract infections in Great Britain and the number of imported psittacine birds. For Finland, the CF sero-positive rate and the number of high (diagnostic) titers have varied extensively despite a very limited import of psittacine birds into the country, suggesting that *C. psittaci* infections caught from birds cannot be considered a major source of chlamydial CF antibody activity in that country (Puolakkainen et al., 1988).

Improved diagnostic tests for *C. psittaci* infections are needed. ELISA tests that detect chlamydial genus-specific antibodies have been introduced, and their value must be established (Lewis et al., 1977; Puolakkainen et al., 1985).

Therapy

The fatality rate in psittacosis was high, i.e., up to 20%, in the preantibiotic era. After the introduction of antibiotic therapy (tetracycline), it dropped to less than 1%.

Tetracycline is now recommended as the standard drug of treatment for psittacosis/ornithosis except in pregnant women and children. In the latter groups of patients, erythromycin or other macrolides should be used instead. The recommended dosages for these drugs are the same as those used in the therapy of complicated genital *C. trachomatis* infections, i.e., doxycycline 100 mg twice daily, lymecycline 300 mg twice daily, tetracycline hydrochloride 250 mg four times daily, or 500 mg erythromycin twice to four times daily. Treatment should continue for at least 2 weeks. A prolonged tetracycline course of 3 weeks has sometimes been recommended to avoid relapse. Resolution of psittacosis/ornithosis after the institution of therapy usually occurs in 1–6 days but sometimes occurs later. Relapses sometimes occur.

Experience with other drugs in the treatment of chlamydial pneumonia, e.g., chloramphenicol and rifampicin, is not extensive.

When the etiology of assumed cases of psittacosis/ornithosis is uncertain, therapy should also be effective against *M. pneumoniae* and *Legionella* spp., since the clinical picture in these cases may be similar to that of parrot fever.

PLACENTITIS AND ABORTION

A pathogenic role of *C. psittaci* in human abortion had not been well established earlier (Roberts et al., 1967), but current studies from the United

Kingdom seem to firmly support such an etiological relationship (Johnson et al., 1985; Wong et al., 1986; Helm et al., 1987). Thus a women who had been exposed to aborting ewes developed a mild febrile disease in her 28th week of pregnancy. Subsequently, she became severely ill and aborted. *Chlamydia psittaci* was isolated from fetal tissue and chlamydial inclusions were demonstrated in placental trophoblast (Johnson et al., 1985; Wong et al., 1986). Another case occurred in a 30-year-old primigravida, a member of a sheep-farming family. She had assisted in lambing a flock of sheep, but only by wiping the lambs after delivery. There was no history of abortion among the sheep. The woman developed thrombocytopenia, renal failure, and spontaneous miscarriage at the 27th gestational week (Helm et al., 1987).

Chlamydia psittaci placentitis is characterized by an intense inflammatory cell reaction in the intervillous space and by focal fine fibrin deposits. Upon initial inspection of the placentas, one has the impression of focal microinfarcts. There can also be mild inflammation in the decidual bed. No signs of chorioamnionitis have been seen in cases diagnosed so far. In one case, the fetal stem vessels displayed a focal early perivasculitis (Wong et al., 1986).

Chlamydia psittaci seems to have a predilection for the human trophoblast where it multiplies rapidly and is released into the intervillous spaces, infecting more chorionic villi and inducing intense inflammation. This can result in placental insufficiency and fetal death (Wong et al., 1986).

The cases of placentitis resulting in abortion diagnosed so far have all occurred in women involved in sheep farming (in the UK). The aborting women had been dealing not only with aborting animals but with healthy newborn lambs as well. The recommendation would thus be that pregnant women avoid contact with sheep either diseased or healthy. The aborted tissue and feces definitely seem to be sources of infection.

Pregnant women can also inhale infected material from the sheep and subsequently develop psittacosis (Beer et al., 1982). Pregnant women with psittacosis/ornithosis are also at risk of aborting, and the infection can cause severe disease in the women themselves (McKinlay et al., 1985). Thus contact with (*Chlamydia*-infected) birds should be considered a cause of abortion in humans and should be avoided.

Chlamydia psittaci Infection in Birds

EPIDEMIOLOGY

Chlamydia psittaci is a ubiquitous parasite of birds. The organism is known to cause a variety of diseases in birds, involving, e.g., the eye and the respiratory, genital, and gastrointestinal tracts. Systemic infections also occur (cf. Storz, 1971; Pasco, 1985; Grimes and Clark, 1986; Grimes, 1987).

More than 130 species of bird have been found to be infected by *C. psittaci*. Wild and cage birds, pigeons, ducks, and other birds processed in the poultry industry can all be infected.

In a survey of sera (collected between 1974 and 1983) from 6500 English birds studied by complement fixation (CF) test using *C. psittaci* antigen, chickens showed the lowest (1.5%) seropositive rate, while the highest percentage of positive tests occurred in pigeons (47.2%) and collared doves (51.4%). Imported birds of the order *Psittaciformes* (15.9%), geese (22.2%), ducks (23.3%), and game birds (29.0%) were positive less often (Bracewell and Bevan, 1986).

In West Germany, 6133 cases of chlamydial infection in birds or aviaries were diagnosed during the past 15 years (Wachendörfer, 1984). In South Africa, budgerigars and cockatiels are the most common sources of human infection, although transfer from imported Australian finches and South American parrots has also been reported (Gear et al., 1986).

Ducks have been an important source of *C. psittaci* infections in humans (Andrews et al., 1981; Anon, 1981). Such infections were earlier a problem in eastern Europe (Strauss, 1967) and, more recently, in the United Kingdom (Chalmers, 1986). The slaughter of resident flocks has decreased the problem in Czechoslovakia (Strauss, personal communication).

Feathers, feces, nasal secretions, and viscera of infected birds can be sources of infection in humans, either by the handling of such material or by inhalation of infected airborne particles.

CLINICAL FINDINGS

In birds, the primary sites of *C. psittaci* infection are liver, spleen, and pericardium. Thus pericarditis, perihepatitis, and splenomegaly can be seen in infected birds (cf. Chalmers, 1986). The birds might also develop purulent conjunctivitis and keratoconjunctivitis.

Infected birds might present with ruffled feathers, dyspnea, atrophy of the pectoral muscle, and possibly an enlarged liver and spleen. There might be green–yellow fecal material around the vent as a sign of diarrhea. There might be emaciation. *Chlamydia psittaci* infection in birds might also be clinically inapparent.

TREATMENT

The proposed treatment for *C. psittaci*-infected birds is 45 days of feeding with, for example, chlortetracycline-medicated (1%) pellets. For larger birds (e.g., cockatoos, macaws, and parrots), antibiotic-containing pellets are available. Cockatiels, love birds, and budgerigars can be given tetracycline-impregnated seed. Liquid solutions are available for nectar-eating species. In valuable, severely ill birds, intravenous administration of doxycycline is an alternative.

Quaternary ammonium compounds have been recommended as disinfectants for contaminated material and objects that have been infected by *C. psittaci* in birds.

Chlamydia psittaci Infection in Mammals

Chlamydia psittaci can cause a variety of diseases in mammals; the list of manifestations and species affected is growing steadily.

HORSES

Chlamydia psittaci infections in horses have been reported in England, West Germany (Krauss et al., 1988), Russia (cf. Martinov and Popov, 1988), and Australia. In the 1960s, neurological and respiratory tract manifestations and during the 1970s arthritis, abortion, and eye infection were described as manifestations of chlamydial infections in horses. *Chlamydia psittaci* has also been recovered from the genital tract of mares with signs of cervicitis (Krauss et al., 1988). Respiratory tract infections can also occur in foals.

The study of impression smears of infected mucosal surfaces and tissues stained by the Gimenez method is a recommended rapid method for the presumptive diagnosis of equine *C. psittaci* infections (Dilbeck et al., 1986).

CATTLE

A variety of manifestations of chlamydial infection have been described in cattle over the years. Thus neurological complications were described in 1942 followed by descriptions of ocular, intestinal, and respiratory tract infections during the 1950s. During the 1960s arthritis and abortion were added to the list of manifestations that could be attributed to infection by *C. psittaci* (cf. Evermann, 1987).

Inoculation of bovine strains of *C. psittaci* in pregnant cows resulted in pathological parturition in five of six animals (Martel et al., 1983).

Vaccines have been produced against strains of *C. psittaci* that cause abortion in cattle. The best protection is obtained after intradermal challenge.

ELISA tests and immunofluorescence tests were recently introduced as a means for diagnosing bovine chlamydial abortion (Perez-Martinez et al., 1986). Specifically, ELISA was compared with CF and indirect inclusion fluorescence.

Chlamydia-infected cattle from different herds had diverse immune reactions in contrast to cattle exposed to the same serotype of *C. psittaci* (Schmeer et al., 1986b).

PIGS

Chlamydia psittaci can cause disease in pigs, e.g., pericarditis, pneumonia, conjunctivitis, arthritis and reproductive events in both boars and sows. Chlamydial infections occur most commonly in large swine-breeding complexes. Infections have been reported from e.g., United States, United Kingdom, West Germany (Krauss et al., 1988), and eastern Europe (Martinov and Popov, 1988). Serological studies of pigs indicate that subclinical infections may be common (Harris, 1976).

Pericarditis is one manifestation of *C. psittaci* infection in pigs that was recently highlighted (Martinov et al., 1985), thereby confirming older observations (Willigan and Beamer, 1955). The pigs in the study of Martinov and coworkers contracted the disease at the age of 30–70 days. The agent could be isolated from pericardial fluid. The histological examination showed serofibrinous pericarditis.

Pneumonia developed in pigs that had been intranasally or intratracheally inoculated with *C. psittaci* (Harris et al., 1984). The pneumonia was characterized by acute exudative or interstitial pneumonia with peribronchiolar cellular cuffing. The pathological changes started at 4–8 days and peaked at 8–12 days after challenge. Natural infections by *C. psittaci* in pigs can result in pneumonia (Stellmacher et al., 1983; cf. Martinov and Popov, 1988), and the infection often spreads to other organs.

When *Chlamydia*-infected semen was given to sows, the result was the birth of infected piglets. Shedding of the organism can occur for up to 2 years. Abortion and stillbirth may occur in genitally infected sows. Infection in gilts may result in death.

Chlamydial infection in pigs generally has an incubation period of 3–11 days. The body temperature may rise to 39–41°C. There may be eye and respiratory symptoms. Polyarthritis with synovitis may be accompanied by disturbances of gait, and weakness may also be present.

GOATS

Chlamydia psittaci is a major cause of abortion in goats (Staub, 1959; McCauly and Tieken, 1968). The organism has been isolated from goat fetus and placental membranes. Keratoconjunctivitis (Eugster et al., 1977) and pneumonia (Omori et al., 1957) are also manifestations of chlamydial infections in goats.

C. psittaci can infect the gastrointestinal tract of goats without causing clinical signs of gastroenteritis. Shedding from the gastrointestinal tract is believed to be an important source of infection.

Recently, Pépin and associates (1985) described the use of ELISA tests for the detection of chlamydial (IgG) antibodies in caprine sera. They used yolk sac grown antigen, employing strain AB3 of *C. psittaci*. Schmeer and co-workers (1986a) found a difference in the immune response of goats that developed abortion and those that remained clinically healthy. The latter animals did not develop IgG1 antibodies to lipopolysaccharides and other low-weight antigens.

SHEEP

In sheep, *C. psittaci* can cause a variety of manifestations that were documented early in the modern era of *C. psittaci* research. In 1950 abortion, in 1952 respiratory tract, in 1955 ocular, and in 1958 intestinal tract infections were described. In 1960 joint and in 1976 neurological manifestations were added to the list of known manifestations of chlamydial infection in sheep (cf Shewen, 1980).

Ovine enzootic abortion is one of the most common causes of perinatal loss of lambs. The ewes usually become infected during the lambing period. Tests for delayed hypersensitivity to *C. psittaci* antigen distinguished animals that did not develop clinical disease from those that were likely to abort (Wilsmore et al., 1986). The infection can also result in stillbirths. In a West German study (Krauss et al., 1988), *C. psittaci* was isolated from 36 of 66 aborting sheep. In Bulgaria it was found in 43% of 2743 aborting sheep, and in Russia, in 56% of 1425 aborting sheep (cf. Martinov and Popov, 1988).

Chlamydia psittaci (*ovis*) (*Colesiota conjunctivae*) may cause keratoconjunctivitis in sheep, a disease also known as "pink eye" or sheep inclusion keratoconjunctivitis (Bogaard, 1984). It is believed that, as in the case of trachoma, immune factors and secondary bacterial infections play a role in the pathogenesis of this disease. Differential diagnoses include infections with *Mycoplasma conjunctivae* and environmental factors such as dust. Prolonged treatment of infected sheep with tetracyclines is recommended.

Enzootic abortion of ewes is a well-recognized condition caused by *C. psittaci*, which is characterized by placentitis (Storz, 1971). The potential for controlling outbreaks of enzootic abortion in sheep by instituting long-acting oxytetracyclines was tested with a negative result (Grieg and Linklater, 1985). It was concluded that such therapy should be implemented in sheep only to control an actual abortion outbreak.

The possibility of *C. psittaci* being transmitted from infected sheep to humans resulting in abortion was demonstrated by Johnson et al. (1985). Thus pregnant woman in sheep-farming areas should be aware of the potential risk. Healthy sheep and lambs can also spread the infection (see also Chapter 33).

CATS

The feline keratoconjunctivitis (FKC) agent has been isolated from the eyes of young kittens. These animals may show mixed papillary and follicular conjunctivitis with occasional scarring of the conjunctiva and pannus formation (Ostler et al., 1969; Darougar et al., 1977a). In one study (Krauss et al., 1988), 5 of 30 cats with conjunctivitis were culture-positive for *C. psittaci*. Adult cats can also be infected by chlamydiae. Gastritis is a recently considered manifestation of *C. psittaci* infection in cats (Gullard et al., 1984). Cats exposed to isolates of *C. psittaci* from the gastric mucosa of other cats with signs of gastric chlamydiasis as aerosol of material from infected culture medium and by oral installation of such materials developed conjunctivitis, rhinitis, and mild gastritis. The findings are consistent with those associated with the feline pneumonitis agent.

Experimental ocular infection with the feline keratoconjunctivitis or pneumonitis agent resulted in severe conjunctivitis in cats (Wills et al., 1987). In other studies (Darougar et al., 1977a), corneal involvement was reported as well.

Chlamydia psittaci infections can also spread to humans (see also Chapter 33). Thus the feline keratoconjunctivitis (pneumonitis) agent is an uncommon cause of conjunctivitis in cat owners (Johnson, 1983). The agent may also rarely be associated with endocarditis and glomerulonephritis in humans (Regan et al., 1978). Severe systemic infection with the feline chlamydial agent was seen in a renal transplant recipient (Griffith et al., 1978).

Vaccines against the feline keratoconjunctivitis agent have had varying protective effect (Willis et al., 1987). Furthermore, the vaccines do not protect against shedding of the organisms.

DOGS

In 1986, genital and ocular infections in dogs were attributed to *C. psittaci* infection. In one study (Krauss et al., 1988) one of eight dogs with conjunctivitis was infected with *C. psittaci*.

Thus, in addition to birds and domestic mammals, pets are also a potential source of chlamydial infection in humans (Elliot et al., 1985).

KOALAS

Chlamydia psittaci infection is common in koalas and may present as conjunctivitis, urethritis, and cystitis. Koalas can die from the chlamydial infection. Infertility caused by upper genital tract infection with *C. psittaci* is a complication that threatens the existence of the koala species in certain areas. Sexual transmission has been the mode of spread of the organism.

Tetracycline therapy effectively eradicates the organism in koalas and has been instituted to save the animal from extermination in areas where the infection occurs.

TWAR Infections

EPIDEMIOLOGY

As already reported in Chapter 1, there has lately been a renewed interest in a group of chlamydial organisms called TWAR agents or TWAR chlamydiae (Saikku et al., 1985, 1986b; Grayston et al., 1986a,b; Kuo et al., 1986a,b). The first TWAR organisms, i.e., TW-183 and IOL-207, were isolated during the late 1960s. In 1972, these U.S. and English chlamydial isolates were found to be antigenically similar in micro-IF tests (Dwyer et al., 1972).

Antibodies against the TWAR organisms are common in the general adult population. About 25% to 45% of healthy adults (as well as STD clinic patients) have been found to have serum IgG TWAR antibodies, as demonstrated in various parts of the world (e.g., the United States, England, Denmark, and Finland). Men usually have a higher prevalence of TWAR antibodies than women (Grayston et al., 1985). Antibodies to *C. trachomatis*, however, occur more often in females than males.

The prevalence rates of serum micro-IF antibodies to TWAR *Chlamydia* reported from England using IOL-207 as antigen are lower than those reported from the U.S. using TW-183 as antigen (Forsey et al., 1986). The prevalence of antibodies to IOL-207 in the general English population seems to have increased steadily over the last decade. Whether a similar change in the prevalence of TWAR antibodies has occurred in the United States is not known. However, if this is the case, it might explain the difference in the antibody prevalence rates in the European and American populations studied, since the U.S. study was performed one year after the English investigation.

Although antibodies to TWAR chlamydiae have been known to occur frequently in the general population, an association of the organism with clinical illness—except for isolated cases of laboratory infections—was not recognized until 1985. That year, Saikku and co-workers (1985) reported an epidemic of mild pneumonia with serological evidence of TWAR etiology. The cases were diagnosed in two communities in northern Finland in 1977–1978. Prospective studies done between 1985 and 1987 also indicated TWAR epidemics among military trainees in Finland during those same years (Saikku et al., 1986b, 1987; Kleemola et al., 1988). No bird contact could be traced in these cases. Human-to-human spread is considered an important mode of transmission of TWAR chlamydiae.

In a study of Seattle students, serological evidence of TWAR infection was obtained in 12% of those with pneumonia, in 5% of those with bronchitis, and in 1% of those with pharyngitis (Grayston et al., 1986b). TWAR agents could be isolated from pharyngeal swabs of 5, 3, and 1% of the cases, respectively.

TWAR infections have been shown to occur endemically (Mordhorst et al., 1986). In Denmark, the incidence of psittacosis/ornithosis cases diagnosed by CF tests increased sharply in 1979 and during 1982–1983. These findings seem to represent Danish TWAR epidemics. Over 50% of assumed Danish cases of ornithosis turned out to be caused by TWAR chlamydiae, as indicated by micro-IF tests (Mordhorst et al., 1986) (Table 9 and Fig. 67).

In Canada, TWAR organisms were assumed to have been the causative agents of community-acquired pneumonia in elderly people (Marrie et al., 1987). In this study, 6% of pneumonia cases presented serological evidence of a TWAR infection. The mean age of the patients was 64 years.

Children can also develop TWAR pneumonia. In Finland TWAR infections have been diagnosed in a 2-year-old child and in school children (Saikku, personal communication).

C. trachomatis was discussed earlier as a possible etiological agent in adult respiratory tract infections on the basis of serological studies (Komaroff et al., 1981, 1983). However, other investigators have not been able to confirm these results by isolation studies or by direct-specimen antigen detection tests (Huss et al., 1985). Recent data suggest that infection with TWAR organisms might have been responsible for the serologically positive cases (Schachter, 1986a,b). Saikku and co-workers (1988) recently found serological evidence of a possible novel manifestation of TWAR infection, namely chronic coronary heart disease (CCHD) and acute myocardial infarction (AMI). In micro-IF tests, 68% and 50% of patients with AMI and CCHD had elevated titers (IgG$\geq$128; IgM$\geq$32) to TWAR antigen as compared to 17% of controls. Of the 40 patients with AMI 68% showed seroconversion in an ELISA with Re-LPS antigen. Whether TWAR infection is a risk factor, like smoking, for AMI in the middle-aged man remains to be established.

CLINICAL FINDINGS

Symptoms and signs in TWAR infections include cough, sore throat, pulmonary rales, and elevated body temperature (Grayston et al., 1986a,b) (Table

31). The ESR is often elevated whereas the white blood cell count usually remains normal (Grayston et al., 1986a,b; Marrie et al., 1987). Very mild and also asymptomatic TWAR infections can be encountered during epidemics (Ekman et al., 1988). Chest X ray often reveals a single lesion, usually in one of the lower lobes (Grayston et al., 1986b). In the Canadian elderly patients with TWAR pneumonia (Marrie et al., 1987), chest X ray usually showed only one lobe to be involved; usually a lower lobe.

Complications found in generalized chlamydial infections affecting the heart, visceral organs, and the central nervous system seem to occur also in TWAR infections. Reactive skin manifestations (e.g., erythema nodosum) and reactive arthritis may be seen in TWAR infections.

Experience in Finland indicates that TWAR infections in elderly persons can be clinically serious and even fatal (the Mikkeli epidemic). In severely ill patients, assisted ventilation may be necessary (Saikku, personal communication). It is noteworthy that two of the Canadian patients with TWAR pneumonia died, although other potentially pathogenic agents were also identified in these cases. Only three of the 18 TWAR patients showed a rise in antibody titer detectable by CF tests (Marrie et al., 1987).

DIAGNOSIS

Isolation of TWAR agents is difficult. TWAR chlamydiae grow poorly in embryonated hen's egg and in tissue cell cultures. Growth of TWAR organisms in tissue cell cultures can be enhanced by a combination of cycloheximide and DEAE treatment and centrifugation of the cell culture (Kuo et al., 1986). Some studies indicate that HeLa 229 cells are more suitable for isolation of TWAR chlamydiae than McCoy cells, although other studies suggest no difference. Three days incubation at 35°C gave a higher yield of TWAR chlamydiae than 2 or 4 days incubation (Kuo et al., 1986b).

Detection of TWAR antigen (EBs) directly from smears from the respiratory tract with the aid of labeled monoclonal antichlamydial antibodies is possible. However, the method is less sensitive than serology and isolation of the organism in cell cultures (Grayston et al., 1986b).

DNA hybridization studies by nick-translated whole chromosomal DNA from strains of *C. trachomatis, C. psittaci,* and TWAR isolates were used to probe chromosomal DNA from these chlamydial strains have been employed for diagnostic purposes. When TWAR DNA was used as the probe, all TWAR isolates gave a strong hybridization signal in dot blot, in contrast to the *C. trachomatis* and *C. psittaci* strains that had significant homology to the TWAR DNA probe. The whole chromosomal TWAR DNA probe represents a potential diagnostic tool for the direct detection of TWAR chlamydiae from clinical specimens (Campbell et al., 1987a,b).

Antibodies formed against TWAR chlamydiae can be detected in chlamydial genus-specific CF tests, but the method is not considered sensitive (30–50%) enough for clinical use. Patients with TWAR pneumonia often have low titers in CF tests, with values generally considered of no importance in *C. psittaci* infections (<64). CF antibodies in TWAR-infected persons (pneumonia cases) can persist for half a year or longer (Saikku, personal communication). As CF response seems to occur earlier during the course of TWAR infections than M-IF response, an ELISA using bacterial Re-LPS (which is cross-reactive with chlamydial LPS) may be used as a more sensitive screening than CF tests (Leinonen et al., 1988). However, the exact TWAR diagnosis should be confirmed by MIF tests.

Formalinized EBs of TWAR strain AR-39 have been used as antigens in micro-IF tests. The micro-IF test is probably the best serological indicator of TWAR infections, but as in micro-IF tests in general, the results can be difficult to interpret. In primary TWAR infections, a IgG micro-IF antibody response can only be detected after several weeks—in many cases after 6–8 weeks (Wang and Grayston, 1986). The micro-IF IgG titers are generally markedly elevated in TWAR pneumonia cases; in one study the mean titer was 256 (range 16–2024). In recurrent TWAR infections, most often encountered in the elderly, IgG antibodies may appear earlier, i.e., after 2 weeks. IgM antibody response might also be absent in recurring TWAR infections (Grayston et al., 1986a). IgG antibodies to TWAR usually appear within the first or second week after onset of severe disease (pneumonia). In the Finnish military recruits with TWAR pneumonia, three-fourths (143/202) (71%) had IgM TWAR antibodies in samples collected 4 days after the manifestation of disease. Most of the recruits had had diffuse respiratory symptoms for several weeks before the sera had been drawn.

If sera from TWAR cases are collected 10 days or 2 weeks apart, as is conventional, a significant antibody response will not be detected, as antibodies are usually formed later during the course of the disease. This might be one explanation for the fact that TWAR infections remained undiscovered until the mid-1980s. Thus if the diagnosis of TWAR infections is based only on routine serological tests, many TWAR cases could be missed.

Of Seattle college students, only those with positive TWAR serology (micro-IF) were culture-positive. The CF test showed evidence of infection by TWAR chlamydiae in 75% of isolation-positive cases and in 69% of micro-IF-positive students. Direct staining of TWAR EBs from swab material of respiratory tract secretion with specific monoclonal antibodies was successful in 67% of isolation-positive cases (Grayston et al., 1986b).

TREATMENT

Tetracycline is the recommended treatment for TWAR infections. Thus a daily dose of 200 mg of doxycycline or 1 g of a tetracycline hydrochloride for 7–

10 days has resulted in complete recovery from acute respiratory tract infections by TWAR agents (Grayston et al., 1986b). As an alternative, 1 g tetracycline hydrochloride per day for 21 days has been recommended. As with psittacosis, recurrences of TWAR infections can occur in patients given tetracyclines.

Erythromycin for 2 weeks was given to TWAR pneumonia patients in the Finnish military epidemic (see above), and the therapeutic result was generally satisfactory. In another series of upper respiratory tract infections, however, erythromycin therapy of TWAR infections proved less effective, often resulting in continuing or recurrent symptoms (Grayston et al., 1986b).

The outcome of both tetracycline and erythromycin therapy is dependent on dose and length of course given. Shortening the therapy to less than 2 weeks increases the recurrence rate. It is noteworthy that adequate therapy with tetracyclines delays development of an (IgG) antibody response in human TWAR infections. A similar observation was also made in the case of psittacosis (Meyer and Eddie, 1956).

Experience indicates that penicillin therapy does not cure TWAR infections.

Genital *Chlamydia trachomatis* Infections and Associated Conditions
Treatment Guidelines, 1985

U.S. Department of Health and Human Services, Public Health Service, Division of Sexually Transmitted Diseases, Center for Prevention Services, Centers for Disease Control, Atlanta, Georgia 30333.

Excerpted from *Morbidity and Mortality Weekly Report* 34(supp 4): 77S–107S, 1985.

These guidelines for treatment of sexually transmitted diseases (STD) were established after careful deliberation by a group of experts and staff of the Centers for Disease Control (CDC). Commentary received after dissemination of preliminary documents to a large group of physicians was also considered. Certain aspects of these guidelines represent the best judgment of experts. These guidelines should not be construed as rules, but rather as a source of guidance within the United States. This is particularly true for topics that are controversial or based on limited data.

Expert Committee members: MF Rein, MD, School of Medicine, University of Virginia; V Caine, MD, Bellflower Clinic, Indianapolis; JH Grossman III, MD, PhD, George Washington University School of Medicine; LT Gutman, MD, Duke University Medical Center; HH Handsfield, MD, Seattle King County Department of Public Health and University of Washington School of Medicine; KK Holmes, MD, PhD, University of Washington School of Medicine, Seattle; JP Luby, MD, University of Texas Southwestern Medical School, Dallas; Z McGee, MD, University of Utah School of Medicine; RC Reichman, MD, University of Rochester School of Medicine; R Rothenberg, MD, MPH, New York State Health Department.

Abbreviations used: AIDS, acquired immunodeficiency syndrome; APPG, aqueous procaine penicillin G; CMRNG, chromosomally mediated resistant *Neisseria gonorrhoeae;* CMV, cytomegalovirus; CSF, cerebrospinal fluid; DIS, disease intervention specialist(s); HCl, hydrochloride; HPV, human papilloma virus; HSV, herpes simplex virus; HTLV-III/LAV, Human T-cell lymphotropic virus type III/lymphadenopathy-associated virus; IM, intramuscularly; IUD, intrauterine device; IV, intravenously; LGV, lymphogranuloma venereum; NGU, nongonococcal urethritis; PID, pelvic inflammatory disease; PPNG, penicillinase-producing *Neisseria gonorrhoeae;* RPR, rapid plasma reagin; STD, sexually transmitted disease(s).

Chlamydia trachomatis Infection

Chlamydia trachomatis is the most prevalent sexually transmitted bacterial pathogen in the United States today. The importance of serious complications of chlamydial infections has been established. Although laboratory tests for detection of *C. trachomatis* are becoming widely available, diagnosis and treatment of these infections are frequently based on the clinical syndrome. The following guidelines are for laboratory-documented infections caused by non-lymphogranuloma venereum strains of *C. trachomatis*.

Please also see *C. trachomatis* discussions under "Gonococcal Infections."

Treatment of Adults

For uncomplicated urethral, endocervical, or rectal infection:

Recommended Regimens

Tetracycline hydrochloride (HCl) 500 mg by mouth 4 times daily for 7 days

OR

Doxycycline 100 mg by mouth twice daily for 7 days

Alternative Regimens
(for patients in whom tetracyclines are contraindicated or not tolerated)

Erythromycin base or stearate 500 mg by mouth 4 times daily for 7 days OR **erythromycin ethylsuccinate** 800 mg by mouth 4 times daily for 7 days.

Sulfonamides are also active against *C. trachomatis*. Although optimal dosages of sulfonamides for chlamydial infection have not been defined, **sulfamethoxazole** 1.0 g by mouth twice daily for 10 days is probably effective.

Management of Sex Partners

All persons exposed to *C. trachomatis* infection should be examined for STD and promptly treated for exposure to *C. trachomatis* with one of the above regimens.

Follow-Up

When taken as directed, the tetracycline and erythromycin regimens listed above are highly effective (> 95% cure rates). Therefore, post-treatment *C. trachomatis* test-of-cure cultures may be omitted if laboratory resources are limited. Test-of-cure cultures may not become positive until 3-6 weeks after treatment. When they are positive, patients should be re-treated with one of the above regimens and any interim sex partners should be treated.

Treatment for Chlamydial Urogenital Infections During Pregnancy

Treatment should be given to women who have proven infection with *C. trachomatis;* if diagnostic tests are not performed, treatment should be given to women with mucopurulent cervicitis and to women whose sex partners have nongonococcal urethritis or nongonococcal epididymitis.

The suggested treatment is **erythromycin base** 500 mg by mouth 4 times daily for 7 days on an empty stomach OR **erythromycin ethylsuccinate** 800 mg by mouth 4 times daily for 7 days. Erythromycin stearate in the same dosage as base may also be effective, but has not been studied. For women who cannot tolerate these regimens, one-half the daily dose (250 mg base, 400 mg ethylsuccinate) 4 times daily should be used for at least 14 days. The optimal dose and duration of antibiotic therapy for pregnant women has not been established. There are no completely studied alternative regimens for women who are allergic to erythromycin or those who cannot tolerate this antibiotic. Proven treatment failures should be re-treated with erythromycin in either of the dosage schedules outlined above.

Simultaneous treatment of male sex partner(s) with tetracycline or doxycycline is an important component of the therapeutic regimen.

Pregnant women at particular risk for chlamydial infections should undergo diagnostic testing for *C. trachomatis* if possible at their first prenatal visit and during the third trimester. Important risk factors include the following: unmarried, age less than 20 years, residence in a socially disadvantaged community (e.g., inner city), and the presence of other sexually transmitted diseases.

Treatment for Established Chlamydial Conjunctivitis of the Newborn

For all cases of ophthalmia neonatorum appropriate tests should be done to rule out *Neisseria gonorrhoeae* as the cause.

The diagnosis of chlamydial conjunctivitis should be established by a laboratory test. Treatment consists of **oral erythromycin syrup** 50 mg/kg/day in 4 divided doses for 2 weeks. Topical therapy provides no additional benefit. If inclusion conjunctivitis recurs after stopping therapy, erythromycin treatment should be reinstituted for an additional 1-2 weeks.

Treatment for Chlamydial Pneumonia of Infancy

For established cases of lower respiratory disease due to *C. trachomatis*, the recommended therapy is **oral erythromycin syrup** 50 mg/kg/day in 4 divided doses for 14 days. The optimal duration for therapy has not been established.

Parents of newborn infants with chlamydial infection should be treated with one of the recommended regimens for chlamydial infection.

Lymphogranuloma Venereum: Genital, Inguinal, or Anorectal

Infection with a lymphogranuloma venereum (LGV) serotype of *C. trachomatis* should be treated in the following way:

Recommended Regimen

Tetracycline HCl 500 mg by mouth 4 times a day for at least 2 weeks

---

Alternative Regimens

The following drugs are active against LGV serotypes *in vitro* but have not been evaluated extensively in culture-confirmed cases.

Doxycycline 100 mg by mouth twice daily for at least 2 weeks; *OR*

Erythromycin 500 mg by mouth 4 times daily for at least 2 weeks; *OR*

Sulfamethoxazole 1.0 g by mouth twice daily for at least 2 weeks. Other sulfonamides can be used in equivalent dosage.

Management of Sex Partners

Sex partners of patients with LGV should be treated with one of the recommended regimens.

Patient Management and Follow-Up

Fluctuant lymph nodes should be aspirated as needed through healthy adjacent normal skin. Incision and drainage or excision of nodes will delay healing and are contraindicated.

Late sequelae such as stricture and/or fistulae may require surgical intervention.

Nongonococcal Urethritis (NGU)

Urethritis not associated with *N. gonorrhoeae* is usually caused by *C. trachomatis* or *Ureaplasma urealyticum*. NGU requires prompt antimicrobial treatment of the patient and evaluation and treatment of sex partners.

Recommended Regimens

Tetracycline HCl 500 mg by mouth 4 times daily for 7 days

OR

Doxycycline 100 mg by mouth twice daily for 7 days

Alternative Regimen

(for patients in whom tetracyclines are contraindicated or not tolerated)

Erythromycin base or stearate 500 mg by mouth 4 times daily for 7 days; *OR*

Erythromycin ethylsuccinate 800 mg by mouth 4 times daily for 7 days.

Management of Sex Partners

All persons who are sex partners of patients with NGU should be examined for STD and promptly treated with one of the above regimens.

Follow-Up

Patients should be advised to return if symptoms persist or recur.

Persistent or Recurrent NGU

Recurrent NGU may be due to failure to treat the sex partners. Patients with persistent or recurrent objective signs of urethritis after adequate treatment of themselves and their partners warrant further evaluation for less common causes of urethritis.

Prevention of Ophthalmia Neonatorum

Instillation of a prophylactic agent into the eyes of all newborn infants is recommended as required by laws in most states. None of the presently recommended approaches for prophylaxis against gonococcal and chlamydial ophthalmia neonatorum is completely effective. Silver nitrate is effective in preventing gonococcal infections but does not prevent chlamydial disease and frequently causes chemical conjunctivitis. Erythromycin is effective in preventing both gonococcal and chlamydial ophthalmia and does not cause chemical conjunctivitis, but the topical use of this drug does not prevent nasopharyngeal chlamydial infection or pneumonia. Furthermore, erythromycin prophylaxis is considerably more expensive than silver nitrate prophylaxis. Tetracycline ointment has not been as extensively evaluated as has erythromycin but appears to be as effective. Whichever type of prophylaxis is used, it should be implemented no later than 1 hour after birth—preferably immediately after delivery since delayed application may reduce efficacy.

Recommended Regimens

Erythromycin (0.5%) ophthalmic ointment, tetracycline (1%) ointment, OR silver nitrate should be instilled into the eyes of all neonates as soon as possible after delivery and never later than 1 hour after birth. Single-use tubes or ampules are preferable to multiple-use tubes.

The efficacy of tetracycline and erythromycin in the prevention of PPNG ophthalmia is unknown. Bacitracin is NOT recommended.

Acute Pelvic Inflammatory Disease (PID)
(Endometritis, Salpingitis, Parametritis, and/or Peritonitis)

Acute PID refers to the acute clinical syndrome (unrelated to pregnancy or surgery) attributed to the ascent of microorganisms from the vagina and endocervix to the endometrium, fallopian tubes, and/or contiguous structures. Many cases of PID are caused by more than one organism.

Etiologic agents include *N. gonorrhoeae*, *C. trachomatis*, anaerobic bacteria (which include Bacteroides and gram-positive cocci), facultative gram-negative bacilli (such as *Escherichia coli*), *Mycoplasma hominis*, and rarely *Actinomyces israelii*. In the individual patient it is often impossible to differentiate among these agents. Treatment regimens should be used which are active against the broadest possible range of these pathogens.

Hospitalization and Inpatient Treatment

Hospitalization of patients with acute PID is indicated when (1) the diagnosis is uncertain, (2) surgical emergencies such as appendicitis and ectopic pregnancy cannot be excluded, (3) a pelvic abscess is suspected, (4) the patient is pregnant, (5) the patient is a prepubertal child, (6) severe illness precludes outpatient management, (7) the patient is unable to follow or tolerate an outpatient regimen, (8) the patient has failed to respond to outpatient therapy, or (9) clinical follow-up within 72 hours of starting antibiotic treatment cannot be arranged. Many experts recommend that all patients with PID be hospitalized for treatment. Special consideration for hospitalization should be given to adolescents because their compliance with therapy is unpredictable and the long-term sequelae of PID are particularly severe in this group.

Rationale for Selection of Antimicrobials

The treatment of choice is not established. No single agent is active against the entire spectrum of pathogens. Several antimicrobial combinations do provide a broad spectrum of activity against the major pathogens *in vitro*, but none have been adequately evaluated for clinical efficacy in PID.

Examples of Combination Regimens with Broad Activity Against Major Pathogens in PID

Regimen A

Doxycycline 100 mg IV twice daily PLUS **Cefoxitin** 2.0 g IV 4 times daily

Continue drugs IV for at least 4 days and at least 48 hours after the patient improves. Then continue doxycycline 100 mg by mouth twice a day to complete 10-14 days total therapy.

Regimen B

Clindamycin 600 mg IV 4 times daily PLUS **Gentamicin** 2.0 mg/kg IV followed by 1.5 mg/kg 3 times daily in patients with normal renal function

Continue drugs IV for at least 4 days and at least 48 hours after patient improves. Then continue clindamycin 450 mg by mouth 4 times daily to complete 10-14 days total therapy.

Ambulatory Treatment

When the patient is not hospitalized, the following regimen is recommended.

Recommended Regimens

Cefoxitin 2.0 g IM OR **amoxicillin** 3.0 g by mouth OR **ampicillin** 3.5 g by mouth OR **aqueous procaine penicillin G** 4.8 million units IM at 2 sites OR **ceftriaxone** 250 mg IM. Each of these regimens except ceftriaxone is accompanied by **probenecid** 1.0 g by mouth

FOLLOWED BY

Doxycycline 100 mg by mouth twice daily for 10-14 days

Tetracycline HCl 500 mg 4 times daily may be substituted for doxycycline but is less active against certain anaerobes and requires more frequent dosing; these are potentially important drawbacks in the treatment of PID.

Treatment with penicillin, ampicillin, amoxicillin, or
a cephalosporin alone is not recommended

Comment: Cefoxitin or ceftriaxone (or equivalently effective cephalosporins) plus doxycycline (or tetracycline) provide activity against *N. gonorrhoeae*, including PPNG, and *C. trachomatis*. PPNG-associated PID is not adequately treated with the combination of doxycycline with either amoxicillin, ampicillin, or aqueous procaine penicillin. Single doses of penicillin or cephalosporin antibiotic followed by oral tetracycline may not provide sustained activity against many strains of chromosomally mediated resistant *N. gonorrhoeae* or the facultative or anaerobic organisms involved in PID. No data are available on therapy for PID caused by CMRNG. These patients should be followed in consultation with an expert.

Management of Sex Partners

All male sex partners of patients with PID should be examined for STD and promptly treated with a regimen effective against uncomplicated gonococcal and chlamydial infection.

Acute Pelvic Inflammatory Disease in Children

PID in prepubertal children is rare. Data on effective treatment are not available. Adolescents should receive a regimen that treats both *N. gonorrhoeae* and *C. trachomatis* and may receive one of the regimens recommended for adults. Prepubertal children may receive either:

Cefuroxime 150 mg/kg/IV daily OR **ceftriaxone** 100 mg/kg/IV daily

PLUS

Erythromycin 40 mg/kg/day in 4 doses IV OR **sulfasoxazole** 100 mg/kg/day in 4 doses IV OR in children older than 7 years **tetracycline** 30 mg/kg/day in 3 doses IV.

Continue the IV regimen for at least 4 days and at least 2 days after patient shows marked improvement. Thereafter continue the erythromycin, sulfasoxazole, or tetracycline orally to complete at least 14 days of therapy.

Follow-Up

All patients treated as outpatients should be clinically reevaluated within 72 hours. Those not responding favorably should be hospitalized. A culture for test-of-cure should be done 4-7 days after completion of therapy as appropriate for pathogens initially isolated.

Intrauterine Device (IUD)

The IUD is a risk factor for the development of PID. Although the exact effect of removing an IUD on the response of acute salpingitis to antimicrobial therapy and on the risk of recurrent salpingitis is unknown, removal of the IUD is recommended soon after antimicrobial therapy has been initiated. When an IUD is removed, contraceptive counseling is necessary.

Other Genito-Urinary Syndromes

In Men

Acute Epididymo-Orchitis

Acute epididymo-orchitis has two forms: a sexually transmitted form usually associated with urethritis and commonly caused by *C. trachomatis* and/or *N. gonorrhoeae* and a non-sexually transmitted form associated with urinary tract infections caused by Enterobacteriaceae or *Pseudomonas*. Urine should be examined by Gram stain and culture to exclude bacteruria in all patients, including those with urethritis. Testicular torsion is a surgical emergency that should be considered in all cases.

Sexually Transmitted Epididymo-Orchitis

Sexually transmitted epididymo-orchitis occurs in young adults and is associated with presence of urethritis, absence of underlying genito-urinary pathology, and absence of gram-negative rods on Gram stain of urine.

Recommended Regimen

Amoxicillin 3.0 g by mouth OR **ampicillin** 3.5 g by mouth OR **aqueous procaine penicillin G** 4.8 million units IM at 2 sites (each along with **probenecid** 1.0 g by mouth) OR **spectinomycin** 2.0 g IM OR **ceftriaxone** 250 mg IM

FOLLOWED BY

Tetracycline HCl 500 mg by mouth 4 times daily for 10 days

OR

Doxycycline 100 mg by mouth twice daily for 10 days

OR

(for patients for whom tetracyclines are contraindicated or not tolerated)

Erythromycin base or stearate 500 mg by mouth 4 times a day for 7 days OR **erythromycin ethylsuccinate** 800 mg by mouth 4 times a day for 7 days

Alternative Regimens

Alternative regimens have not been well studied. For epididymitis caused by PPNG, clinical experience is limited, but a 10-day course of therapy with oral **trimethoprim/sulfamethoxazole** OR parenteral **ceftriaxone, cefotaxime, cefoxitin**, or **spectinomycin** may be used.

Management of Sex Partners

Sex partners of patients with sexually transmitted acute epididymo-orchitis should be examined for STD and promptly treated with a rogimen effective against uncomplicated gonococcal and chlamydial infection.

Adjuncts to Therapy

Bed rest and scrotal elevation until fever and local inflammation have subsided are recommended.

Follow-Up

Failure to improve within 3 days requires reevaluation of the diagnosis/therapy and consideration for hospitalization.

Nonsexually Transmitted Acute Epididymo-Orchitis

Management includes prompt administration of broad-spectrum antimicrobial therapy. Choice of therapy is initially dictated by the severity of infection and later by results of urine culture and sensitivity. Evaluation for underlying urinary tract disease is indicated. Adjuncts to therapy and follow-up are the same as for sexually transmitted epididymo-orchitis.

Mucopurulent Cervicitis

The presence of mucopurulent endocervical exudate often suggests cervicitis due to chlamydial or gonococcal infection. Criteria for the presumptive diagnosis of mucopurulent cervicitis include: (1) mucopurulent secretion from the endocervix which may appear yellow or green when viewed on a white cotton-tipped swab (positive swab test); (2) greater than 10 polymorphonuclear leukocytes per microscopic oil immersion field (X 1,000) in a gram-stained smear of endocervical secretions; and (3) cervicitis, determined by cervical friability (bleeding when the first swab culture is taken) and/or by erythema or edema within a zone of cervical ectopy.

Treatment of mucopurulent cervicitis:

1. If *N. gonorrhoeae* is found on Gram stain or culture of endocervical or urethral discharge, treatment should be given as recommended for uncomplicated gonorrhea in adults.
2. If *N. gonorrhoeae* is not found, treatment should be given as recommended for chlamydial infection in adults.

Management of Sex Partners

Men exposed to women with mucopurulent cervicitis attributed to gonococcal or chlamydial infection should be evaluated for STD and treated with the same regimen as their sex partners.

Follow-Up

Follow-up cultures for *N. gonorrhoeae* or *C. trachomatis* isolated before therapy should be conducted as outlined in special sections for these organisms.

Urethral Syndrome (Dysuria-Pyuria Syndrome)

Women with dysuria, frequency, pyuria (greater than 10 leukocytes per 400X field on microscopic examination of urinary sediment), and a negative gram-stained smear of unspun urine have the acute urethral syndrome and may be infected with *C. trachomatis* or with *N. gonorrhoeae*. Cultures of the urethra or cervix are needed to identify these agents in individual patients.

Dysuria may also be due to either vaginitis or genital herpes simplex virus (HSV) infection. Patients with dysuria should be evaluated for these infections, as well as for those outlined above.

Recommended Regimens

Initial treatment of patients with dysuria-pyuria syndrome with **tetracycline HCl** 500 mg by mouth 4 times daily for 7 days or **doxycycline** 100 mg by mouth twice daily for 7 days is usually effective. Management of patients should be based on clinical response to therapy.

Special Treatment-Related Discussions

These recommendations are limited to the management of sexually transmitted infections. Appropriate management of medical-legal aspects, potential pregnancy, and physical and psychological trauma are also an integral part of management.

There are no firm data with which to estimate the risk of a sexually assaulted person's contracting a sexually transmitted infection. Based on the prevalence of infections in the general population, the most likely diseases for which these patients are at risk appear to be chlamydial infections, gonorrhea, genital herpes, cytomegalovirus, and trichomoniasis. If the offender is at high risk for having syphilis and hepatitis B, there is an increased risk of the victim's acquiring these diseases.

Rape

Initial examination of the rape victim should include:

- Cultures for *N. gonorrhoeae* from any potentially infected sites.
- If available, cultures for *C. trachomatis* from any potentially infected sites.
- Examination of vaginal specimens for *T. vaginalis* by wet mount and, if available, by culture.
- A bimanual pelvic examination for women.
- A serologic test for syphilis.
- A sample of serum to be frozen and saved for future testing.

The risk of infection after rape, while unknown, is thought to be low. If prophylaxis is to be administered because the physician feels it is indicated or because the patient requests it, the following should be used: **Tetracycline** 500 mg by mouth 4 times daily for 7 days or **doxycycline** 100 mg by mouth twice daily for 7 days.

Patients who are allergic to tetracycline and pregnant women should be treated with **amoxicillin** 3.0 g or **ampicillin** 3.5 g, each given with 1.0 g of **probenecid** as a single oral dose.

Patients should be seen for medical follow-up in 7 days, and the aforementioned studies repeated, except for the serologic test for syphilis. A serologic test for syphilis, 6 weeks after the incident, is important in cases of assault by individuals who are at high risk for syphilis.

Every effort should be made to establish whether the assailant is infected with an STD. Victims should receive treatment for exposure to an STD which is documented in the assailant.

Sexual Abuse of Children

Sexual abuse (including incest) of children is one aspect of the larger problem of child abuse and neglect. Diagnosis of any sexually transmitted infection in a child who is prepubertal but not neonatal raises the strong possibility of sexual abuse unless proven otherwise. The presence of an STD may be the major or only physical evidence of sexual abuse and may be asymptomatic. Therefore, particular care in the evaluation of a child for STD is appropriate.

Sexually abused children are best assessed and managed by a team of professionals who are experienced in addressing their medical, social, and psychological needs. Members of such a team commonly include a pediatrician, gynecologist, and social worker who coordinate their efforts and function as a part of the child protection services for their community.

The assessment and management of children suspected of having been sexually abused is beyond the scope of this statement (see references below). However, several common issues should be noted:

a. An internal pelvic examination is not necessarily indicated unless there is evidence of trauma or a foreign body. If an internal pelvic examination is to be performed, many children will require general anesthesia.

b. The results of cultures may be required to be legally admissible as evidence in court proceedings resulting from a diagnosis of sexual abuse. Accordingly, the physician caring for the child is responsible for ensuring that correct procedures are used in identifying specimens and conveying them to the laboratory and that accurate identification of isolates has occurred.

c. In all states, reporting of suspected as well as confirmed cases of sexual abuse to the social services department of city, county, and/or state governments is legally mandatory.

d. The safety and welfare of the child is of paramount concern. If sexual abuse or incest has occurred or is suspected, it may be necessary to hospitalize the child pending an investigation into the safety of the household for the child.

Children with known or suspected sexual abuse should be assessed for the following infections from the following body sites:

Females

- *N. gonorrhoeae* culture from pharynx, anal canal, and vagina.
  NOTE: Endocervical cultures are not necessary.
- *C. trachomatis* culture from pharynx, vagina, and rectum.
- Trichomonas from urine and vagina.
- Herpes simplex culture from vagina, rectum, urethra, or eye area if inflammation is present.
- Serologic tests for syphilis.
- Examination for venereal warts.
- Examination for vaginitis with a wet mount for clue cells.
- Examination for pregnancy if appropriate.

Males

- *N. gonorrhoeae* culture from pharynx, rectum, and urethra.
- *C. trachomatis* culture from rectum, pharynx, and urethra.
- Herpes simplex culture from areas of genital tract which show inflammation.
- Serologic tests for syphilis.
- Examination for venereal warts.

Treatment is indicated when disease is present. Prophylactic treatment prior to diagnosis is usually not indicated unless there is evidence that the assailant is infected. Follow-up cultures and a serology are required in cases of acute assault or molestation.

References

Sgroi S. Handbook of Clinical Intervention in Child Sexual Abuse. Lexington, Massachusetts: Lexington Books, D.C. Health & Co., 1982.

White ST, Loda FA, Ingram DL, Parson A. Sexually transmitted diseases in sexually abused children. Pediatrics 1983;72:16-21.

Rimsza ME, Niggemann EH. Medical evaluation of sexually abused children: A review of 311 cases. Pediatrics 1982;69:8-14.

Neinstein LS, Goldenring J, Carpenter S. Nonsexual transmission of sexually transmitted diseases: An infrequent occurrence. Pediatrics 1984;74:67-76.

References

Adger, H.; Shafer, M.A.; Sweet, R.L.; Schachter, J. Screening for *Chlamydia trachomatis* and *Neisseria gonorrhoeae* in adolescent males: value of first-catch urine examination. Lancet ii:944–945, 1984.

Adler, M.W.; Belsey, E.H.; O'Connor, B.H. Morbidity associated with pelvic inflammatory disease. Br. J. Vener. Dis. 58:151–157, 1982.

Ahlqvist, J.; Andersson, L. Methyl green-pyronin staining: Effects of fixation; use in routine pathology. Stain Technol. 47:17–22, 1972.

Alani, M.D.; Darougas, S.; MacBurns, D.C.; Thin, R.N.; Dunn, H. Isolation of *Chlamydia trachomatis* from the male urethra. Br. J. Vener. Dis. 53:88–92, 1977.

Alexander, E.R.; Chiang, W.T. Infection of pregnant monkeys and their offspring with TRIC agents. Am. J. Ophthalmol. 63:1145–1153, 1967.

Alexander, E.R.; Harrison, H.R. Role of *Chlamydia trachomatis* in perinatal infection. Rev. Infect. Dis. 5:713–719, 1983.

Alexander, E.R.; Wang, S.-P.; Grayston, J.T. Further classification of TRIC agents from ocular trachoma and other sources by mouse toxicity prevention test. Am. J. Ophthalmol. 63:1469–1478, 1967.

Alexander, E.R.; Skahen, P.; Holmes, K.K. Antibiotic susceptibility of *Chlamydia trachomatis* in cell culture. In: Nongonococcal Urethritis and Related Infections. Hobson, D.; Holmes, K.K. Washington, D.C.: American Society for Microbiology, 1977, pp. 223–226.

Alexander, E.R.; Harrison, H.R.; Lewis, M.; Sim, D.A.; Podgore, J.K. Strategies for prevention of infant chlamydial disease. In: Chlamydial Infections. Mårdh, P.-A.; Holmes, K.K.; Oriel, J.D.; Piot, P.; Schachter, J. eds. Amsterdam: Elsevier Biomedical Press, 1982, pp. 225–228.

Alexander, I.; Paul, I.D.; Caul, E.O. Evaluation of a genus reactive monoclonal antibody in rapid identification of *Chlamydia trachomatis* by direct immunofluorescence. Genitourin. Med. 61:252–254, 1985.

Allan, I. Chlamydial antigenic structure and genetics. In: Chlamydial Infections. Oriel, D.; Ridgway, G.; Schachter, J.; Taylor-Robinson, D.; Ward, M., eds. Cambridge: Cambridge University Press, 1986, pp. 73–80.

Allan, I.; Cunningham, T.M.; Lovett, M.A. Molecular cloning of the major outer membrane protein of *Chlamydia trachomatis*. Infect. Immun. 45:637–641, 1984.

Allen, J.H. Inclusion blennorrhea. Am. J. Ophthalmol. 27:833–846, 1944.

Amman, R.; Zehender, O.; Jenny, S.; Bass, G. Die Perihepatitis acuta Gonorrhoica (Fitz-Hugh–Curtis Syndrome) (in German). Deutsche Med. Wsch. 96:1515–1519, 1971.

Amor, B.; Kahan, A.; Lecoq, F.; Delbarre, F. Le test de transformation lymphoblastique par des antigènes bedsonieus (TTL Bedsonieu) (in French). Rev. Rhum. 39:671–676, 1972.

Amortegui, A.J.; Meyer, M.P. Enzyme immunoassay for detection of *Chlamydia trachomatis* from the cervix. Obstet. Gynecol. 65:523–526, 1985.

Amsel, R.; Totten, P.A.; Spiegel, C.A.; Chen, K.C.S.; Eschenbach, D.A.; Holmes, K.K. Nonspecific vaginitis: Diagnostic criteria and microbial and epidemiological associations. Am. J. Med. 74:14–22, 1983.

Andersen, P.; Møller, B.R. Autoantibodies in patients with acute salpingitis caused by *Chlamydia trachomatis*. Scand. J. Infect. Dis. 14:19–21, 1982.

Andrews, B.E.; Major, R.; Palmer, S.R. Ornithosis in poultry workers. Lancet i:632–634, 1981.

Anon, J. Ornithosis in poultry workers. Vet. Record. 108:155, 1981.

Aral, S.O.; Cates, W. The increasing concern with infertility. Why now? JAMA 250:2327–2331, 1983.

Aral, S.O.; Mosher, W.D.; Cates, W. Contraceptive use, pelvic inflammatory disease, and fertility problems among American women: 1982. Am. J. Obstet. Gynecol. 157:59–64, 1987.

Arya, O.P.; Mallinson, H.; Goddard, A.D. Epidemiological and clinical correlates of chlamydial infection of the cervix. Br. J. Vener. Dis. 57:118–124, 1981.

Arya, O.P.; Mallison, H.; Andrews, B.E.; Sillis, M. Diagnosis of urethritis: role of polymorphonuclear counts in gram-stained urethral smears. Sex. Transm. Dis. 11:10–17, 1984.

Arya, O.P.; Hobson, D.; Hart, C.A.; Bartozokas, C.; Pratt, B.C. Evaluation of ciprofloxacin 500 mg twice daily for one week in treating uncomplicated gonococcal chlamydial and non-specific urethritis in men. Genitourin. Med. 62:170–174, 1986.

Ashley, C.R.; Richmond, S.J.; Caul, E.O. Identification of the elementary bodies of *Chlamydia trachomatis* in the electron microscope by an indirect immunoferritin technique. J. Clin. Microbiol. 2:327–331, 1975.

Assaad, F.A.; Maxwell-Lyons, F. The application of clinical scoring systems to trachoma research. Am. J. Ophthalmol. 63:1327–1356, 1967.

Attenburrow, A.A.; Baker, C.M. Chlamydial pneumonia in the low birth weight neonate. Arch. Dis. Child. 60:1169–1172, 1985.

Attiah, M.A.H.; El Togby, A.F. Factors influencing the course of trachoma. Bull. Ophth. Soc. Egypt. 30:137–142, 1937.

Ballard, R.C. The epidemiology and immunopathology of chlamydial infections in southern Africa. Academic dissertation. University of Witwatersrand, 1982.

Banck, G.; Forsgren, A. Many bacterial species are mitogenic for human blood B lymphocytes. Scand. J. Immunol. 8:347–354, 1978.

Barbucci, M.B.; Spence, M.R.; Kappus, E.W.; Burkman, R.C.; Rao, L.; Quinn, T.C. Postabortal endometritis and isolation of *Chlamydia trachomatis*. Obstet. Gynecol. 68:686–690, 1986.

Bard, J.; Levitt, D. *Chlamydia trachomatis* stimulates human peripheral blood B lymphocytes to proliferate and secrete polyclonal immunoglobulins in vitro. Infect. Immun. 43:84–92, 1984.

Barnes, R.C.; Roddy, R.E.; Stamm, W.E. Serovars of *Chlamydia trachomatis* causing repeated genital infection. In: Chlamydial Infections. Oriel, D.; Ridgway, G.; Schachter, J.; Taylor-Robinson, D.; Ward, M. eds. Cambridge: Cambridge University Press, 1986, pp. 503–506.

Barron, A.A. Contributions of animal models to the study of human chlamydial infections. In: Chlamydial Infections. Mårdh, P.-A.; Holmes, K.K.; Oriel, J.D.; Piot, P; Schachter, J. eds. Amsterdam: Elsevier Biomedical Press, 1982, pp. 357–366.

Barron, A.L.; White, H.J.; Rank, R.G.; Soloff, B.L. Target tissues associated with genital infection of female guinea pigs by the chlamydial agent of guinea pig inclusion conjunctivitis. J. Infect. Dis. 139:60–68, 1979.

Barron, A.L.; White, H.J.; Rank, R.G.; Soloff, B.L.; Moses, E.B. A new animal model for the study of *Chlamydia trachomatis* genital infections: Infection of mice with the agent of mouse pneumonitis. J. Infect. Dis. 143:63–66, 1981.

Barron, A.L.; Rank, R.G.; Moses, E.B. Immune response in mice infected in the genital tract with mouse pneumonitis agent (*Chlamydia trachomatis* biovar). Infect. Immun. 44:82–85, 1984.

Barry, W.C.; Teare, E.L.; Uttby, A.H.C.; Wilson, S.A.; McManus, T.J.; Lim, K.S.; Gdmsu, H.; Price, J.F. *Chlamydia trachomatis* as a cause of neonatal conjunctivitis. Arch. Dis. Child. 61:797–799, 1986.

Barsoum, I.S.; Mostafa, M.S.E.; Shibab, A.A.; El Alamy, M.; Habib, M.A.; Colley, D.G. Prevalence of trachoma in school children and ophthalmological outpatients in rural Egypt. Am. J. Trop. Med. Hyg. 36:97–101, 1987.

Barton, S.E.; Thomas, B.J.; Taylor-Robinson, D.; Goldmeier, D. Detection of *Chlamydia trachomatis* in the vaginal vault of women who have had hysterectomies. Br. Med. J. 291:250, 1985.

Barwell, C.F. Some observations on the antigenic structure of psittacosis and lymphogranuloma venereum viruses. I. Preparation and use in complement-fixation tests of antisera from different sources. Br. J. Exp. Pathol. 33:258–267, 1952.

Barwell, C.F.; Dunlop, E.M.C.; Race, J.W. Results of complement-fixation and intradermal tests for Bedsoniae in genital infection, disease of the eye and Reiter's disease. Am. J. Ophthalmol. 63:1527–1534, 1967.

Batteiger, B.E.; Rank, R.G. Antigenic specificity of the humoral immune response to chlamydial genital infection in guinea pigs. In: Chlamydial Infections. Oriel, D., Ridgway, G., Schachter, J.; Taylor-Robinson, D.; Ward, M. eds. Cambridge: Cambridge University Press, 1986, pp. 453–456.

Baum, J.L. Current concepts in ophthalmology. Ocular infections. N. Engl. J. Med. 299:28–31, 1978.

Bavoil, P.; Ohlin, A.; Schachter, J. Role of disulfide bonding in outer membrane structure and permeability in *Chlamydia trachomatis*. Infect. Immun. 44:479–485, 1984.

Becker, Y. The chlamydiae: molecular biology of procaryotic obligate parasites of eucaryotes. Microbiol. Rev. 42:274–306, 1978.

Bedson, S.P.; Western, G.T.; Levy-Simpson, S. Observations of the aetiology of psittacosis. Lancet i:235–236, 1930.

Beem, M.O.; Saxon, E.M. Respiratory-tract colonization and a distinctive pneumonia syndrome in infants infected with *Chlamydia trachomatis*. N. Engl. J. Med. 296:306–310, 1977.

Beem, M.O.; Saxon, E.M. *Chlamydia trachomatis* infections in infants. In: Chlamydial Infections. Mårdh, P.-A.; Holmes, K.K.; Oriel, J.D.; Piot, P.; Schachter, J. eds. Amsterdam: Elsevier Biomedical Press, 1982, pp. 199–212.

Beem, M.O.; Saxon, E.M.; Tipple, M.A. Treatment of chlamydial pneumonia of infancy. Pediatrics 63:198–203, 1979.

Beer, R.J.S.; Bradford, W.P.; Hart, R.J.S. Pregnancy complicated by psittacosis acquired from sheep. Br. Med. J. 284:1156–1157, 1982.

Van der Bel-Kahn, J.M.; Watanakunakorn, C.; Menefee, M.G.; Long, H.D.; Dicter, R. *Chlamydia trachomatis* endocarditis. Am. Heart J. 95:627–636, 1978.

Bell, T.A. Major sexually transmitted diseases of children and adolescents. Ped. Infect. Dis. 2:153–161, 1983.

Bell, T.A. *Chlamydia trachomatis, Mycoplasma hominis* and *Ureaplasma urealyticum* infections of infants. Sem. Perinatol. 9:29–37, 1985.

Bell, T.A.; Kuo, C.-C.; Stamm, W.F.; Tam, M.R.; Stephens, R.S.; Holmes, K.K.; Grayston, J.T. Direct fluorescent monoclonal antibody stain for rapid detection of infant *Chlamydia trachomatis* infections. Pediatrics 74:224–228, 1984.

Bell, T.A.; Hein, K. Adolescents and sexually transmitted diseases. In: Sexually Transmitted Diseases. Holmes, K.K.; Mårdh, P.-A.; Sparling, P.F.; Wiesner, P.J. eds. New York: McGraw-Hill, 1984, pp. 73–84.

Bell, T.A.; Stamm, W.E.; Kuo, C.C.; Holmes, K.K.; Grayston, J.T. Chronic *Chlamydia trachomatis* infections in infants. In: Chlamydial Infections. Oriel, D.; Ridgway, G.; Schachter, J.; Taylor-Robinson, D.; Ward, M. eds. Cambridge: Cambridge University Press, 1986, pp. 305–308.

Benedict, A.A.; O'Brien, E. A passive hemagglutination reaction for psittacosis. J. Immunol. 80:94–99, 1958.

Bengtsson, A.; Ahlstrand, C.; Lindström, F.D.; Kihlström, E. Bacteriological findings in 25 patients with Reiter's syndrome (reactive arthritis). Scand. J. Rheumatol. 12:157–160, 1983.

Berger, R.E. Epididymitis. In: Sexually Transmitted Diseases. Holmes, K.K.; Mårdh, P.A.; Sparling, F.; Wiesner, P. eds. New York: McGraw-Hill, 1984, pp. 650–662.

Berger, R.E.; Alexander, E.R.; Monda, G.D.; Ansell, J.; McCormick, G.; Holmes, K.K. *Chlamydia trachomatis* as a cause of acute "idiopathic" epididymitis. N. Engl. J. Med. 298:301–304, 1978.

Berger, R.E.; Alexander, E.R.; Harnisch, J.P.; Paulsen, C.A.; Monda, G.D.; Ansell, J.; Holmes, K.K. Etiology, manifestations and therapy of acute epididymitis: prospective study of 50 cases. J. Urol. 121:750–754, 1979.

Berger, R.E.; Holmes, K.K.; Mayo, M.E.; Reed, R. The clinical use of epididymal aspiration cultures in the management of selected patients with acute epididymitis. J. Urol. 124:60–61, 1980.

Bernkopf, H. The susceptibility of white mice to a strain of trachoma virus and their use in neutralization tests. Bull. Res. Council Israel 8E:25–29, 1959.

Bernstein; D.I.; Hubbard, T.; Wenman, W.M.; Johnson, B.L.; Holmes, K.K.; Liebhaber, H.; Schachter, J.; Barnes, R.; Lovett, M.A. Mediastinal and supraclavicular lymphadenitis due to *Chlamydia trachomatis* serovars L1 and L2. N. Engl. J. Med. 311:1543–1546, 1984.

Bhopal, R.S.; Thomas, G.O. Psittacosis presenting with Reiter's syndrome. Br. Med. J. 284:1606, 1982.

Bialasiewicz, A.A.; Jahn, G.J. Mehrjähriger Verlaufeiner Oculogenitalen Chlamydieninfektion (in German). Klin. Mbl. Augenheilk. 190:50–52, 1987.

Bienenstock, J.; Befus, A.D. Some thoughts on the biologic role of immunoglobulin A. Gastroenterology 84:178–185, 1983.

Bietti, G.B.; Guerra, P.; Vozza, R.; Felici, A.; Ghione, M.; Lolli, B.; Buogo, A.; Saolomons, R.; Kebreth, Y. Results of a large scale vaccination against trachoma in East Africa (Ethiopia) 1960–1965. Am. J. Ophthalmol. 61:1010–1029, 1966.

Bietti, G.B.; Soldati, M.; Isetta, A.M.; Intini, C.; Ghione, M. Some aspects of immunity in trachoma. Israel. J. Med. Sci. 8:1124–1129, 1972.

Birkhead, J.S.; Apostolov, K. Endocarditis caused by a psittacosis agent. Br. Heart J. 36:728–731, 1974.

Bischoff, W. Ofloxacin: therapeutic results in *Chlamydia trachomatis* urethritis. Infection, 14 Suppl. 4:S316–317, 1986.

Black, S.B.; Grossman, M.; Cles, L.; Schachter, J. Serologic evidence of chlamydial infection in children. J. Pediatr. 98:65–67, 1981.

Blyth, W.; Taverne, J. Cultivation of TRIC agents: a comparison between the use of BHK 21 and irradiated McCoy cells. J. Hyg. (Cambr.) 72:121–128, 1974.

Bogaard, A.E. Jr. Inclusion keratoconjunctivitis ("pink eye") in sheep. A proposal for a new name for chlamydial keratoconjunctivitis in sheep and comment on recent clinical trials. Vet. Q. 6:229–235, 1984.

von Bogaert, L.J. Diagnostic aid of endometrium biopsy. Gynecol. Obstet. Invest. 10:289–297, 1979.

Bollerup, A.C.; Kristensen, G.B.; Mårdh, P.-A.; Livel, I. Laboratory diagnosis of *Chlamydia trachomatis* infection in patients with acute salpingitis. In: Chlamydial Infections. Mårdh, P.-A.; Holmes, K.K.; Oriel, J.D.; Piot, P.; Schachter, J. eds. Amsterdam: Elsevier Biomedical Press, 1982, pp. 171–174.

Bone, N.L.; Greene, R.R. Histologic study of uterine tubes with tubal pregnancy. Am. J. Obstet. Gynecol. 82:1166–1170, 1961.

Bowie, W.R. Comparison of gram stain and first-voided urine sediment in the diagnosis of urethritis. Sex. Transm. Dis. 5:39–42, 1978.

Bowie, W.R. Treatment of chlamydial infections. In: Chlamydial Infections. Mårdh, P.-A.; Holmes, K.K.; Oriel, J.D.; Piot, P.; Schachter, J. eds. Amsterdam: Elsevier Biomedical Press, 1982, pp. 231–244.

Bowie, W.R. Urethritis in males. In: Sexually Transmitted Diseases. Holmes, K.K.; Mårdh, P.-A.; Sparling, P.F.; Wiesner, P.J. eds. New York: McGraw-Hill, 1984, pp. 638–650.

Bowie, W.R.; Wang, S.-P.; Alexander, E.R.; Floyd, J.; Forsyth, P.S.; Pollock, H.M.; Lin J.L.; Buchanan, T.M.; Holmes, K.K. Etiology of nongonococcal urethritis: evidence for *Chlamydia trachomatis* and *Ureaplasma urealyticum*. J. Clin. Invest. 59:735–742, 1977a.

Bowie, W.R.; Alexander, E.R.; Holmes, K.K. Chlamydial pharyngitis? Sex. Transm. Dis. 4:140–141, 1977b.

Bowie, W.R.; Jones, H. Acute pelvic inflammatory disease in outpatients: association with *Chlamydia trachomatis* and *Neisseria gonorrhoeae*. Ann. Intern. Med. 95:685–688, 1981.

Bowie, W.R.; Alexander, E.R.; Holmes, H.H. Eradication of *Chlamydia trachomatis* from the urethra of men with nongonococcal urethritis. Sex. Transm. Dis. 8:79–81, 1981.

Bowie, W.R.; Manzon, L.M.; Borrie-Hume, C.J.; Fawcett, A.; Jones, H.D. Efficacy of treatment regimens for lower urogenital *Chlamydia trachomatis* infections in women. Am. J. Obstet. Gynecol. 142:125–129, 1982.

Bowie, W.R.; Willets, V., Sibau, L. Failure of norfloxacin to eradicate *Chlamydia trachomatis* in non-gonococcal urethritis. Antimicrob. Agents Chemother. 30:594–597, 1986a.

Bowie, W.R.; Yu, J.S.; Jones, H.D. Partial efficacy of clindamycin against *Chlamydia trachomatis* in men with non-gonococcal urethritis. Sex. Transm. Dis. 13:76–80, 1986b.

Bracewell, C.D.; Bevan, B.J. Chlamydiosis in birds in Great Britain. Serological reactions to *Chlamydia* in birds sampled between 1974 and 1983. J. Hyg. (Lond.) 96:447–451, 1986.

Brade, H.; Brunner, H. Serological cross-reactions between *Acinetobacter calcoaceticus* and chlamydiae. J. Clin. Microbiol. 10:819–822, 1979.

Brade, L.; Nurminen, M.; Mäkelä, P.H.; Brade, H. Antigenic properties of *Chlamydia trachomatis* lipopolysaccharide. Infect. Immun. 48:569–572, 1985.

Bradley, M.G.; Hobson, D.; Kee, N.; Tait, I.A.; Rees, E. Chlamydial infections of the urethra in women. Genitourin. Med. 61:371–375, 1985.

Braley, A.E. Inclusion blennorrhea. A study of the pathologic changes in the conjunctiva and cervix. Am. J. Ophthalmol. 21:1203–1208, 1938.

Braun, P.; Lee, Y.H.; Klein, J.O.; Marcy, S.M.; Klein, T.A.; Charles, D.; Levy, P.; Kass, E.H. Birth weight and genital mycoplasmas in pregnancy. N. Engl. J. Med. 284:167–171, 1971.

Brayden, R.; Paisley, J.W.; Lower, B.A. Apné in infants with *Chlamydia trachomatis* pneumonia. Ped. Infect. Dis. 6:423–425, 1987.

Brewerton, D.A.; Caffrey, M.; Nichols, A.; Walters, D.; Oates, J.K.; James, D.C.O. Reiter's disease and HL-A 27. Lancet ii:996–998, 1973.

Briggs, R.M.; Paavonen, J. Cervical intraepithelial neoplasia. In: Sexually Transmitted Diseases. Holmes, K.K.; Mårdh, P.-A.; Sparling, P.F.; Wiesner, P.J. eds. New York: McGraw-Hill, 1984: pp. 589–615.

Brihmer, C.; Kallings, I.; Nord, C.E.; Brundin, J. Salpingitis; aspects of diagnosis and etiology: a 4-year study from a Swedish capital hospital. Eur. J. Obstet. Gynecol. Reprod. Biol. 24:211–220, 1987.

Broholm, K.A.; Böttiger, M.; Jernelius, H.; Johannisson, M.; Grandien, M.; Sölver, K. Ornithosis as a nosocomial infection. Scand. J. Infect. Dis. 9:263–267, 1977.

Brown, A.S.; Grice, R.G. Experimental transmission of *Chlamydia psittaci* in the koala. In: Chlamydial Infections. Oriel, D.; Ridgway, G.; Schachter, J.; Taylor-Robinson, D.; Ward, M. eds. Cambridge: Cambridge University Press, 1986, pp. 349–352.

Brudenell, J.M. Chronic endometritis and plasma cell infiltration of the endometrium. J. Obstet. Gynecol. Br. Emp. 62:269–274, 1955.

Brunham, R.C. Therapy for acute pelvic inflammatory disease: a critique of recent treatment trials. Am. J. Obstet. Gynecol. 148:235–240, 1984.

Brunham, R.C.; Martin, D.H.; Kuo, C.-C.; Wang, S.-P.; Stevens, C.E.; Hubbard, T.; Holmes, K.K. Cellular immune response during uncomplicated genital infection with *Chlamydia trachomatis* in humans. Infect. Immun. 34:98–104, 1981.

Brunham, R.C.; Kuo, C.-C.; Hubbard, T.; Holmes, K.K. Further studies of the lymphocyte transformation response during genital infection with *Chlamydia trachomatis*. In: Chlamydial Infections. Mårdh, P.-A.; Holmes, K.K.; Oriel, J.D.; Piot, P.; Schachter, J. eds. Amsterdam: Elsevier Biomedical Press, 1982a, pp. 349–354.

Brunham, R.C.; Kuo, C.C.; Stevens, C.E.; Holmes, K.K. Treatment of concomitant *Neisseria gonorrhoeae* and *Chlamydia trachomatis* infections in women: Comparison of trimethoprim-sulfamethoxazole with ampicillin-probenecid. Rev. Infect. Dis. 4:491–499, 1982b.

Brunham, R.C.; Kuo, C.C.; Stevens, C.E.; Holmes, K.K. Therapy of cervical chlamydial infection. Ann. Intern. Med. 97:216–219, 1982c.

Brunham, R.C.; Kuo, C.-C.; Cles, L.; Holmes, K.K. Correlation of host immune response with quantitative recovery of *Chlamydia trachomatis* from the human endocervix. Infect. Immun. 39:1491–1494, 1983.

Brunham, R.C.; Paavonen, J.; Stevens, C.; Kiviat, N.; Kuo, C.C.; Critchlow, C.W.; Holmes, K.K. Mucopurulent cervicitis: the ignored counterpart in women of urethritis in men. N. Engl. J. Med. 311:1–6, 1984.

Brunham, R.C.; Kuo, C.C.; Chen, W.J. Systemic *Chlamydia trachomatis* infection in mice: comparison of lymphogranuloma venereum and trachoma biovars. Infect. Immun. 48:78–82, 1985a.

Brunham, R.C.; Maclean, I.W.; Binns, B.; Peeling, R.W. *Chlamydia trachomatis:* its role in tubal infertility. J. Infect. Dis. 152:1275–1282, 1985b.

Brunham, R.C.; Binns, B.; McDowell, J.; Paraskevas, M. *Chlamydia trachomatis* infection in women with ectopic pregnancy. Obstet. Gynecol. 67:722–726, 1986.

Brunham, R.C.; Peeling, R.; Maclean, I.; McDowell, J.; Persson, K.; Osser S. Postabortal *Chlamydia trachomatis* salpingitis: correlating risk with antigen-specific serological responses and with neutralization. J. Infect. Dis. 155:749–755, 1987.

Bump, R.C. *Chlamydia trachomatis* as a cause of prepubertal vaginitis. Obstet. Gynecol. 65:384–388, 1985.

Burke, R.K.; Hertig, A.T.; Miele, C.A. Prognostic value of subacute focal inflammation of the endometrium, with special reference to pelvic adhesions as observed on laparoscopic examination. J. Reprod. Med. 30:646–650, 1985.

Burns, D.C.; Darougar, S.; Thin, R.N.; Lothian, L.; Nichol, C.S. Isolation of *Chlamydia trachomatis* from women attending a clinic for sexually transmitted disease. Br. J. Vener. Dis. 51:314–319, 1975.

Butler, C. Surgical pathology of acute salpingitis. Human Pathol. 12:870–878, 1981.

Buus, D.R., Pflugfelder, S.C., Schachter, J.; Miller, D.; Forster, R.K. Lymphogranuloma venereum conjunctivitis with a marginal corneal perforation. Ophthalmology 95:799–802, 1988.

Byrne, G.I.; Moulder, J.W. Parasite-specified phagocytosis of *Chlamydia psittaci* and *Chlamydia trachomatis* by L and HeLa cells. Infect. Immun. 19:598–606, 1978.

Byrne, G.I.; Lehmann, L.K.; Landry, G.J. Induction of tryptophan catabolism is the mechanism for gamma-interferon-mediated inhibition of intracellular *Chlamydia psittaci* replication in T24 cells. Infect. Immun. 53:347–351, 1987.

Byrne, G.I; Williams, D.M.; Schobert, C.S.; Krueger, D.A. Persistent infections and the immune response to chlamydiae. In: Proceedings of the Eur. Soc. for Chlamydia Research, 1st Meeting, Bologna, Italy, May 30–June 1, 1988, pp. 113–116.

Caldwell, H.D.; Kuo, C.-C. Serologic diagnosis of lymphogranuloma venereum by counterimmunoelectrophoresis with a *Chlamydia trachomatis* protein antigen. J. Immunol. 118:442–445, 1977.

Caldwell, H.D.; Judd, R.C. Structural analysis of chlamydial major outer membrane proteins. Infect. Immun. 38:960–968, 1982.

Caldwell, H.D.; Perry, L.J. Neutralization of *Chlamydia trachomatis* infectivity with antibodies to the major outer membrane protein. Infect. Immun. 38:745–754, 1982.

Caldwell, H.D.; Schachter, J. Antigenic analysis of the major outer membrane protein of *Chlamydia* spp. Infect. Immun. 35:1024–1031, 1982.

Caldwell, H.D.; Schachter, J. Immunoassay for detecting *Chlamydia trachomatis* major outer membrane protein. J. Clin. Microbiol. 18:539–545, 1983.

Caldwell, H.D.; Hitchcock, P.J. Monoclonal antibody against a genus-specific antigen of *Chlamydia* species: location of the epitope on chlamydial lipopolysaccharide. Infect. Immun. 44:306–314, 1984.

Caldwell, H.D.; Kuo, C.-C.; Kenny, G.E. Antigenic analysis of Chlamydiae by two-dimensional immunoelectrophoresis. I. Antigenic heterogeneity between *C. trachomatis* and *C. psittaci*. J. Immunol. 115:963–968, 1975a.

Caldwell, H.D.; Kuo, C.-C.; Kenny, G.E. Antigenic analysis of Chlamydiae by two-dimensional immunoelectrophoresis. II. A trachoma-LGV-specific antigen. J. Immunol. 115:969–975, 1975b.

Caldwell, H.D.; Kromhout, J.; Schachter, J. Purification and partial characterization of the MOMP of *Chlamydia trachomatis*. Infect. Immun. 31:1161–1176, 1981.

Caldwell, H.D.; Stewrat, S.; Johnson, S.; Taylor, H. Tear and serum antibody response to *Chlamydia trachomatis* antigens during acute chlamydial conjunctivitis in monkeys as determined by immunoblotting. Infect. Immun. 55:93–98, 1987.

Campbell, L.A.; Kuo, C.C.; Grayston, J.T. Characterization of the new Chlamydia agent, TWAR, as a unique organism by restriction endonuclease analysis and DNA-DNA hybridization. J. Clin. Microbiol. 25:1911–1916, 1987a.

Campbell, L.A.; Kuo, C.C.; Grayston, J.T. Use of whole chromosomal DNA probe for differentiation on the new Chlamydia TWAR agent from *C. trachomatis* and *C. psittaci*. In Abstracts of the 1987 ICAAC, Abstract No. 728, p. 224, 1987b.

Carlson, E.M.; Peterson, E.M.; de la Maza, L.M. Identification of *Chlamydia* glycoproteins. In: Chlamydial Infections. Oriel, D.; Ridgway, G.; Schachter, J.; Taylor-Robinson, D.; Ward, M. eds. Cambridge: Cambridge University Press, 1986, pp. 118–121.

Carr, M.C.; Hanna, L.; Jawetz, E. Chlamydiae, cervicitis and abnormal Papanicolaou smears. Obstet. Gynecol. 53:27–30, 1979.

Cassell, G.H.; Davis, R.O.; Waites, K.B.; Brown, M.B.; Marriott, P.A.; Stagno, S.; Davis, J.K. Isolation of *Mycoplasma hominis* and *Ureaplasma urealyticum* from amniotic fluid at 16–20 weeks of gestation: Potential effect on outcome of pregnancy. Sex. Transm. Dis. 10(Suppl):294–302, 1983.

Cates, W. Sexually transmitted organisms and infertility: the proof of the pudding. Sex. Transm. Dis. 11:113–116, 1984.

Cates, W.; Farley, T.M.M.; Rowe, P.J. Worldwide patterns of infertility: Is Africa different? Lancet ii:596–598, 1985.

Catterall, R.D. The situation of gonococcal and non-gonococcal infections in the United Kingdom. In: Genital Infections and Their Complications. Danielsson, D.; Juhlin, L.; Mårdh, P.-A. eds. Stockholm: Almqvist & Wiksell International, 1975, pp. 5–8.

Caul, E.O.; Paul, I.D. Monoclonal antibody based ELISA for detecting *Chlamydia trachomatis*. Lancet i:279, 1985.

Cevenini, R.; Costa, S.; Rumpianesi, F.; Donati, M.; Guerra, B.; Diana, R.; Antonini, M.P. Cytological and histopathological abnormalities of the cervix in genital *Chlamydia trachomatis* infections. Br. J. Vener. Dis. 57:334–337, 1981.

Cevenini, R.; Possati, G.; La Placa, M. *Chlamydia trachomatis* infection in infertile women. In: Chlamydial Infections. Mårdh, P.-A.; Holmes, K.K.; Oriel, J.D.; Piot, P.; Schachter, J. eds. Amsterdam: Elsevier Biomedical Press, 1982, pp. 189–192.

Cevenini, R.; Sarov, I.; Rumpianesi, F.; Donati, M.; Melega, C.; Varotti, C.; La Placa, M. Serum specific IgA antibody to *Chlamydia trachomatis* in patients with chlamydial infections detected by ELISA and an immunofluorescence test. J. Clin. Pathol. 37:686–691, 1984.

Cevenini, R.; Rumpianesi, F.; Sambri, V.; La Placa, M. Antigenic specificity of serological response in *Chlamydia trachomatis* urethritis detected by immunoblotting. J. Clin. Pathol. 39:325–327, 1986a.

Cevenini, R.; Rumpianesi, F.; Donati, M.; Moroni, A.; Samori, V.; La Placa, M. Class specific immunoglobulin response to individual polypeptides of *Chlamydia trachomatis*, elementary bodies and reticulate bodies in patients with chlamydial infection. J. Clin. Pathol. 39:1313–1316, 1986b.

Cevenini, R.; Sambri, V.; La Placa, M. Comparative in vitro activity of Ru 28965 against *Chlamydia trachomatis*. Eur. J. Clin. Microbiol. 5:598–600, 1986c.

Chacko, M.R.; Lovchik, J.C. *Chlamydia trachomatis* infection in sexually active adolescents: prevalence and risk factors. Pediatrics 73:836–840, 1984.

Chalmers, W.S.K. Duck ornithosis and related zoonosis in the U.K. In: Chlamydial Infections. Oriel, D.; Ridgway, G.; Schachter, J.; Taylor-Robinson, D.; Ward, M. eds. Cambridge: Cambridge University Press, 1986: pp. 345–348.

Chandiok, S. Incidence of prostatitis as a complication of nongonococcal urethritis. Eur. J. Sex. Transm. Dis. 2:197–205, 1985.

Chandler, J.W.; Alexander, E.R.; Pheiffer, T.A.; Wang, S.-P.; Holmes, K.K.; English, M. Ophthalmia neonatorum associated with maternal chlamydial infections. Trans. Am. Acad. Ophthalmol. Otolaryngol. 83:302–308, 1977.

Chang, M.J.; Rodriguez, W.; Mohla, C. *Chlamydia trachomatis* in otitis media in children. Ped. Infect. Dis. 1:95–97, 1982.

Chen, W.J.; Kuo, C.C. A mouse model of pneumonitis induced by *Chlamydia trachomatis*: morphologic, microbiologic and immunologic studies. Am. J. Pathol. 100:365–377, 1980.

Chernesky, M.A.; Mahony, J.B.; Castriciano, S.; Mores, M.; Stewart, I.O.; Landis, S.J.; Seidelman, W.; Sargeant, E.J.; Leman, C. Detection of *Chlamydia trachomatis* antigens by enzyme immunoassay and immunofluorescence in genital specimens from symptomatic and asymptomatic men and women. J. Infect. Dis. 154:141–148, 1986.

Chi, E.Y.; Kuo, C.C.; Grayston, J.T. Unique ultrastructure in the elementary body of *Chlamydia* sp. strain TWAR. J. Bacteriol. 169:3757–3763, 1987.

Chow, A.W.; Jewesson, P.J. Pharmacokinetics and safety of antimicrobial agents during pregnancy. Rev. Infect. Dis. 7:287–313, 1985.

Christensen, K.K.; Högerstrand, I.; Mårdh, P.A. Late spontaneous abortion associated with *Mycoplasma hominis* infection of the fetus. Scand. J. Infect. Dis. 14:73–74, 1982.

Christiansson, A.; Mårdh, P.A. Tetracycline resistance in *Mycoplasma hominis*. Sex. Transm. Dis. 10(Suppl):371–373, 1983.

Christophersen, J.; Gräm, N.; Dahlgård, T. Hemorrhagic proctitis in male homosexuals caused by *Chlamydia trachomatis*. Ugeskr. Laeger. 147:1407–1409, 1985.

Clark, R.B.; Nachamkin, I.; Schatzki, P.F.; Dalton, H.P. Localization of distinct surface antigens on *Chlamydia trachomatis* HAR-13 by immune electron microscopy with monoclonal antibodies. Infect. Immun. 38:1273–1278, 1982.

Clark, R.B.; Schneider, V.; Gentile, F.G.; Pechan, B.; Dalton, H.P. Cervical chlamydial infections: diagnostic accuracy of the Papanicolaou smear. Southern Med. J. 78:1301–1303, 1985.

Cleary, R.E.; Jones, R.B. Recovery of *Chlamydia trachomatis* from the endometrium in infertile women with serum antichlamydial antibodies. Fertil. Steril. 44:233–235, 1985.

Colaert, J.; Denef, M.; Piot, P. Isolation of *Trichomonas vaginalis* from cycloheximide-treated McCoy cells. Eur. J. Clin. Bacteriol. 6:320, 1987.

Coleman, P.; Varitek, V.; Grier, T.; Kurpiewski, G.; Hauseu, J.; Safford, J.; Marchlewicz, B.; Mushawar, I.K. Testback Chlamydia: a new rapid assay for the detection of *Chlamydia trachomatis*. In: Proceedings of the Eur. Soc. for Chlamydia Research, 1st Meeting, Bologna, Italy, May 30–June 1, 1988, p. 950.

Colleen, S.; Mårdh, P.-A. Complicated infections of the male genital tract with emphasis on *Chlamydia trachomatis* as an etiological agent. In: *Chlamydia trachomatis* in genital and related infections. Mårdh, P.-A.; Møller, B.R.; Paavonen, J. eds. Scand. J. Infect. Dis. Suppl. 32:93–99, 1982.

Colleen, S.; Mårdh, P.-A. Prostatitis. In: Sexually Transmitted Diseases. Holmes, K.K.; Mårdh, P.-A.; Sparling, P.F.; Wiesner, P.J. eds. New York: McGraw-Hill, 1984, pp. 662–671.

Colleen, S.; Mårdh, P.-A.; Schytz, A. Magnesium and zinc in seminal fluid of healthy males and patients with non-acute prostatitis with and without gonorrhoea. Scand. J. Nephrol. Urol. 9:192–197, 1975.

Colley, D.G.; Goodman, T.G.; Barsoum, I.S. Ocular sensitization of mice with live (but not irradiated) *Chlamydia trachomatis* serovar A. Infect. Immun. 55:93–98, 1986.

Collier, L.H. Experimental infection of baboons with inclusion blennorrhoea and trachoma. Ann. N.Y. Acad. Sci. 81:188–196, 1962.

Collier, L.H. Some aspects of trachoma control and personal estimates of the cost of vaccine production. Israel. J. Med. Sci. 8:1114–1123, 1972.

Collins, A.R.; Barron, A.L. Demonstration of group- and species-specific antigens of chlamydial agents by gel diffusion. J. Infect. Dis. 121:1–8, 1970.

Committee on Drugs, Committee on Fetus and Newborn, Committee on Infectious Diseases, American Society of Pediatrics. Prophylaxis and treatment of neonatal gonococcal infections. Pediatrics 65:1047, 1980.

Conway, D.; Glazener, C.M.A.; Caul, E.O.; Hodgson, J.; Hull, M.G.R.; Clarke, S.K.R.; Stirrat, G.M. Chlamydial serology in fertile and infertile women. Lancet i:191–193, 1984.

Coutts, W.E. Lymphogranuloma venereum: a general review. Bull. WHO 2:545–562, 1950.

Cox, H.R. Use of yolk sac of developing chick embryo as medium for growing rickettsiae of Rocky Mountain spotted fever and typhus groups. Publ. Health Reports (Wash.) 53:2241–2247, 1938.

Cramer, D.W. Tubal infertility and the intrauterine device. N. Engl. J. Med. 312:941–949, 1985.

Croy, T.R.; Kuo, C.C.; Wang, S.P. Comparative susceptibility of eleven mammalian cell lines to infection with trachoma organisms. J. Clin. Microbiol. 1:434–439, 1975.

Csonka, G.W. Recurrent attacks of Reiter's syndrome. Arthr. Rheum. 3:164–169, 1960.

Curtis, A.H. A cause of adhesions in the right upper quadrant. J. Am. Med. Assoc. 94:1221–1222, 1930.

Czernobilsky, B. Endometritis and infertility. Fertil Steril. 30:119–130, 1978.

Dalaker, K.; Gjønness, H., Kvile, G.; Urnes, G.; Ånestad, G.; Bergan, T. *Chlamydia trachomatis* as a cause of acute perihepatitis associated with pelvic inflammatory disease. Br. J. Vener. Dis. 57:41–43, 1981.

Dalgaard, J. Ornithose familieepidemi med interhuman smitta (in Norwegian). Tidskr. Nor. Laegeforen. 77:47–50, 1957.

Danielsson, D.; Forslin, L.; Moi, H.; Ingvarsson, A.; Parkhede, U. A comparative study between cell culture and a new enzyme immunoassay for detection of genital *Chlamydia* infection. Fifth International Symposium on Rapid Methods and Automation in Microbiology and Immunology, Florence. 4–6 November, 1987, p. 305.

Darougar, S.; Kinnison, J.R.; Jones, B.R. Chlamydial isolates from the rectum in association with chlamydial infection of the eye or genital tract. I. Laboratory aspects. In: Trachoma and Related Disorders caused by Chlamydial Agents. Nichols, R.L. ed. Amsterdam: Excerpta Medica, 1971a, pp. 501–506.

Darougar, S.; Treharne, J.D.; Dwyer, R.St.C.; Kinnison, J.R.; Jones, B.R. Isolation of TRIC agent (*Chlamydia*) in irradiated McCoy cell culture from endemic trachoma in field studies in Iran. Comparison with other laboratory tests for detection of *Chlamydia*. Br. J. Ophthalmol. 55:591–599, 1971b.

Darougar, S.; Monnickendam, M.A.; El-Sheikh, H.; Treharne, J.D.; Woodland, R.M.; Jones, B.R. Animal models for the study of chlamydial infections of the eye and genital tract. In: Nongonococcal Urethritis and Related Infections. Hobson, D.; Holmes, K.K. eds. Washington, D.C.: American Society for Microbiology, 1977a, pp. 186–198.

Darougar, S.; Woodland, R.M.; Forsey, T.; Cubitt, S.; Allami, J.; Jones, B.R. Isolation of Chlamydia from ocular infections. In: Nongonococcal Urethritis and Related Infections. Hobson, D.; Holmes, K.K. eds. Washington, D.C.: American Society for Microbiology, 1977b, pp. 295–298.

Darougar, S.; Treharne, J.D.; Minassian, D.; El-Sheikh, H.; Dines, R.J.; Jones, B.R. Rapid serological test for the diagnosis of chlamydial ocular infections. Br. J. Ophthalmol. 62:503–508, 1978.

Darougar, S.; Jones, B.R.; Daghfous, T.; Hejazi, R. Isolation of *Chlamydia trachomatis* from different areas of conjunctiva in relation to intensity of hyperendemic trachoma in school children in Southern Tunisia. Br. J. Ophthalmol. 63:110–112, 1979.

Darougar, S.; Forsey, T.; Wood, J.J.; Bolton, J.P.; Allan, A. Chlamydia and the Curtis–Fitz-Hugh syndrome. Br. J. Vener. Dis. 57:391–194, 1981.

Darougar, S.; Aramesh, B.; Gibson, J.A.; Treharne, J.D.; Jones, B.R. Chlamydial infection in prostitutes in Iran. Br. J. Vener. Dis. 59:53–55, 1983.

Darougar, S.; Jones, B.R. Trachoma. Br. Med. Bull. 39:117–122, 1983.

Dawson, C.R. Eye disease with chlamydial infections. In: Chlamydial Infections. Oriel, D.; Ridgway, G.; Schachter, J.; Taylor-Robinson, D.; Ward, M. eds. Cambridge: Cambridge University Press, 1986, pp. 135–144.

Dawson, C.R.; Schachter, J. TRIC agent infections of the eye and genital tract. Am. J. Ophthalmol. 63:1288–1289, 1967.

Dawson, C.R.; Schachter, J. Strategies for treatment and control of blinding trachoma: cost-effectiveness of topical or systemic antibiotics. Rev. Infect. Dis. 7:768–773, 1985.

Dawson, C.R.; Jawetz, E.; Hanna, L.; Rose, L.; Wood, T.R.; Thygeson, P. Experimental inclusion conjunctivitis in man. II. Partial resistance to reinfection. Am. J. Epidemiol. 84:411–425, 1966.

Dawson, C.; Wood, T.R.; Rose, L.; Hanna, L. Experimental inclusion conjunctivitis in man. III. Keratitis and other complications. Arch. Ophthalmol. 78:341–349; 1967.

Dawson, C.R.; Schachter, J.; Ostler, H. B.; Gilbert, R. M.; Smith, D.E.; Engleman, E.P. Inclusion conjunctivitis and Reiter's syndrome in a married couple. Chlamydial infections in a series of both diseases. Arch. Ophthalmol. 83:300–306; 1970.

Dawson, C.R.; Jones, B.R.; Darougar, S. Blinding and non-blinding trachoma: assessment of intensity of upper tarsal inflammatory disease and disabling lesions. Bull. WHO 52:279–282; 1975.

Dawson, C.R.; Dagfous, T.; Messadi, M.; Hoshiwara, I.; Schachter, J. Severe endemic trachoma in Tunisia. Br. J. Ophthalmol. 60:245–252, 1976.

Dawson, C.R.; Jones, B.R.; Tarizzo, M.L. Guide to trachoma control. Geneva: World Health Organization, 1981.

Dhir, S.P.; Boatman, E.E. Location of polysaccharide on *Chlamydia psittaci* by silver-methenamine staining and electron microscopy. J. Bacteriol. 111:267–271, 1972.

Dhir, S.P.; Hakomori, S.; Kenny, G.E.; Grayston, J.T. Immunochemical studies on chlamydial group antigen (presence of a 2-keto-3-deoxycarbohydrate as immunodominant group). J. Immunol. 109:116–122, 1972.

Dick, D.C.; McGregor, C.G.A.; Michell, K.G. Sommerville, R.G.; Wheatley, D.J. Endocarditis as a manifestation of chlamydial B infections (psittacosis). Br. Heart J. 39:914–916, 1977.

DiGiacomo, R.F.; Gale, J.L.; Wang, S.P.; Kiviat, M.D. Chlamydial infection of the male baboon urethra. Br. J. Vener. Dis. 51:310–313, 1975.

Dilbeck, P.M.; Evermann, J. F.; Kraft, S.; Tyler, S. Equine chlamydial infections: comparative and diagnostic aspects with bovine and ovine chlamydiosis. Proc. Am. Assoc. Vet. Lab. Diag. 28:285–296, 1986.

Dimitrov, K.; Martinov, S.; Popov, G. Klinisch ätiologische Befunde bei Chlamydienurethritiden bei Männern (In German). Z. Hautkr. 59(18):1229–1236, 1984.

Donath, E.M.; Schrage, R.; Hoyme, U.B. *Chlamydia trachomatis*-Untersuchungen zur Wertigkeit des Nachweises im Papanicolaou-Präparat (in German). Geburtsh. u Frauenheilk. 45:402–405, 1985.

Dorman, S.A.; Danos, L.M.; Wilson, D.J.; Noller, K.L.; Malkasian, G.D.; Goellner, J.R.; Smith, T.F. Detection of chlamydial cervicitis by Papnicolaou stained smear and culture. Am. J. Clin. Pathol. 79:421–425, 1983.

Drach, G.W.; Fair, W.; Meares, E.M.; Stamey, T.A. Classification of benign disease with prostatic pain: Prostatitis: prostatodynia? J. Urol. 120:266, 1978.

Duke-Elder, S. A system of ophthalmology. In: Diseases of the Outer Eye, Vol. 8. London: Henry Kimpton, 1965, pp. 267–.

Dumoulin, J.G.; Hughesdon, P.E. Chronic endometritis. J. Obstet. Gynecol. 58:222, 1951.

Duncan, M.O.; Fehler, H.G.; de L' Exposto, F.; Dangor, Y.; Ballard, R.C. Lymphogranuloma venereum among migrant mine workers in Southern Africa. In: Chlamydial Infections. Oriel, D.; Ridgway, G.; Schachter, J.; Taylor-Robinson, D.; Ward, M. eds. Cambridge: Cambridge University Press, 1986, pp. 263–265.

Dunlop, E.M.C.; Jones, B.R.; Al-Hussaini, M.K. Genital infection in association with TRIC virus infection of the eye. Br. J. Vener. Dis. 40:33–42, 1964.

Dunlop, E.M.C.; Harper, I.A.; Jones, B.R. Seronegative polyarthritis. The Bedsoniae (*Chlamydiae*) group of agents in Reiter's disease. Ann. Rheum. Dis. 27:234–240, 1968.

Dunlop, E.M.C.; Vaughan-Jackson, J.D.; Darougar, S.; Jones, B.R. Chlamydial infection. Incidence of "non-specific" urethritis. Br. J. Vener. Dis. 48:425–428, 1972.

Dwyer, R. StC.; Treharne, J.D.; Jones, B.R.; Herring, J. Chlamydial infection. Results of micro-immunofluorescence test for detection of type-specific antibody in certain chlamydial infections. Br. J. Vener. Dis. 48:452–459, 1972.

Eb, F.; Orfila, J.; Milon, A.; Géral, M.F. Intérêt épidémiologique du typage par immunofluorescence de *Chlamydia psittaci* (in French). Ann. Inst. Pasteur/Microbiol. 137 B:77–93, 1986.

Editorial. Chlamydial endocarditis. Lancet i:132, 1980.

Eilard, T.; Bronsson, J.R.; Hamark, B.; Forsman, L. Isolation of chlamydia in acute salpingitis. Scand. J. Dis. Suppl. 9:82–84, 1976.

Ekman, M.R.; Saikku, P.; Kleemola, M.; Visakorpi, R.; Kuo, C.C.; Grayston, J.T. Mild and asymptomatic respiratory infections with *Chlamydia* TWAR during a military pneumonia epidemic. In: Proceedings of the Eur. Soc. of Chlamydia Research, 1st Meeting, Bologna, Italy, May 30–June 1, 1988, p. 56.

Elbagir, A.N.; Stenberg, K.; Mårdh, P.-A. Notes on anti-chlamydial activity of tear fluid. In: Proceedings of the Eur. Soc. for Chlamydia Research, 1st Meeting, Bologna, Italy, May 30–June 1, 1988, p. 56.

Elliot, D.L.; Tolle, S.W.; Goldberg, L.; Miller, J.B. Pet-associated illness. N. Engl. J. Med. 313:985–995, 1985.

Eschenbach, D.A. Epidemiology and diagnosis of acute pelvic inflammatory disease. Obstet. Gynecol. 55(Suppl):142–153, 1980.

Eschenbach, D.A. Fitz-Hugh–Curtis syndrome. In: Sexually Transmitted Diseases. Holmes, K.K.; Mårdh, P.-A.; Sparling, P.F.; Wiesner, P.J. eds. New York: McGraw-Hill, 1984, pp. 633–638.

Eschenbach, D.A. Acute pelvic inflammatory disease. In: Gynecology and Obstetrics, Vol. 1. Sciarra, J. ed. New York: Harper and Row, 1986, pp. 1–20.

Eschenbach, D.A.; Daling, J.R. Ectopic pregnancy. JAMA 249:1759–1769, 1983.

Eschenbach, D.A.; Buchanan, T.M.; Pollock, H.M.; Forsyth, P.S.; Alexander, E.R.; Lin, J.S.; Wang, S.P.; Wentworth, B.B.; McCormack, W.M.; Holmes, K.K. Polymicrobial etiology of acute pelvic inflammatory disease. N. Engl. J. Med. 293:166–171, 1975.

Eschenbach, D.A.; Harnisch, J.P.; Holmes, K.K. Pathogenesis of acute pelvic inflammatory disease: Role of contraception and other risk factors. Am. J. Obstet. Gynecol. 128:838–850, 1977.

Eugster, A.K.; Jones, L.P.; Gayle, L.G. Epizootics of chlamydial abortions and keratoconjunctivitis in goats. Proceedings of the 20th annual meeting of the American Association of Veterinary Laboratory Diagnosticians, Madison, WI, 20:69–78, 1977.

Evans, R.T.; Taylor-Robinson, D. Comparison of various McCoy cell treatment procedures used for detection of C. trachomatis. J. Clin. Microbiol. 10:198–201, 1979.

Evans, R.T.; Taylor-Robinson, D. Development and evaluation of an enzyme-linked immunosorbent assay (ELISA), using chlamydial group antigen, to detect antibodies to Chlamydial trachomatis. J. Clin. Pathol. 35:1122–1128, 1982.

Evermann, J.F. Chlamydia psittaci: zoonotic potential worthy of concern. Clin. Microbiol. Newslett. 9(1):1–3, 1987.

Falk, V. Treatment of acute nontuberculous salpingitis with antibiotics alone and in combination with glucocorticoids. Acta Obstet. Gynecol. Scand. 44 (Suppl 6):1–118, 1965.

Finn, M.P.; Ohlin, A.; Schachter, J. Enzyme-linked immunosorbent assay for immunoglobulin G and M antibodies to Chlamydia trachomatis in human sera. J. Clin. Microbiol. 17:848–852, 1983.

Fitz-Hugh, T. Acute gonococcic peritonitis of the right upper quadrant in women. J. Am. Med. Assoc. 102:2094–2096, 1934.

Fluhmann, C.F. The endometrium in so-called idiopathic uterine hemorrhage. J. Am. Med. Assoc. 93:1136–1929.

Forsey, T.; Darougar, S. Acute conjunctivitis caused by an atypical chlamydial strain: Chlamydia IOL-207. Br. J. Ophthalmol. 68:409–411, 1984.

Forsey, T.; Darougar, S.; Treharne, J.D. Prevalence in human beings of antibodies to Chlamydia IOL-207, an atypical strain of chlamydia. J. Infect. Dis. 12:145–152, 1986.

Forslin, L.; Danielsson, D.; Kjellander, J.; Falk, V. Antibiotic treatment of acute salpingitis. A study of plasma concentrations of two tetracyclines (doxycycline and lymecycline). Acta Obstet. Gynecol. Scand. 61:59–64, 1982.

Forster, G.; Jha, R.; Cheetham, D.; Munday, P.; Coleman, D.; Taylor-Robinson, D. Cytological diagnosis of chlamydial infection of female genital tract. Lancet ii:578–579, 1983.

Foulkes, S.J.; Deighton, R.; Feeney, A.R.B.; Mohanty, K.C.; Freeman, C.W.J. Comparison of direct immunofluorescence and cell culture for detecting *Chlamydia trachomatis*. Genitourin. Med. 61:255–257, 1985.

Francis, R.A.; Abbas, A.M.A. Fluorescein-conjugated monoclonal antibodies to detect *Chlamydia trachomatis* in smears. Lancet ii:222, 1985.

Fransen, L.; Nsanze, H.; Klauss, V.; Van der Stuyft, P.; D'Costa, L.; Brunham, R.C.; Piot, P. Ophthalmia neonatorum in Nairobi, Kenya: the roles of *Neisseria gonorrhoeae* and *Chlamydia trachomatis*. J. Infect. Dis. 5:862–869, 1986.

Fraser, J.J.; Rettig, P.J.; Kaplan, D.W. Prevalence of cervical *Chlamydia trachomatis* and *Neisseria gonorrhoeae* in female adolescents. Pediatrics 71:333–336, 1983.

Freedman, A.; Al-Hussaini, M.K.; Dunlop, E.M.C.; Emarah, M.H.M.; Garland, J.A.; Harper, I.A.; Jones, B.R.; Race, J.W.; du Toit, M.S.; Treharne, J.D.; Wright, D.J.M. Infections by TRIC agent and other members of the Bedsonia group; with a note on Reiter's disease. II. Ophthalmia neonatorum due to TRIC agent. Tr. Ophthalmol. Soc. UK. 86:313–320, 1966.

Friberg, J.; Gleicher, N.; Suarez, M.; Confino, E. Chlamydia attached to spermatozoa. J. Infect. Dis. 152:854, 1985.

Friis, R.R. Interaction of L cells and *Chlamydia psittaci:* entry of the parasite and host responses to its development. J. Bacteriol. 110:706–721, 1972.

Fritsch, H.O.; Hofstätter, A.; Lindner, K. Experimentelle Studien zur Trachomfrage (in German). Graefe's Archiv für Ophthalmologie 76:547, 1910.

Frommel, G.R.; Rothenberg, R.; Wang, S.P.; McIntosh, K. Chlamydial infection of mothers and their infants. J. Pediatr. 95:28–32, 1979.

Frost, E.; Collet, M.; Reniers, J.; Leclerc, A.; Ivanoff, B.; Meheus, A. Importance of antichlamydial antibodies in acute salpingitis in central Africa. Genitourin. Med. 63:176–178, 1987.

Fuster, C.D.; Neinstein, L.S. Vaginal *Chlamydia trachomatis* prevalence in sexually abused prepubertal girls. Pediatrics 79:235–238, 1987.

Gale, J.L.; Wang, S.P.; Grayston, J.T. Chronic trachoma in two Taiwan monkeys ten years after infection. In: Trachoma and Related Disorders caused by Chlamydial Agents. Nichols, R.L. ed. Amsterdam: Excerpta Medica, 1971, pp. 489–493.

Gale, J.L.; DiGiacomo, R.F.; Kiviat, M.D.; Wang, S.P.; Bowie, W.R. Experimental nonhuman primate urethral infection with *Chlamydia trachomatis* and *Ureaplasma urealyticum* (T-mycoplasma). In: Nongonococcal Urethritis and Related Infections. Hobson, D.; Holmes, K.K. eds. Washington, D.C.: American Society for Microbiology, 1977, pp. 205–213.

Garrett, A.J.; Harrison, M.J.; Manire, G.P. A search for the bacterial mucopeptide component, muramic acid, in *Chlamydia*. J. Gen. Microbiol. 80:315–318, 1974.

Gatt, D.; Jantet, G. Perisplenitis and perinephritis in the Curtis–Fitz-Hugh syndrome. Br. J. Surg. 74:110–112, 1987.

Gear, J.H.; Miller, G.B.; Woolf, M.; Patz, I.M. Psittacosis in the RSA. S. Afr. Med. J. 69:689–693, 1986.

Geerling, S.; Nettum, J.A.; Lindner, L.E.; Miller, S.L.; Dutton, L.; Wechter, S. Sensitivity and specificity of the Papanicolaou-stained cervical smear in the diagnosis of *Chlamydia trachomatis* infection. Acta Cytol. 29:671–675, 1985.

Gerber, M.A.; Ryan, R.W.; Tilton, R.C.; Watson, J.E. Role of *Chlamydia trachomatis* in acute pharyngitis in young adults. J. Clin. Microbiol. 20:993–994, 1984.

Gerber, M.A.; Randolph, M.F.; Chanatry, J.; Mayo, D.R.; Schachter, J.; Tilton, R.C. Role of *Chlamydia trachomatis* and *Mycoplasma pneumoniae* in acute pharyngitis in children. Diagn. Microbiol. Infect. Dis. 6:263–265, 1987.

Gerloff, R.K.; Watson, R.O. The radioisotope precipitation test for psittacosis group antibody. Am. J. Ophthalmol. 63:1492–1498, 1967.

Ghione, M.; Brivio, R.; Saufilippo, A.; Schioppacassi, G. Research on factors influencing experimental chemotherapy tests in trachoma. Am. J. Ophthalmol. 63:547–551, 1967.

Gibbs, R.S.; Blanco, J.D.; St. Clair, P.J.; Castaneda, Y.S. *Mycoplasma hominis* and intrauterine infection in late pregnancy. Sex. Transm. Dis. 10(Suppl):303–306, 1983.

Gibson, M.; Gump, D.; Ashigane, T.; Hall, B. Patterns of adnexal inflammatory damage: Chlamydia, the intrauterine device, and history of pelvic inflammatory disease. Fertil. Steril. 41:47–51, 1984.

Givner, L.B.; Rennels, M.B.; Woosward, C.L.; Huang, S.W. *Chlamydia trachomatis* infection in infants delivered by cesarean section. Pediatrics 68:420–421, 1981.

Gjønnaess, H.; Dalaker, K.; Urnes, A.; Noeling, B.; Kvile, J.; Mårdh, P.-A.; Ånestad, G.; Bergan, T. Treatment of pelvic inflammatory disease. Effects of lymecycline and clindamycin. Curr. Ther. Res. 29:885–892, 1982a.

Gjønnaess, H.; Dalaker, K.; Ånestad, G., Mårdh, P.-A.; Kvile, G.; Bergan, T. Pelvic inflammatory disease: etiological studies with emphasis on chlamydial infection. Obstet. Gynecol. 59:550–555, 1982b.

Golden, N.; Hammerschlag, M.R.; Neuhoff, S.; Gleyzer, A. Prevalence of *Chlamydia trachomatis* cervical infection in female adolescents. Am. J. Dis. Child. 138:562–564, 1984.

Gordon, F.B.; Quan, A. Drug susceptibilities of the psittacosis and trachoma agents. Ann. N.Y. Acad. Sci. 981:261–270, 1962.

Gordon, F.B.; Quan, A.L. Isolation of the trachoma agent in cell culture. Proc. Soc. Exp. Biol. Med. 118:354–359, 1965.

Gordon, F.B.; Quan, A.L.; Steinman, T.I.; Phillips, R.N. Chlamydial isolates from Reiter's syndrome. Br. J. Vener. Dis. 49:376–380, 1973.

Graham, D.M. Growth and neutralization of the trachoma agent in mouse lungs. Nature 207:1379–1380, 1965.

Graham, D.M. Growth and immunogenicity of TRIC agents in mice. Am. J. Ophthalmol. 63:1173–1190, 1967.

Grant, J.B.F.; Brooman, P.J.C.; Chowdbury, S.D.; Sequeira, P.O.; Blacklock, N.J. The clinical presentation of *Chlamydia trachomatis* in a urological practice. Br. J. Urol. 57:218–221, 1985.

Gravett, M.G.; Hummel, D.; Eschenbach, D.A.; Holmes, K.K. Preterm labor associated with subclinical amniotic fluid infection and with bacterial vaginosis. Obstet. Gynecol. 67:229–237, 1986a.

Gravett, M.G.; Nelson, H.P.; DeRouen, T.; Critchlow, C.; Eschenbach, D.A.; Holmes, K.K. Independent associations of bacterial vaginosis and *Chlamydia trachomatis* infection with adverse pregnancy outcome. J. Am. Med. Assoc. 256:1899–1903, 1986b.

Gray, J.W.; Hovelius, B.; Mårdh, P.-A. Antibody response to *Chlamydia trachomatis* in sera of children; a seroepidemiological study. Eur. J. Clin. Microbiol. 5:576–580, 1986.

Grayston, J.T. Trachoma vaccine (discussion). Vaccines against viral, rickettsial and bacterial diseases of man. PAHO/WHO Sci. Publ. 226:311–315, 1971.

Grayston, J.T.; Wang, S.-P. New knowledge of chlamydiae and the diseases they cause. J. Infect. Dis. 132:87–105, 1975.

Grayston, J.T.; Wang, S.-P. The potential for vaccine against infection of the genital tract with *Chlamydia trachomatis*. Sex. Transm. Dis. 5:73–77, 1978.

Grayston, J.T.; Wang, S.-P.; Woolridge, R.L.; Alexander, E.R. Prevention of trachoma with vaccine. Arch. Environ. Health. 8:518–526, 1964.

Grayston, J.T.; Kim, K.S.W.; Alexander, E.R.; Wang, S.-P. Protective studies in monkeys with trivalent and monovalent trachoma vaccines. In: Trachoma and Related Disorders caused by Chlamydial Agents. Nichols, R.L. ed. Amsterdam: Excerpta Medica, 1971, pp. 377–385.

Grayston, J.T.; Yeh, L.J.; Wang, S.P.; Kuo, C.C.; Beasley, R.P.; Gale, J.L. Pathogenesis of ocular *Chlamydia trachomatis* infections in humans. In: Nongonococcal Urethritis and Related Infections. Hobson, D.; Holmes, K.K. eds. Washington, D.C.: American Society for Microbiology, 1977, pp. 113–125.

Grayston, J.T.; Wang, S.-P.; Foy, H.M.; Kuo, C.-C. Seroepidemiology of *Chlamydia trachomatis* infection. In: Chlamydial Infections. Mårdh, P.-A.; Holmes, K.K.; Oriel, J.D.; Piot, P., Schachter, J. eds. Amsterdam: Elsevier Biomedical Press, 1982, pp. 405–419.

Grayston, J.T.; Wang, S.-P.; Kuo, C.-C.; Mordhorst, C.H.; Saikku, P.; Marrie, T.J. Seroepidemiology with TWAR, a new group of *Chlamydia psittaci*. Abstr. 24th Intersci. Congr. Antimicrob. Agents Chemother. Washington, D.C., 290, 1984.

Grayston, J.T.; Wang, S.P.; Yeh, L.J.; Kuo, C.C. Importance of reinfection in the pathogenesis of trachoma. Rev. Infect. Dis. 7:717–725, 1985a.

Grayston, J.T.; Kuo, C.-C.; Wang, S.-P.; Altman, J. Isolation of TWAR strains, a human *Chlamydia psittaci*, from acute respiratory disease. Abstr 25th Intersci Congr Antimicrob Agents Chemoth, Minneapolis, 257, 1985b.

Grayston, J.T.; Kuo, C.-C.; Wang, S.-P.; Cooney, M.K.; Altman, J.; Marrie, T.J.; Marshall, J.G.; Mordhorst, C.H. Clinical findings in TWAR respiratory tract infections. In: Chlamydial Infections. Oriel, D.; Ridgway, G.; Schachter, J.; Taylor-Robinson, D.; Ward, M. eds. Cambridge: Cambridge University Press, 1986a, pp. 337–340.

Grayston, J.T.; Kuo, C.C.; Wang, S.P.; Altman, J. A new *Chlamydia psittaci* strain, TWAR, isolated in acute respiratory tract infections. N. Engl. J. Med. 315:161–168, 1986b.

Greenberg, S.B.; Harris, D.; Giles, P.; Martin, R.R.; Wallace, R.J. Inhibition of *Chlamydia trachomatis* growth in McCoy, HeLa, and human prostate cells by zinc. Antimicrob. Agents Chemother. 27:953–957, 1985.

Greenwood, S.M.; Moran, J.J. Chronic endometritis: morphologic and clinical observations. Obstet. Gynecol. 58:176–184, 1981.

Gregory, W.W.; Gardner, M.; Byrne, G.I.; Moulder, J.W. Arrays of hemispheric projections on *Chlamydia psittaci* and *Chlamydia trachomatis* observed by scanning electron microscopy. J. Bacteriol. 138:241–244, 1979.

Grieg, A.; Linklater, K.A. Field studies on the efficiency of a long acting preparation of oxytetracycline in controlling outbreaks of enzootic abortion of sheep. Vet. Rec. 117:627–628, 1985.

Griffith, P.D.; Lechler, R.I.; Treharne, J.D. Unusual chlamydial infection in a human renal allograft recipient. Br. Med. J. 2:1264, 1978.

Grimes, J.E. Chlamydiosis in psittacine birds. J. Am. Vet. Med. Assoc. 190:394–397, 1987.

Grimes, J.E.; Clark, F.D. Pet psittacine birds; a continuing potential source of psittacosis for humans. Tex. Med. 82:46–47, 1986.

Grimes, D.A.; Blount, J.H.; Patrick, J. Antibiotic treatment of pelvic inflammatory disease. Trends among private physicians in the United States, 1966 through 1983. J. Am. Med. Assoc. 256:3223–3226, 1986.

Grossman, C.J. Interactions between the gonadal steroids and the immune system. Science 227:257–261, 1985.

Grossman, M.; Schachter, J.; Sweet, R.; Bishop, E.; Jordan, C. Prospective studies in newborns. In: Chlamydial Infections. Mårdh, P.A.; Holmes, K.K.; Oriel, J.D.; Piot, P.; Schachter, J. eds. Amsterdam: Elsevier Biomedical Press, 1982, pp. 213–216.

Guerra, P.; Buogo, A.; Marubini, E.; Ghione, M. Analysis of clinical and laboratory data of an experiment with trachoma vaccine in Ethiopia. Am. J. Ophthalmol. 63:1631–1638, 1967.

Guillard, E.T.; Harris, A.M.; Prieur, D.J.; Everman, J.D.; Dhillon, A.S. Pathogenesis of feline gastric chlamydial infection. Am. J. Vet. Res. 45:2314–2321, 1984.

Gump, D.W.; Dickenstein, S.; Gibson, M. Endometritis related to *Chlamydia trachomatis* infection. Ann. Intern. Med. 95:61–63, 1983a.

Gump, D.W.; Gibson, M.; Ashikaga, T. Evidence of prior pelvic inflammatory disease and its relationship to *Chlamydia trachomatis* antibody and intrauterine contraceptive device use in infertile women. Am. J. Obstet. Gynecol. 146:153–159, 1983b.

Gupta, P.K.; Lee, E.F.; Erozan, Y.S.; Frost, J.K.; Geddes, S.T.; Donovan, P.A. Cytologic investigation in *Chlamydia* infection. Acta Cytol. 23:315–320, 1979.

Hager, W.D.; Eschenbach, D.A.; Spence, M.R.; Sweet, R.L. Criteria for diagnosis and grading of salpingitis. Obstet. Gynecol. 61:113–114, 1983.

Hahon, N.; Cooke, K.O. Fluorescent cell-counting neutralization test for psittacosis. J. Bacteriol. 89:1465–1471, 1965.

Haight, J.B.; Ockner, S.A. *Chlamydia/trachomatis* perihepatitis with ascites. Am. J. Gastroenterol. 83:323–325, 1988.

Halberstaedter, L.; von Prowazek, S. Zur Ätiologie des Trachoms (in German). Deutsch. Med. Wochenschr. 33:1285–1287, 1907.

Halberstaedter, L., von Prowazek, S. Üeber Chlamydozoenbefunde bei Blennorrhoe neonatorum non-gonorrhoica (in German). Berlin. Klin. Wochenschr. 46:1839–1840, 1909.

Hallberg, A.; Mårdh, P.A.; Persson, K.; Ripa, K.T. Pneumonia-associated with *Chlamydia trachomatis* infection in an infant. Acta Paediatr. Scand. 68:765–767, 1979.

Hallberg, T.; Wølner-Hanssen, P.; Mårdh, P.-A. Pelvic inflammatory disease in patients infected with *Chlamydia trachomatis:* in vitro cell mediated immune response to chlamydial antigens. Genitourin. Med. 61:247–251, 1985.

Hamark, B.; Brorsson, J.E.; Eilard, T.; Forssman, L. Salpingitis and *Chlamydia* subgroup A. Acta Obstet. Gynecol. Scand. 55:377–378, 1976.

Hambling, M.H.; Kurtz, J.B. Preliminary evaluation of an enzyme immunoassay test for the detection of *Chlamydia trachomatis*. Lancet i:53, 1985.

Hammerschlag, M.R.; Anderka, M.; Semine, D.Z.; McComb, D.; McCormack, W.M. Prospective study of maternal and infantile infection with *Chlamydia trachomatis*. Pediatrics 64:142–148, 1979.

Hammerschlag, M.R.; Chandler, J.W.; Alexander, E.R.; English, M.; Chiang, W.T.; Koutsky, L.; Eschenbach, D.A.; Smith, J.R. Erythromycin ointment in ocular prophylaxis of neonatal conjunctivitis. J. Am. Med. Assoc. 244:2291–2293, 1980a.

Hammerschlag, M.R.; Hammerschlag, P.E.; Alexander, E.R. The role of *Chlamydia trachomatis* in middle ear effusions in children. Pediatrics 66:615–617, 1980b.

Hammerschlag, M.R.; Doraiswamy, B.; Alexander, E.R.; Cox, P.; Price, W.; Gleyzer, A. Are rectogenital chlamydial infections a marker of sexual abuse in children? Ped. Infect. Dis. 3:100–104, 1984.

Hammerschlag, M.R.; Herrmann, J.E.; Cox, P.; Worku, M.; Lanx, R.; Howard, L.V. Enzyme immunoassay for diagnosis of neonatal chlamydial conjunctivitis. J. Ped. 107:741–743, 1985.

Handsfield, H.H.; Jasman, L.L.; Roberts, P.L.; Hanson, V.W.; Kothenbeutel, R.L.; Stamm, W.E. Criteria for selective screening for *Chlamydia trachomatis* infection in women attending family planning clinics. J. Am. Med. Assoc. 255:1730–1734, 1986.

Hanna, L.; Dawson, C.R.; Briones, O.; Thygeson, P.; Jawetz, E. Latency in human infections with TRIC agents. J. Immunol. 101:45–50, 1968.

Hanna, L.; Jawetz, E.; Briones, O.; Antibodies to TRIC agents in matched human tears and sera. J. Immunol. 110:1464–1469, 1973.

Hanna, L.; Schmidt, L.; Sharp, M.; Stites, D.P.; Jawetz, E. Human cell-mediated immune responses to chlamydial antigens. Infect. Immun. 23:412–417, 1979.

Hanna, L.; Keshishyan, H.; Brooks, G.F.; Stites, D.P.; Jawetz, E. Effect of seminal plasma on *Chlamydia trachomatis* strain LB-1 in cell culture. Infect. Immun. 32:404–406, 1981.

Hanna, L.; Jawetz, E.; Dawson, C.R.; Thygeson, P. Long-term clinical microbiological and immunological observations of the volunteer repeatedly infected with *Chlamydia trachomatis*. J. Clin. Microbiol. 16:895–900, 1982.

Hardy, D. The diagnosis of trachoma by the cytology of conjunctival smears. Med. J. Aust. 2:339–341, 1966.

Hardy, D.; Surman, P.G.; Howarth, W. H. A system of representation of cytologic features of external eye infections with special reference to trachoma. Am. J. Ophthalmol. 63:1535–1537, 1967.

Hardy, P.H.; Hardy, J.B.; Nell, E.E.; Graham, D.A.; Spence, M.R.; Rosenbaum, R.C. Prevalence of six sexually transmitted disease agents among pregnant inner-city adolescents and pregnancy outcome. Lancet ii:333–337, 1984.

Hare, M.J.; Toone, E.; Taylor-Robinson, D.; Evans, R.T.; Furr, P.M.; Cooper, P.; Oates, J.K. Follicular cervicitis—Colposcopic appearances and association with *Chlamydia trachomatis*. Br. J. Obstet. Gynecol. 88:174–180, 1981.

Harnisch, J.P.; Berger, R.E.; Alexander, E.R.; Mouda, G.D.; Holmes, K.K. Etiology of acute epididymitis. Lancet i:819–821, 1977.

Harris, J.W. Chlamydial antibodies in pigs in Scotland. Vet. Rec. 98:505–506, 1976.

Harris, J.W.; Hunter, A.R.; Martin, D.A. Experimental chlamydial pneumonia in pigs. Comp. Immun. Microbiol. Infect. Dis. 7:19–26, 1984.

Harrison, H.R. Chlamydial infection in neonates and children. In: Chlamydial Infections. Oriel, D.; Ridgway, G.; Schachter, J.; Taylor-Robinson, D.; Ward, M. eds. Cambridge: Cambridge University Press, 1986, pp. 283–292.

Harrison, H.R.; Riggin, R.T. Infection of untreated primary human amnion monolayers with *Chlamydia trachomatis*. J. Infect. Dis. 140:968–971, 1979b.

Harrison, H.R.; English, M.G.; Lee, C.K.; Alexander, E.R. *Chlamydia trachomatis* infant pneumonitis: Comparison with matched controls and other infant pneumonitis. N. Engl. J. Med. 298:225–228, 1978.

Harrison, H.R.; Alexander, E.R.; Chiang, W.T.; Giddens, W.E.; Boyce, J.T.; Bejamin, D.; Gale, J.L. Experimental nasopharyngitis and pneumonia caused by *Chlamydia trachomatis* in infants baboons: histopathologic comparison with a case in a human infection. J. Infect. Dis. 139:141–146, 1979a.

Harrison, H.R.; Taussig, L.M.; Fulginetti, V.A. *Chlamydia trachomatis* and chronic respiratory disease in childhood. Ped. Infect. Dis. 1:29–33, 1982.

Harrison, H.R.; Alexander, E.R.; Weinstein, L.; Lewis, M.; Nash, M.; Sim, D.A. Cervical *Chlamydia trachomatis* and mycoplasma infections in pregnancy. J. Am. Med. Assoc. 250:1721–1727, 1983a.

Harrison, H.R.; Boyce, W.T.; Haffner, W.H.J. The prevalence of genital *Chlamydia trachomatis* and mycoplasmal infections during pregnancy in an American Indian population. Sex. Transm. Dis. 10:184–186, 1983b.

Harrison, H.R.; Riggins, R.M.; Alexander, E.R.; Weinstein, L. In vitro activity of clindamycin against strains of *Chlamydia trachomatis, Mycoplasma hominis* and *Ureaplasma urealyticum* isolated from pregnant women. Am. J. Obstet. Gynecol. 149:477–480, 1984.

Harrison, H.R.; Boyce, W.T.; Wang, S.-P.; Gibb, G.N.; Cox, J.E.; Alexander, E.R. Infection with *Chlamydia trachomatis* immunotype J associated with trachoma in an area previously endemic for trachoma. J. Infect. Dis. 151:1034–1036, 1985.

Harwick, H.J.; Purcell, R.H.; Iuppa, J.B.; Fekety, F.R. *Mycoplasma hominis* and abortion. J. Infect. Dis. 121:260–268, 1970.

Hatch, T.P. Competition between *C. psittaci* and L cells for host isoleucine pools: a limiting factor in chlamydial multiplication. Infect. Immun. 12:211–219, 1975.

Hatch, T.P.; Vance, D.W., Jr.; Al-Hossainy, E. Identification of a major envelope protein in *Chlamydia* spp. J. Bacteriol. 146:426–429, 1981.

Hawkins, D.A.; Taylor-Robinson, D.; Thomas, B.J.; Osborn, M.F.; Harris, J.R.W. *Chlamydia trachomatis* in acute epididymitis: aspirations without aspirates. In: Chlamydial Infections. Oriel, D.; Ridgway, G.; Schachter, J.; Taylor-Robinson, D.; Ward, M. eds. Cambridge: Cambridge University Press, 1986, pp. 259–262.

Heggie, A.D.; Lumicao, G.G.; Stuart, L.A.; Gyves, M.T. *Chlamydia trachomatis* infection in mothers and infants. Am. J. Dis. Child. 135:507–511, 1981.

Heggie, A.D.; Jaffe, A.C.; Stuart, L.A.; Thrombe, P.S.; Sorensen, R.V. Topical sulfacetamide vs. oral erythromycin for neonatal chlamydial conjunctivitis. Am. J. Dis. Child. 139:556–564, 1985.

Heggie, A-D.; Wentz, W.B.; Reagan, J.W.; Anthony, D.D. Roles of cytomegalovirus and *Chlamydia trachomatis* in the induction of cervical neoplasia in the mouse. Cancer Res. 46:5211–5214, 1986.

Heinonen, P.K.; Teisala, K.; Punnonen, R.; Lehtinen, M.; Miettinen, A.; Paavonen, J. Treatment of pelvic inflammatory disease with doxycycline plus metronidazole or penicillin plus metronidazole. Genitourin. Med. 62:235–239, 1986.

Helm, C.W.; Smart, G.E.; Groy, J.A.; Cunning, A.D.; Lambie, A.T.; Smith, I.W.; Allan, N.C. Exposure to *Chlamydia psittaci* in pregnancy. Lancet i:1144–1145, 1987.

Helmy, N.; Fowler, W. Intensive and prolonged tetracycline therapy in non-specific urethritis. Br. J. Vener. Dis. 51:336–339, 1975.

Henry-Suchet, J.; Catalan, F.; Loffredo, V.; Serfaty, D.; Siboulet, A.; Perol, Y.; Sanson, M.J.; Debache, C.; Pigeau, F.; Coppin, R.; de Brux, J.; Poynard, T. Microbiology of specimens obtained by laparoscopy from controls and from patients with pelvic inflammatory disease or infertility with tubal obstruction: *Chlamydia trachomatis* and *Ureaplasma urealyticum*. Am. J. Obstet. Gynecol. 138:1022–1025, 1980.

Henry-Suchet, J.; Catalan, F.; Loffredo, V.; Sanson, M.J.; Debache, C.; Pigeau, F.; Coppin, R. *Chlamydia trachomatis* associated with chronic inflammation in abdominal specimens from women selected for tuboplasty. Fertil. Steril. 36:599–605, 1981.

Henry-Suchet, J.; Utzmann, C.; De Brux, J.; Ardoin, P.; Catalan, F. Microbiologic study of chronic inflammation associated with tubal factor infertility: role of *Chlamydia trachomatis*. Fertil. Steril. 47:274–277, 1987.

Higashi, N.; Notake, K.; Fukuda, T. Growth characteristics of the meningopneumonitis virus in strain L cells. Annu. Rep. Inst. Virus Res. Kyoto Univ. 2:23–56, 1959.

Hilton, A.A.; Richmond, S.J.; Milne, J.D.; Hindley, F.; Clarke, S.K.R. *Chlamydia* A in the female genital tract. Br. J. Vener. Dis. 50:1–10, 1974.

Hipp, S.S.; Kirkwood, M.W.; Han, Y. Recovery of *Chlamydia trachomatis* by inoculation of McCoy cell suspension. Curr. Microbiol. 9:141–144, 1983.

Hipp, S.S.; Han, Y.; Murphy, D. Assessment of enzyme immunoassay and immunofluorescence tests for detection of *Chlamydia trachomatis*. J. Clin. Microbiol. 25:1938–1943, 1987.

Hobson, D. Tissue culture procedures for the isolation of *Chlamydia trachomatis* from patients with nongonococcal genital infection. In: Nongonococcal Urethritis and Related Infections. Hobson, D.; Holmes, K.K. eds. Washington, D.C.: American Society for Microbiology, 1977, pp. 286–294.

Hobson, D.; Johnson, F.W.; Rees, E.; Tait, I.A. Simplified method for diagnosis of genital and ocular infections with *Chlamydia*. Lancet ii:555–556, 1974.

Hobson, D.; Karayiannis, P.; Byng, R.E.; Rees, E.; Tait, I.A.; Davies, J.A. Quantitative aspects of chlamydial infection of the cervix. Br. J. Vener. Dis. 56:156–162, 1980.

Hobson, D.; Lee, N.; Quayle, E.; Beckett, E.E. Growth of *Chlamydial trachomatis* in Buffalo green monkey cells. Lancet i:872–873, 1982a.

Hobson, D.; Lee, N.; Bushell, A.A.; Withana, N. The activity of β-lactam antibiotics against *Chlamydia trachomatis* in McCoy cell cultures. In: Chlamydial Infections. Mårdh, P.A.; Holmes, K.K.; Oriel, J.D.; Piot, P.; Schachter, J. eds. Amsterdam: Elsevier Biomedical Press, 1982b, pp. 249–252.

Holmes, K.K. Acute epididymitis. Curr. Ther. Res. 26:738–744, 1979.

Holmes, K.K. The *Chlamydia* epidemic. J. Am. Med. Assoc. 245:1718–1723, 1981.

Holmes, K.K. Lower genital tract infections in women: cystitis/urethritis, vulvovaginitis and cervicitis. In: Sexually Transmitted Diseases. Holmes, K.K.; Mårdh, P.-A.; Sparling, P.F.; Wiesner, P.J. eds. New York: McGraw-Hill, 1984, pp. 557–589.

Holmes, K.K.; Mårdh, P.-A. eds. International Perspective on Neglected Sexually Transmitted Diseases: Impact on Venereology, Fertility and Maternal and Infant Health. Hemisphere Publishing, Washington, D.C., 1983.

Holmes, K.K.; Johnson, D.W.; Floyd, T.M. Studies of venereal disease. II. Observations on the incidence, etiology and treatment of the post-gonococcal urethritis syndrome. J. Am. Med. Assoc. 202:131–137, 1967a.

Holmes, K.K.; Johnson, D.W.; Floyd, T.M. Studies in venereal disease. III. Double-blind comparison of tetracycline hydrochloride and placebo in treatment of non-gonococcal urethritis. J. Am. Med. Assoc. 202:138–140, 1967b.

Holmes, K.K.; Handsfield, H.H.; Wang, S.-P.; Wentworth, B.B.; Turck, M.; Anderson, J.B.; Alexander, E.R. Etiology of nongonococcal urethritis. N. Engl. J. Med. 292:1199–1205, 1975.

Holmes, K.K.; Eschenbach, D.A.; Knapp, J.S. Salpingitis: Overview of etiology and epidemiology. Am. J. Obstet. Gynecol. 138:893–900, 1980.

Holst, E.; Svensson, L.; Skarin, A.; Weström, L.; Mårdh, P.-A. Vaginal colonization with Gardnerella vaginalis and anaerobic curved rods. In: Bacterial Vaginosis. Mårdh, P.-A.; Taylor-Robinson, D. eds. Almqvist & Wiksell International, Stockholm, 1984a, pp. 147–152.

Holst, E.; Mårdh, P.A.; Thelin, I. Recovery of anaerobic curved rods and Gardnerella vaginalis from the urethra of men, including male heterosexual consorts of female carriers. In: Bacterial Vaginosis. Mårdh, P.-A.; Taylor-Robinson, D. eds. Almqvist & Wiksell International, Stockholm, 1984b, pp. 173–177.

Holst, E.; Wathne, B.; Hovelius, B.; Mårdh, P.A. Bacterial vaginosis: Microbiological and clinical findings. Eur. J. Clin. Microbiol. 6:536–541, 1987.

Holt, S.; Pedersen, A.H.B.; Wane, S.P.; Kenny, G.E.; Foy, H.M.; Grayston, J.T. Isolation of TRIC agents and mycoplasma from the genitourinary tracts of patients of a venereal disease clinic. Am. J. Ophthalmol. 63:1057–1064, 1967.

Horn, J.E.; Hammer, M.L.; Falkow, S.; Quinn, T.C. Detection of Chlamydia trachomatis in tissue culture and cervical scrapings by in situ DNA hybridization. J. Infect. Dis. 153:1155–1159, 1986.

Hoshiwara, I.; Powers, D.K.; Krutz, G. Comprehensive trachoma control program among the southwestern American Indians. In: Ophthalmology, Proceedings of the XII International Congress, International Congress Series no. 222. Amsterdam: Excerpta Medica, 1971, pp. 1935–1939.

Howard, H. A short history of TRIC agent infection of the conjunctiva in Australia and the results of recent virological investigations. Med. J. Aust. 53:337–341, 1966.

Howard, L.V.; Coleman, P.F.; England, B.J.; Herrmann, J.E. Evaluation of Chlamydiazyme® for the detection of genital infections caused by Chlamydia trachomatis. J. Clin. Microbiol. 23:329–332, 1986.

Hoyme, U.B.; Kiviat, N.; Eschenbach, D.A. Microbiology and treatment of late postpartum endometritis. Obstet. Gynecol. 68:226–232, 1986.

Hull, M.G.R.; Glazener, C.M.A.; Kelly, N.J.; Conway, D.I.; Foster, P.A.; Hinton, R.A.; Coulson, C.; Lambert, P.A.; Watt, E.M.; Desai, K.M. Population study of causes, treatment and outcome of infertility. Br. Med. J. 291:1693–1697, 1985.

Hunter, J.M.; Sommerville, R.G. Erythromycin stearate in treating chlamydial infection of the cervix. Br. J. Vener. Dis. 60:387–389, 1984.

Huss, H.; Jungkind, D.; Amadio, P.; Rubenfield, I. Frequency of *Chlamydia trachomatis* as the cause of pharyngitis. J. Clin. Microbiol. 22:858–860, 1985.

Hutchinson, G.R.; Taylor-Robinson, D.; Dourmashkin, R.R. Growth and effect of chlamydiae in human and bovine oviduct cultures. Br. J. Vener. Dis. 55:194–202, 1979.

Hyypiä, T.; Larsen, S.H.; Ståhlberg, T., Terho, P. Analysis and detection of chlamydial DNA. J. Gen. Microbiol. 130:3159–3164, 1984.

Hyypiä, T.; Jalava, A.; Larsen, S.H.; Terho, P.; Hukkanen, V. Detection of *Chlamydia trachomatis* in clinical specimens by nucleic acid spot hybridization. J. Gen. Microbiol. 131:975–978; 1975.

Idtse, F.S. Chlamydia and chlamydial disease of cattle: a review of literature. Vet. Med. 63:543–550, 1984.

Ingerslev, H.J.; Møller, B.R.; Mårdh, P.-A. *Chlamydia trachomatis* in acute and chronic endometritis. In: *Chlamydia trachomatis* in genital and related infections. Mårdh, P.-A.; Møller, B.R.; Paavonen, J. eds. Scand. J. Infect. Dis. Suppl. 32:59–63, 1982.

Ingram, D.L.; Runyan, D.K.; Collins, A.D.; White, S.T.; Durfee, M.F.; Pearson, A.W.; Occhiuti, A.R. Vaginal *Chlamydia trachomatis* infection in children with sexual contact. Ped. Infect. Dis. 3:97–99, 1984.

Isaacs, D. Psittacosis. Br. Med. J. 289:510–511, 1984.

Ismail, M.A.; Chandler, A.E.; Beem, M.O.; Moawad, A.H. Chlamydial colonization of the cervix in pregnant adolescents. J. Reprod. Med. 30:549–553, 1985.

Jacobs, N.F.; Arum, E.S.; Kraus, S.J. Experimental infection of the chimpanzee urethra and pharynx with *Chlamydia trachomatis*. Sex. Transm. Dis. 5:132–136, 1978.

Jacobson, L.; Weström, L. Objectivized diagnosis of acute pelvic inflammatory disease. Am. J. Obstet. Gynecol. 105:1088–1098, 1969.

Jansson, E. Ornithosis in Helsinki and some other localities in Finland. A serological and clinical study. Ann. Med. Exp. Biol. 38, Suppl. 4:1–110, 1960.

Johannisson, G. Studies on *Chlamydia trachomatis* as a cause of lower urogenital tract infection. Academic dissertation. University of Gothenborg, 1981.

Johannisson, G.; Sernryd, A.; Lycke, E. Susceptibility of *C. trachomatis* to antibiotics in vitro and in vivo. Sex. Transm. Dis. 6:50–57, 1979.

Johannisson, G.; Löwhagen, G.B.; Lycke, E. Genital *Chlamydia trachomatis* infection in women. Obstet. Gynecol. 56:671–675, 1980.

Johannisson, G.; Löwhagen, G.B.; Nilsson, S. *Chlamydia trachomatis* and urethritis in men. In: *Chlamydia trachomatis* in genital and related infections. Mårdh, P.-A.; Møller, B.R.; Paavonen, J. eds. Scand. J. Infect. Dis. Suppl. 32:87–92, 1982.

Johansson, E.; Moi, H.; Forslin, H.; Danielsson, D. Prevalence of chlamydial infection, gonorrhoea and non-specific urethritis in regular sexual partners of women with acute salpingitis. In: Abstracts of the Scandinavian Society for Genitourinary Medicine, 4th meeting, Elsinore, 11–13 September, 1987.

John, J. Efficacy of prolonged regimens of oxytetracycline in the treatment of nongonococcal urethritis. Br. J. Vener. Dis. 47:266–268, 1971.

Johnson, A.P.; Hetherington, C.M.; Osborn, M.F.; Thomas, B.J.; Taylor-Robinson, D. Experimental infection of the marmoset genital tract with *Chlamydia trachomatis*. Br. J. Exp. Pathol. 61:291–295, 1980.

Johnson, A.P.; Hare, M.J.; Wilbanks, G.D.; Cooper, P.; Hertherington, C.M.; Al-Kurdi,

M.; Osborne, M.F.; Taylor-Robinson, D. A colposcopic and histological study of experimental chlamydial cervicitis in marmosets. Br. J. Exp. Pathol. 65:59–65, 1984.

Johnson, F.W.A. Zoonoses in practical: chlamydiosis. Br. Vet. J. 139:93–96, 1983.

Johnson, F.W.A.; Hobson, D. The effect of penicillin on genital strains of *C. trachomatis* in tissue culture. J. Antimicrob. Chemother. 3:49–56, 1977.

Johnson, F.W.A.; Matheson, B.A.; Williams, H.; Laing, A.G.; Jandial, V.; Davidson-Lamb, R.; Halliday, G.J.; Hobson, D.; Wong, S.Y.; Hadley, K.M.; Moffat, M.A.; Postletwaithe, R. Abortion due to infection with *Chlamydia psittaci* in a sheep farmer's wife. Br. Med. J. 290:592–594, 1985.

Jones, B.R. Ocular syndromes of TRIC virus infection and their possible genital significance. Br. J. Vener. Dis. 40:3–15, 1964.

Jones, B.R. Laboratory tests for chlamydial infection. Their role in epidemiological studies of trachoma and its control. Br. J. Ophthalmol. 58:438–454, 1974.

Jones, B.R. The prevention of blindness from trachoma. Trans. Ophthalmol. Soc. UK 95:16–33, 1975.

Jones, B.R.; Collier, L.H.; Smith, C.H. Isolation of virus from inclusion blennorrhoea. Lancet i:902–905, 1959.

Jones, B.R.; Al-Hussaini, M.K.; Dunlop, E.M.C.; Emarah, M.H.M.; Freedman, A.; Garland, J.A.; Harper, I.A.; Race J.W.; Du Toit, M.S.; Treharne, J.D. Infection by TRIC agent and other members of the Bedsonia group; with a note on Reiter's disease. I. Ocular disease in the adult. Tr. Ophthalmol. Soc. UK 86:291–312, 1966.

Jones, M.F.; Smith, T.F.; Houglum, A.J.; Herrmann, J.E. Detection of *Chlamydia trachomatis* in genital specimens by the Chlamydiazyme® test. J. Clin. Microbiol. 20:465–467, 1984.

Jones, R.B.; Batteiger, B.E. Human immune response to *Chlamydia trachomatis* infections. In: Chlamydial Infections. Oriel, D.; Ridgway, G.; Schachter, J.; Taylor-Robinson, D.; Ward, M. eds. Cambridge: Cambridge University Press, 1986, pp. 423–432.

Jones, R.B.; Batteiger, B.; Newhall, V.W.J. Cross-reactive antigenic determinants in the major surface proteins of *Chlamydia trachomatis*. In: Chlamydial Infections. Mårdh, P.-A.; Holmes, K.K.; Oriel, J.D.; Piot, P.; Schachter, J. eds. Amsterdam: Elsevier Biomedical Press, 1982a, pp. 61–64.

Jones, R.B.; Ardeny, B.R.; Hui, S.L.; Cleary, R.E. Correlation between serum anti-chlamydial antibodies and tubal factor infertility. Fertil. Steril. 38:533–538, 1982b.

Jones, R.B.; Bruins, S.C.; Newhall, W.J. Comparison of reticulate and elementary body antigens in detection of antibodies against *Chlamydia trachomatis* by an enzyme-linked immunosorbent assay. J. Clin. Microbiol. 17:466–471, 1983.

Jones, R.B.; Rabinowitch, R.A.; Katz, B.P.; Batteiger, B.E.; Quinn, T.A.; Terho, P.; Lapworth, M.A. *Chlamydia trachomatis* in the pharynx and rectum of heterosexual patients at risk for genital infection. Ann. Intern. Med. 102:757–762, 1985.

Jones, R.B.; Katz, B.P.; van der Pol, B.; Caine, V.A.; Batteiger, B.E.; Newhall, V.W.J. Effect of blind passage and multiple sampling on recovery of *Chlamydia trachomatis* from urogenital specimens. J. Clin. Microbiol. 24:1029–1033, 1986a.

Jones, R.B.; Mammel, J.B.; Shepard, M.K.; Fisher, R.R. Recovery of *Chlamydia tra-*

chomatis from the endometrium of women at risk for chlamydial infection. Am. J. Obstet. Gynecol. 155:35–39, 1986b.

Jones, R.B.; Harrison, H.R.; Quinn, T.C.; Stamm, W.E.; Katz, B.P. Susceptibility of *Chlamydia trachomatis* to clindamycin, erythromycin and tetracycline. In Abstracts of the 1987 ICAAC, abstract no. 732, p. 224, 1987.

Jordan, J.A.; Singer, A. The Cervix. London: W.B. Saunders, Ltd., 1976.

Joseph, T.; Nano, F.E.; Garon, C.F.; Caldwell, H.D. Molecular characterization of *Chlamydia trachomatis* and *Chlamydia psittaci* plasmids. Infect. Immun. 51:699–703, 1986.

Judson, F.N.; Assessing the number of genital chlamydial infections in the United States. J. Reprod. Med. 30(Suppl.):269–272, 1985.

Kallings, I.; Mårdh, P.-A. Sampling and specimen handling in the diagnosis of genital *Chlamydia trachomatis* infections. In: *Chlamydia trachomatis* in Genital and Related Infections. Mårdh, P.-A.; Møller, B.R.; Paavonen, J. eds. Scand. J. Infect. Dis. Suppl. 32:21–24, 1982.

Kane, J.L.; Woodland, R.N.; Forsey, T. *Chlamydia trachomatis* and infertility. Lancet i:736, 1984a.

Kane, J.L.; Woodland, R.M.; Forsey, T.; Darougar, S.; Elder, M.G. Evidence of chlamydial infection in infertile women with and without fallopian tube obstruction. Fertil. Steril. 42:843–848, 1984b.

Kaper, J.B.; Moseley, S.L.; Falkow, S. Molecular characterization of environmental and nontoxigenic strains of *Vibrio cholerae*. Infect. Immun. 32:661–667, 1981.

Karney, W.W.; Pedersen, A.H.B.; Nelson, M.; Adams, H.; Pfeifer, R.T.; Holmes, K.K. Spectinomycin versus tetracycline for the treatment of gonorrhea. N. Engl. J. Med. 296:899–894, 1977.

Kass, E.H.; McCormack, W.M.; Lin, J.S. Genital mycoplasmas as a cause of excess premature delivery. Trans. Assoc. Am. Phys. 94:261–266, 1981.

Kaufman, R.E.; Wiesner, P.J. Non-specific urethritis. N. Engl. J. Med. 291:1175–1177, 1974.

Keat, A.C. Reiter's syndrome and reactive arthritis in perspective. N. Engl. J. Med. 309:1606–1615, 1983.

Keat, A.C.; Maini, R.N.; Nkwazi, G.C.; Pegrum, G.D.; Ridgway, O.L.; Scott, J.T. Role of *Chlamydia trachomatis* and HLA-B27 in sexually acquired reactive arthritis. Br. Med. J. 1:605–607, 1978.

Keat, A.C.; Thomas, B.J.; Taylor-Robinson, D.; Pegrum, G.D.; Maini, R.N.; Scott, J.T. Evidence of *Chlamydia trachomatis* infection in sexually acquired reactive arthritis. Ann. Rheum. Dis. 39:431–437, 1980.

Keat, A.; Thomas, B.J.; Taylor-Robinson, D. Chlamydial infection in the aetiology of arthritis. Br. Med. Bull. 39:168–174, 1983.

Keat, A.; Thomas, B.; Dixey, J.; Osborn, M.; Sonnex, C.; Taylor-Robinson, D. *Chlamydia trachomatis* and reactive arthritis: the missing link. Lancet i:72–74, 1987.

Keene, F.E.; Payne, F.L. Functional uterine bleeding. South. Med. J. 27:108, 1934.

Khurana, C.M.; Deddish, P.A.; DelMundo, F. Prevalence of *Chlamydia trachomatis* in the pregnant cervix. Obstet. Gynecol. 66:241–243, 1985.

Kihlström, E.; Bogosian, G.; Bassford, P.J. Jr.; Wyrick, P. B. Molecular cloning and expression of proteins of *Chlamydia psittaci*. In: Chlamydial Infections. Oriel, D.; Ridgway, G.; Schachter, J.; Taylor-Robinson, D.; Ward, M. eds. Cambridge: Cambridge University Press, 1986, pp. 101–104.

Kimball, M.W.; Knee, S. Gonococcal perihepatitis in a male. N. Engl. J. Med. 282:1082–1083, 1970.

Kingborn, G.R.; Waugh, M.A. Oral contraceptive use and prevalence of infection with *Chlamydia trachomatis* in women. Br. J. Vener. Dis. 57:187–190, 1981.

Kingsbury, D.T.; Weiss, E. Lack of deoxyribonucleic acid homology between species of the genus *Chlamydia*. J. Bacteriol. 96:1421–1423, 1968.

Kirshon, B.; Faro, S.; Phillips, L.E.; Pruett, K. Correlation of ultrasonography and bacteriology of the endocrine and posterior cul-de-sac of patients with severe pelvic inflammatory disease. Sex. Trans. Dis. 15:103–107, 1988.

Kiviat, N.B.; Paavonen, J.A.; Brockway, J.; Critchlow, C.W.; Brunham, R.C.; Stevens, C.E.; Stamm, W.E.; Kuo, C.-C.; DeRouen, T.; Holmes, K.K. Cytologic manifestations of cervical and vaginal infections. I. Epithelial and inflammatory cellular changes. J. Am. Med. Assoc. 253:989–996, 1985a.

Kiviat, N.B.; Peterson, M.; Kinney-Thomas, E.; Tam, M.; Stamm, W.E.; Holmes, K.K. Cytologic manifestations of cervical and vaginal infections. II. Confirmation of *Chlamydia trachomatis* infection by direct immunofluorescence using monoclonal antibodies. J. Am. Med. Assoc. 253:997–1000; 1985b.

Kiviat, N.; Paavonen, J.; Wølner-Hanssen, P.; Critchlow, C.; DeRouen, T.; Douglas, J.; Stevens, C.; Holmes, K.K. Histologic manifestations of chlamydial cervicitis. In: Chlamydial Infections. Oriel, D.; Ridgway, G.; Schachter, J.; Taylor-Robinson, D.; Ward, M. eds. Cambridge: Cambridge University Press, 1986a; pp. 209–212.

Kiviat, N.B.; Wølner-Hanssen, P.; Peterson, M.; Wasserheit, J.; Stamm, W.E.; Eschenbach, D.A.; Paavonen, J.; Lingenfelter, J.; Bell, T.; Zabriskie, V.; Kirby, B.; Holmes, K.K. Localization of *Chlamydia trachomatis* infection by indirect immunofluorescence and culture in pelvic inflammatory disease. Am. J. Obstet. Gynecol. 154:865–873; 1986b.

Kleemola, M.; Saikku, P.; Visakorpi, R.; Wang, S.P.; Grayston, J.T. Pneumonia epidemics in military trainees in Finland caused by TWAR, a new chlamydia organism. J. Infect. Dis., 157:230–236; 1988.

von Knorring, J.; Nieminen, J. Gonococcal perihepatitis in a surgical ward. Ann. Clin. Res. 11:66–70, 1979.

Komaroff, A.L. Acute dysuria in women. N. Engl. J. Med. 310:368–375, 1984.

Komaroff, A.L.; Aronson, M.D.; Schachter, J. *Chlamydia trachomatis* infection in adults with community-acquired pneumonia. J. Am. Med. Assoc. 245:1319–1322, 1981.

Komaroff, A.L.; Aronson, M.D.; Pass, T.M.; Ervin, C.T.; Branch, W.T. Jr.; Schachter, J. Serologic evidence of chlamydial and mycoplasmal pharyngitis in adults. Science 222:927–929, 1983.

Kordova, N.; Witt, J.C. Effect of trypsinization on susceptibility of primary human amniotic cells to *Chlamydia trachomatis* TW⁻³ strain. Curr. Microbiol. 4:27–30, 1980.

Koss, L.G. Diagnostic Cytology and Its Histopathologic Bases, 3rd ed. Philadelphia: JB Lippincott, 1979.

Kousa, M. Clinical observations on Reiter's disease with special reference to the venereal and non-venereal etiology. Acta Dermatovener. (Stockh) 58, Suppl. 81:1–36, 1978.

Kousa, M. Evidence of chlamydial involvement in the development of arthritis. In: *Chlamydia trachomatis* in Genital and Related Infections. Mårdh, P.-A.; Møller, B.R.; Paavonen, J. eds. Scand. J. Infect. Dis. Suppl. 32:116–121, 1982.

Kousa, M.; Saikku, P.; Richmond, S.; Lassus, A. Frequent association of chlamydial infection with Reiter's syndrome. Sex. Transm. Dis. 5:57–61, 1978.

Kousa, M.; Saikku, P.; Kanerva, L. Erythema nodosum in chlamydial infections. Acta dermatovener. (Stockh) 60:319–322, 1980.

Koutsky, L.; Stamm, W.E.; Brunham, R.C.; Stevens, C.E.; Cole, B.; Hale, J.; Davick, P.; Holmes, K.K. Persistence of *Mycoplasma hominis* after therapy: Importance of tetracycline resistence and of coexisting vaginal flora. Sex. Transm. Dis. 10(Suppl):374–381, 1983.

Kramer, D.G.; Jason, J. Sexually abused children and sexually transmitted diseases. Rev. Infect. Dis. 4(Suppl):883–890, 1982.

Krauss, H.; Schmeer, N.; Wittenbrink, M.M. Significance of *Chlamydia psittaci* infections in animal in the F.R.G. In: Proceedings of the Eur. Soc. for Chlamydia Research, Bologna, Italy, May 30–June 1, 1988, p. 65.

Krech, T.; Gerhard-Fsadni, D.; Hofman, N.; Miller, S.M. Interference of *Staphylococcus aureus* in the detection of *Chlamydia trachomatis* by monoclonal antibodies. Lancet i:1161–1162, 1985.

Kristensen, G.B.; Bollerup, A.C.; Lind, K.; Mårdh, P.-A.; Ladehoff, P.; Larsen, S.; Marushak, A.; Rasmussen, P.; Rolschau, J.; Skoven, I.; Sorensen, I.; Lind, I. Infection with *Neisseria gonorrhoeae* and *Chlamydia trachomatis* in women with acute salpingitis. Genitourin. Med. 61:179–184; 1985.

Kristensen, J.K.; Scheibel, J.H. Etiology of acute epididymitis presenting in a venereal disease clinic. Sex. Transm. Dis. 11:32–33; 1984.

Kristensen, J.K.; Schmid, G.P.; Potter, M.E.; Anderson, D.C.; Kaufmann, A.F. Psittacosis. A diagnostic challenge. J. Occup. Med. 26:731–733; 1984.

Kunimoto, D.; Brunham, R.C. Human immune response and *Chlamydia trachomatis* infection. Rev. Infect. Dis. 7:665–673; 1985.

Kuo, C.-C. Cultures of *Chlamydia trachomatis* in mouse peritoneal macrophages: factors affecting organism growth. Infect. Immun. 20:439–445; 1978.

Kuo, C.-C.; Grayston, J.T. Factors affecting viability and growth in HeLa cells of *Chlamydia* sp. strain TWAR. J. Clin. Microbiol. 28:812–815; 1988.

Kuo, C.-C.; Kenny, G.E.; Wang, S.-P. Trachoma and psittacosis antigens in agar gel double immunodiffusion. In: Trachoma and Related Disorders Caused by Chlamydial Agents. Nichols, R.L. ed. Amsterdam: Excerpta Medica, 1971; pp. 113–123.

Kuo, C.-C.; Wang, S.-P.; Wentworth, B.B.; Grayston, J.T. Primary isolation of TRIC organism in HeLa 229 cells treated with DEAE-dextran. J. Infect. Dis. 125:665–668; 1972.

Kuo, C.-C.; Wang, S.-P.; Grayston, J.T. Effect of polycations, polyanions, and neuraminidase on the infectivity of trachoma-inclusion conjunctivitis and lymphogranuloma venereum organisms in HeLa cells; sialic acid residues as possible receptors for trachoma-inclusion conjunctivitis. Infect. Immun. 8:74–79, 1973.

Kuo, C.-C.; Wang, S.-P.; Grayston, J.T. Antimicrobial activity of several antibiotics and a sulfonamide against *Chlamydia trachomatis* organisms in cell culture. Antimicrob. Agents Chemother. 12:80–83, 1977.

Kuo, C.-C.; Chen, W.J.; Brunham, R.C.; Stephens, R.S. A mouse model of *Chlamydia trachomatis* infection. In: Chlamydial Infections. Mårdh, P.-A.; Holmes, K.K.; Oriel, J.D.; Piot, P.; Schachter, J. eds. Amsterdam: Elsevier Biomedical Press, 1982, pp. 379–382.

Kuo, C.-C.; Chen, H.H.; Wang, S.-P.; Grayston, J.T. Characterization of TWAR strains, a new group of *Chlamydia psittaci*. In: Chlamydial Infections. Oriel, D.; Ridgway, G.; Schachter, J.; Taylor-Robinson, D.; Ward, M. eds. Cambridge: Cambridge University Press, 1986a, pp. 321–324.

Kuo, C.-C.; Chen, H.H.; Wang, S.P.; Grayston, J.T. Identification of a new group of *Chlamydia psittaci* strains called TWAR. J. Clin. Microbiol. 24:1034–1037, 1986b.

Kuritsky, J.N.; Scheibel, J.H. Etiology of acute epididymitis presenting in a venereal disease clinic. Sex. Transm. Dis. 11:32–33, 1984.

Landis, S.J.; Stewart, I.O.; Chernesky, M.A.; Mahony, J.B.; Cunningham, A.I.; Grenier-Landis, M.N.; Seidelman, W.E. Value with urethritis. Sex. Trans. Dis. 15:78–84, 1988.

Langham, J.G.; Doyle, D.V., Reactive arthritis following psittacosis. Br. J. Rheumatol. 23:225–226, 1984.

Lannigan, R.; Hardy, G.; Tanton, R.; Marrie, T.J. *Chlamydia trachomatis* peritonitis and ascites following appendectomy. Can. Med. Assoc. 123:295–296, 1980.

Lassus, A.; Mustakallio, K.K.; Wager, O. Autoimmune serum factors and IgA elevation in lymphogranuloma venereum. Ann. Clin. Res. 2:51–56, 1970.

Lassus, A.; Paavonen, J.; Kousa, M.; Saikku, P. Erythromycin and lymecycline treatment in chlamydia-positive and chlamydia-negative nongonococcal urethritis: a partner-controlled study. Acta Dermatovener. (Stockh) 59:278–281, 1979.

Lee, C.K.; Moulder, J.W. Persistent infection of mouse fibroblasts (McCoy cells) with a trachoma strain of *Chlamydia trachomatis*. Infect. Immun. 32:822–829, 1981.

Lehtinen, M.; Rantala, I.; Aine, R.; Miettinen, A.; Laine, S.; Heinonen, P.; Teisala, K.; Punnonen, R.; Paavonen, J. B cell response in *Chlamydia trachomatis* endometritis. Eur. J. Clin. Microbiol. 5:596–598, 1986.

Leinonen, M.; Saikku, P.; Ekman, M.R.; Suomalainen, R.; Kerttula, Y. Demonstration of antibody responses to Re-lipopolysaccharide as a diagnostic tool for chlamydial pneumonia. In: Proceedings of the Eur. Soc. for Chlamydia Research, 1st Meeting, Bologna, Italy, May 30–June 1, 1988, p. 269.

Leirisalo, M.; Skylv, G.; Kousa, M.; Voipio-Pulkki, L.M.; Suoranta, H.; Nissilä, M.; Hvidman, L.; Damm Nielsen, E.; Svejgard, A.; Tiilikainen, A.; Laitinen, O. Follow-up study on patients with Reiter's disease and reactive arthritis, with special reference to HLA-B27. Arthr. Rheum. 25:249–259, 1982.

Levison, D.A.; Ward, C.; Guthrie, W.; Green, D.M.; Robertson, P.G.C. Infective endocarditis as part of psittacosis. Lancet ii:844–847, 1971.

Levitt, D.; Bard, J. Chlamydiae as polyclonal B cell activators in humans and mice. In: Chlamydial Infections. Oriel, D.; Ridgway, G.; Schachter, J.; Taylor-Robinson, D.; Ward, M. eds. Cambridge: Cambridge University Press, 1986, pp. 449–452.

Levitt, D.; Barol. J. The immunobiology of Chlamydia. Immunol. Today 8:246–251, 1987.

Levitt, D.; Newcomb, R.S.; Beem, M.O. Excessive numbers and activity of peripheral blood B cells in infants with Chlamydia trachomatis pneumonia. Clin. Immunol. Immunopathol. 29:429–432, 1983.

Levy, N.J.; McCormack, W.M. Detection of serum antibody to Chlamydia with ELISA. In Chlamydial Infections. Mårdh, P.-A.; Holmes, K.K.; Oriel, J.D.; Piot, P.; Schachter, J. eds. Amsterdam: Elsevier Biomedical Press, 1982, pp. 341–344.

Lewis, J.; Kraus, S.; Hambie, E.; Harrison, H. Detection of Neisseria gonorrhoeae and Chlamydia trachomatis by enzyme immunoassay of urine sediment. Abstracts of the 1987 ICAAC. Abstract no. 427, p. 171, 1987.

Lewis, V.J.; Thacker, W.L.; Mitchell, S.H. Enzyme-linked immunosorbent assay for chlamydial antibodies. J. Clin. Microbiol. 6:507–510, 1977.

Liebowitz, L.D.; Saunders, J.; Fehler, G.; Ballard, R.C.; Koornhof, H.J. In vitro activity of A-56619 (difloxacin), A-56620, and other new quinolone antimicrobial agents against genital pathogens. Antimicrob. Agents Chemother. 30:948–950, 1986.

Lindner, K. Zur Ätiologie der gonokokkenfreien Urethritis (in German). Wien. Klin. Wochenschr. 8:283–284, 1910.

Lindner, K. Gonoblenorrhoe. Einschlussblenorrhoe und Trachom (in German). Albert von Graefes Arch. Klin. Exp. Ophthalmol. 78:345–380, 1911.

Lindner, L.E.; Geerling, S.; Nettum, J.A.; Miller, S.L.; Altman, K.H. The cytologic features of chlamydial cervicitis. Acta Cytol. 29:676–682, 1985.

Lipkin, E S.; Moncada, J.V.; Shafer, M.A.; Wilson, T.E.; Schachter, J. Comparison of monoclonal antibody staining and culture in diagnosing cervical chlamydial infection. J. Clin. Microbiol. 23:114–117, 1986.

Litt, I.F.; Cohen, M.I. Perihepatitis associated with salpingitis in adolescents. J. Am, Med. Assoc. 240:1253–1254, 1978.

Longhi, S. Efficacia clinica di minociclina miocamicina e norfloxacin nelle infezioni urogenitali da Chlamydia trachomatis e sua incidenza (in Italian). Poster of Cong. Naz. sulle Malattie a Transmissione Sessuale, Bologna, Nov. 23–25, 1987.

Lovett, M.; Kuo, C.-C.; Holmes, K.K.; Falkow, S. Plasmids of the genus Chlamydia. In: Current Chemotherapy and Infectious Diseases, Vol. 2. Nelson, J.D.; Grassai, C. eds. Washington, D.C.: American Society for Microbiology, 1980, pp. 1250–1252.

Lycke, E. Assaying antichlamydial drugs in vitro. In: Chlamydia trachomatis in genital and related infections. Mårdh, P.-A.; Møller, B.R.; Paavonen, J. eds. Scand. J. Infect. Dis. Suppl. 32:38–41, 1982.

Lycke, E.; Peterson, M. Hemolysis-in-gel test for demonstration of chlamydia antibodies. J. Clin. Microbiol. 4:450–452, 1976.

Mabey, D.C.W.; Ogbaselassie, G.; Robertson, J.N.; Heckels, J.E.; Ward, M.E. Tubal infertility in the Gambia: chlamydial and gonococcal serology in women with tubal occlusion compared with pregnant controls. Bull. WHO 63:1107–1113, 1985.

Mabey, D.C.W.; Robertson, J.N.; Ward, M.E. Detection of Chlamydia trachomatis by enzyme immunoassay in patients with trachoma. Lancet ii:1491–1492, 1987.

MacCallan, A.F. Trachoma. London: Butterworth, 1936, pp. 8–26.

Macfarlane, J.T.; Macrae, A.D. Psittacosis. Br. Med. Bull. 39:163–167, 1983.

Maclachlan, W.W.G.; Crum, G.E.; Kleinschmidt, R.F.; Wehrle, P.F. Psittacosis. Am. J. Med. Sci. 226:157–163, 1953.

Maffei, C.; Di Stanislao, F.; Pauri, P.; Clementi, M. Psittacosis of non-avian origin. Lancet i:806–807, 1984.

Maffei, C.; Marracino, A.; di Stanislao, F.; Pauri, P.; Clementi, M.; Varaldo, P.E. Psittacosis in a highly endemic area in Italy. Epidemiol. Inf. 99:413–419, 1987.

Mahony, J.B.; Chernesky, M.A. Effect of swab type and storage temperature on the isolation of *Chlamydia trachomatis* from clinical specimens. J. Clin. Microbiol. 22:865–867, 1985.

Mahony, J.B.; Schachter, J.; Chernesky, M.A. Detection of antichlamydial immunoglobulin G and M antibodies by enzyme-linked immunosorbent assay. J. Clin. Microbiol. 18:270–275, 1983.

Malaty, R.; Zaki, S.; Said, M.E.; Vastine, D.W.; Dawson, C.R.; Schachter, J. Extraocular infections in children in areas with endemic trachoma. J. Infect. Dis. 143:853, 1981.

Manire, G.P.; Galasso, G.J. Persistent infection of HeLa cells with meningopneumonitis virus. J. Immunol. 83:529–533, 1959.

Manire, G.P.; Tamura, A. Preparation and chemical composition of the cell walls of mature infectious dense forms of meningopenumonitis organisms. J. Bacteriol. 94:1178–1183, 1967.

Marbet, U.A.; Stalder, G.A.; Vögtlin, J.; Loosli, J.; Frei, A.; Althaus, B.; Gyr, K. Diffuse peritonitis and chronic ascites due to infection with *Chlamydia trachomatis* in patients without liver disease: new presentation of the Fitz-Hugh-Curtis syndrome. Br. Med. J. Clin. Res. 293:5–6, 1986.

Mårdh, P.-A. An overview of infectious agents of salpingitis, their biology and recent advances in methods of detection. Am. J. Obstet. Gynecol. 138:933–951, 1980.

Mårdh, P.-A. Some constituents of body fluids influencing the capability of *Chlamydia trachomatis* to multiply in McCoy cell cultures. In: Proc. of the 4th Meeting of the Int. Soc. for STD Res. Heidelberg, Oct. 18–20, 1981, Abstract 82.

Mårdh, P.-A. Influence de choix du tampon de prélèvement et de l'eprovelte de transport sur le résultat des cultures chlamydiales (in French). Rev. Int. de Trachome 2–3:41–47, 1982.

Mårdh, P.-A. Laboratory diagnosis of STD. Bacteria, chlamydiae and mycoplasmas. In: Sexually Transmitted Diseases. Holmes, K.K.; Mårdh, P.A.; Sparling, F.; Wiesner, P. eds. McGraw-Hill, New York, 1984, pp. 829–855.

Mårdh, P.-A. Ascending chlamydial infection in the female genital tract. In: Chlamydial Infections. Oriel, J.; Ridgway, G.; Schachter, J.; Taylor-Robinson, D.; Ward, M. eds. Cambridge: Cambridge University Press, 1986, pp. 173–184.

Mårdh, P.-A. The importance of chlamydial infections in gynecology and the need for programs for control and prevention. In Le Malattie a Transmissione Sessuale. Danesino, V.; Montemagno, U.; Orlando, C. eds. Bologna: Farmacie comunali AFM, 1987, pp. 43–47.

Mårdh, P.-A. The chlamydial epidemic, with special emphasis on European perspectives. In: Proceedings of the Eur. Soc. for Chlamydia Research, 1st Meeting, Bologna, Italy, May 30–June 1, 1988, pp. 3–6.

Mårdh, P.-A.; Colleen, S. Lysozyme in seminal fluid of healthy males and patients with prostatitis and in tissues of the male urogenital tract. Scand. J. Nephrol. Urol. 8:179–189, 1974.

Mårdh, P.-A.; Colleen, S. Antimicrobial activity of human seminal fluid. Scand. J. Nephrol. 9:17–23, 1975.

Mårdh, P.-A.; Møller, B.R.; Ingerslev, H.J.; Nüssler, E.; Weström, L.; Wølner-Hanssen, P. Endometritis caused by *Chlamydia trachomatis*. Br. J. Vener. Dis. 57:191–195, 1981a.

Mårdh, P.-A.; Svensson, L. Chlamydial salpingitis. In: *Chlamydia trachomatis* in genital and related infections. Mårdh, P.-A.; Møller, B.R.; Paavonen, J. eds. Scand. J. Infect. Dis. Suppl. 32:64–72, 1982.

Mårdh, P.-A.; Wølner-Hanssen, P. Periappendicitis and chlamydial salpingitis. Surg. Gynecol. Obstet. 160:304–306, 1985.

Mårdh, P.-A.; Zeeberg, B. The toxic effect of sampling swabs and transportation test tubes on the formation of intracytoplasmic inclusions of *Chlamydia trachomatis*. Br. J. Vener. Dis. 57:268–272, 1981.

Mårdh, P.-A., Stormby, N.; Weström, L. Mycoplasma and vaginal cytology. Acta Cytol. 15:310–314, 1971.

Mårdh, P.-A.; Ripa, T.; Svensson, L.; Weström, L. *Chlamydia trachomatis* infection in patients with acute salpingitis. N. Engl. J. Med. 296:1377–1379, 1977a.

Mårdh, P.-A.; Ripa, K.T.; Wang, S.-P.; Weström, L. *Chlamydia trachomatis* as an etiologic agent in acute salpingitis. In: Nongonococcal Urethritis and Related Infections. Hobson, D.; Holmes, K.K. Washington, D.C.: American Society for Microbiology, 1977b, pp. 77–83.

Mårdh, P.-A.; Ripa, K.T., Colleen, S.; Treharne, J.D.; Darougar, S. Role of *Chlamydia trachomatis* in non-acute prostatitis. Br. J. Vener. Dis. 54:330–334, 1978.

Mårdh, P.-A.; Colleen, S.; Sylwan, J. Inhibitory effect on the formation of chlamydial inclusions in McCoy cells by seminal fluid and some of its components. Invest. Urol. 17:510–513, 1980a.

Mårdh, P.-A.; Helin, I.; Bobeck, S. Colonization of pregnant and puerperal women and neonates with *Chlamydia trachomatis*. Br. J. Vener. Dis. 56:96–100, 1980b.

Mårdh, P.-A.; Weström, L.; Colleen, S.; Wølner-Hanssen, P. Sampling, specimen handling and isolation techniques in diagnosis of chlamydial and other genital infections. Sex. Transm. Dis. 8:280–285, 1981b.

Mårdh, P.-A.; Lind, I.; Svensson, L.; Weström, L.; Møller, B.R. Antibodies to *Chlamydia trachomatis, Mycoplasma hominis,* and *Neisseria gonorrhoeae* in sera from patients with acute salpingitis. Br. J. Vener. Dis. 57:125–129, 1981c.

Mårdh, P.-A.; Møller, B.R.; Paavonen, J. Chlamydial infection of the female genital tract with emphasis on pelvic inflammatory disease. Sex. Transm. Dis. 8:140–155, 1981d.

Mårdh, P.-A.; Stenberg, K.; Herrmann, B.; Väänänen, P. Comparison of two tests in the diagnosis of chlamydial conjunctivitis. Fifth International Symposium on Rapid Methods and Automation in Microbiology and Immunology, Florence, 4–6 November, 1987, p. 495.

Marrie, T.J.; Grayston, J.T.; Wang, S.P.; Kuo, C.C. Pneumonia associated with the TWAR strain of *Chlamydia*. Ann. Intern. Med. 106:507–511, 1987.

Martel, J.L.; Perrin, M.; Rodolakis, A.; Russo. P.; Deschanel, J.P.; Garnier, F. Infection expérimentale de la vache gestante par *Chlamydia psittaci* (in French). Ann. Rech. Vet. 14:117–120, 1983.

Martin, D.H.; Koutsky, L.; Eschenbach, D.A.; Daling, J.R.; Alexander, E.R.; Benedetti, J.K.; Holmes, K.K. Prematurity and perinatal mortality in pregnancies complicated by maternal *Chlamydia trachomatis* infections. J. Am. Med. Assoc. 247:1585–1588, 1982.

Martin, D.A.; Pollock, S.; Kuo, C.C.; Wang, S.P.; Brunham, R.C.; Holmes, K.K. *Chlamydia trachomatis* infections in men with Reiter's syndrome. Ann. Intern. Med. 100:207–213, 1984.

Martin, D.H.; Pastorek, J.G. 2nd; Faro, S. In vitro and in vivo activity of parenterally administered beta-lactam antibiotics against *Chlamydia trachomatis*. Sex. Transm. Dis. 13:81–87, 1986a.

Martin, D.H.; Pastorek, J.G.; Faro, S. Risk factors for *Chlamydia trachomatis* infection in a high risk population of pregnant women. In: Chlamydial Infections. Oriel, D.; Ridgway, G.; Schachter, J.; Taylor-Robinson, D.; Ward, M. eds. Cambridge: Cambridge University Press, 1986b, pp. 189–192.

Martinov, S.P.; Popov, G.V. *Chlamydia psittaci* infections in animals in Eastern Europe. In: Proceedings of the Eur. Soc. For Chlamydia Research, 1st Meeting, Bologna, Italy, May 30–June 1, 1988, p. 69.

Martinov, S.; Shoilev, K.H.; Popov, G. Prouchvaniia na klamidinata infektsiia pre perikarditi po prasetata (Chlamydial infection in pericarditis in pigs) (in Bulgarian). Vet. Med. Nauki 22:20–26, 1985.

Martinov, S.P.; Popov, G.W.; Dimitrov, K.D. Untersuchungen über die Chlamydieninfektion beim Reiter's syndrom (RS) (in German). Z. Hautkr. 62(3):216–219, 1987.

Matikainen, M.T. *Chlamydia trachomatis* lymphogranuloma venereum strains. Immunodetection and biochemical characterization. Academic dissertation. University of Turku, 1984.

Matsumoto, A. Recent progress of electron microscopy in microbiology and its development in future: from a study of the obligate intracellular parasites. Chlamydia organisms. J. Electron. Microsc. 28(Suppl):57–64, 1979.

Matsumoto, A.; Manire, G.P. Electron microscopic observations on the effects of penicillin on the morphology of *Chlamydia psittaci*. J. Bacteriol. 101:278–285, 1970.

McCauly, E.H.; Tieken, E.L. Psittacosis-lymphogranuloma venereum agent isolated during an abortion epizootics in goats. J. Am. Vet. Med. Assoc. 152:1758–1765, 1968.

McComb, R.E.; Nichols, R.L. Antibodies to trachoma in eye secretions of Saudi Arab children. Am. J. Epidemiol. 90:278–282, 1969.

McComb, D.E.; Nichols, R.L. Antibody specificity to trachoma in eye secretions of Saudi Arab children. Infect. Immun. 2:65–68, 1970.

McComb, D.E.; Nichols, R.L.; Semine, D.Z.; Evrad, J.R.; Alpert, S.; Crockett, V.A.; Rosner, B.; Zinner, S.H.; McCormack, W.M. *Chlamydia trachomatis* in women: antibody in cervical secretions as a possible indicator of genital infection. J. Infect. Dis. 139:628–633, 1979.

McCormack, W.M.; Alpert, S.; McComb, D.E.; Nichols, R.L.; Semine, Z.; Zinner, S.H. Fifteen-month follow-up study of women infected with *C. trachomatis*. N. Engl. J. Med. 300:123–125, 1979.

McCutchan, J.A. Epidemiology of venereal urethritis: comparison of gonorrhoea and non-gonococcal urethritis. Rev. Infect. Dis. 6:669–688, 1984.

McDonald, A.B.; McComb, D.; Howard, L. Immune response of owl monkeys to topical vaccination with irradiated Chlamydia trachomatis. J. Infect. Dis. 149:439–442, 1984.

McDonald, P.C.; Porter, J.C.; Schwartz, B.E.; Johnston, J.M. Initiation of parturition in the human female. Semin. Perinatol. 2:273–286, 1978.

McKercher, D.G.; Crenshaw, G.L.; Theis, J.H.; Wada, E.M.; Mauris, C.M. Experimentally induced immunity to chlamydial abortion of cattle. J. Infect. Dis. 128:231–234, 1973.

McKinlay, A.W.; White, N.; Buxton, D.; Inglis, J.M.; Johnson, F.W.A.; Kurtz, J.B.; Brettle, R.P. Severe Chlamydia psittaci sepsis in pregnancy. Q. J. Med. 57:689–696, 1985.

McMillan, A.; Sommerville, R.G.; McKie, P.M.K. Chlamydial infection in homosexual men: frequency of isolation of Chlamydia trachomatis from the urethra, ano-rectum, and pharynx. Br. J. Vener. Dis. 57:47–49, 1981.

Meheus, A.; van Dycke, E.; Ursi, J.P.; Ballard, R.C.; Piot, P.E. Etiology of genital ulcers in Swaziland. Sex. Transm. Dis. 10:33–35, 1983.

Meheus, A.; Reniers, J.; Collet, M.; Frost, E.; Leclerc, A.; Gass, R.; Ivanoff, B. Chlamydia trachomatis in women with acute salpingitis and infertility in Central Africa. In: Chlamydial Infections. Oriel, D.; Ridgway, G.; Schachter, J.; Taylor-Robinson, D.; Ward, M. eds. Cambridge: Cambridge University Press, 1986, pp. 241–244.

Menke, H.E.; Schuller, J.I.; Stolz, E. Treatment of lymphogranuloma venereum with rifampicin. Br. J. Vener. Dis. 55:379, 1979.

Meurman, O.; Terho, P.; Sonck, C.E. Type-specific IgG and IgA antibodies in old lymphogranuloma venereum determined by solid-phase radioimmunoassay. Med. Microbiol. Immunol. 170:279–286, 1982.

Meyer, K.F.; Eddie, B. Human carrier of the psittacosis virus. J. Infect. Dis. 88:109–125, 1953.

Meyer, K.F.; Eddie, B. The influence of tetracycline compounds on the development of antibodies in psittacosis. Am. Rev. Tuberc. Pulm. Dis. 74:566–571, 1956.

Miller, B.R.; Arthur, J.D.; Parry, W.H.; Perez, T.R.; Mosman, P.L. Atypical croup and Chlamydia trachomatis. Lancet i:1022, 1982.

Minkoff, H. Prematurity: Infection as an etiologic factor. Obstet. Gynecol. 62:137–144, 1983.

Minkoff, H.; Grunebaum, A.N.; Schwarz, R.H.; Feldman, J.; Cummings, M.; Crobleholme, W.; Clark, L.; Pringle, G.; McCormack, W.M. Risk factors for prematurity and premature rupture of membranes: A prospective study of the vaginal flora in pregnancy. Am. J. Obstet. Gynecol. 150:965–972, 1984.

Miyagawa, Y.; Mitamura, T.; Yaoi, H.; Ishi, N.; Nakajima, N.; Okanishi, T.; Watanabe, S.; Sato, K. First report: studies on the virus of lymphogranuloma inguinale Nicolas, Favre and Durand. Cultivation of the virus on the chorio-allantoic membrane of the chicken embryo. Jap. J. Exp. Med. 13:733–738, 1935.

Moi, H.; Danielson, D. Diagnosis of genital Chlamydia trachomatis infection in males by cell culture and antigen detection test. Eur. J. Clin. Microbiol. 5:563–568, 1986.

Møller, B.R. The grivet monkey as animal model for inflammation of the lower genital tract caused by *Chlamydia trachomatis*. In: Chlamydial Infections. Oriel, D.; Ridgway, G.; Schachter, J.; Taylor-Robinson, D.; Ward, M. Cambridge: Cambridge University Press, 1986, pp. 375–379.

Møller, B.R.; Mårdh, P.-A. Experimental salpingitis in grivet monkeys by *Chlamydia trachomatis*. Modes of spread of infection to the fallopian tubes. Acta Pathol. Microbiol. Scand. (B) 88:107–114, 1980a.

Møller, B.R.; Mårdh, P.-A. Experimental epididymitis and urethritis in grivet monkeys provoked by *Chlamydia trachomatis*. Fertil. Steril. 34:275–279, 1980b.

Møller, B.R.; Mårdh, P.A. Animal models for the study of chlamydial infections of the urogenital tract. In: *Chlamydia trachomatis* in Genital and Related Infections. Mårdh, P.-A.; Møller, B.R.; Paavonen, J. eds. Scand. J. Infect. Dis. Suppl. 32:103–108, 1982.

Møller, B.R.; Cramers, M.; From, E. Pivampicillin in treating genital infection with *Chlamydia trachomatis*. Genitourin. Med. 61:264–265, 1985.

Møller, B.R.; Weström, L.; Ahrons, S.; Ripa, K.T.; Svensson, L.; von Mecklenburg, C.; Henriksson, H.; Mårdh, P.-A. *Chlamydia trachomatis* infection of the fallopian tubes. Histological findings in two patients. Br. J. Vener. Dis. 55:422–428, 1979.

Møller, B.R.; Freundt, E.A.; Mårdh, P.A. Experimental pelvic inflammatory disease provoked by *Chlamydia trachomatis* and *Mycoplasma hominis* in grivet monkey. Am. J. Obstet. Gynecol. 138:990–995, 1980.

Møller, B.R.; Ahrons, S.; Laurin, J.; Mårdh, P.A. Pelvic infection after elective abortion associated with *Chlamydia trachomatis*. Obstet. Gynec. 59:210–212, 1982.

Moncada, J.V.; Schachter, J.; Wofsy, C. Prevalence of *Chlamydia trachomatis* lung infection in patients with acquired immunodeficiency syndrome. J. Clin. Microbiol. 23:986, 1986.

Monnickendam, M.; Pearce, J.H. Immune responses and chlamydial infections. Br. Med. Bull. 39:187–193, 1983.

Moore, D.E.; Spadoni, L.R.; Foy, H.M.; Wang, S.P.; Daling, J.R.; Kuo, C.C.; Grayston, J.T.; Eschenbach, D.A. Increased frequency of serum antibodies to *Chlamydia trachomatis* in infertility due to distal tubal obstruction. Lancet 2:574–577, 1982.

Morbidity and Mortality Weekly Report, *Chlamydia trachomatis* infections. Policy guidelines for prevention and control. MMWR 34:53s–74s, 1985.

Morbidity and Mortality Weekly Report, Ectopic pregnancy–United States, 1981–1983. MMWR 35:289–291, 1986.

Mordhorst, C.H. Isolation of the TRIC agent from 3 cases of neonatal inclusion blennorrhoea and from the cervix of one of the mothers. Acta Pathol. Microbiol. Scand. 63:301–302, 1964.

Mordhorst, C.H.; Dawson, C. Sequelae of neonatal inclusion conjunctivitis and associated disease in parents. Am. J. Ophthalmol. 71:861–867, 1971.

Mordhorst, C.H.; Hegazy, N. Laboratory study of trachoma in Egyptian rural school children. Bull. WHO 51:167–171, 1974.

Mordhorst, C.H.; Wang, S.P.; Grayston, J.T. Epidemic "ornithosis" and TWAR infection, Denmark 1976–85. In: Chlamydial Infections. Oriel, J.; Ridgway, G.;

Schachter, J.; Taylor-Robinson, D.; Ward, M. eds. Cambridge: Cambridge University Press, 1986, pp. 326–328.

Morgan, H.R.; Bader, J.P. Latent viral infection of cells in tissue culture. IV. Latent infection of L cells with psittacosis virus. J. Exp. Med. 106:39–44, 1957.

Moritz, E. Wurmvorsatzveränderungen nach Tubernentzündungen (in German). Z. Geburtsh. Gynekol. 70:404–416, 1912.

Moseley, S.L.; Echeverria, P.; Seriwatana, J.; Tirapat, C.; Chaicumpa, W.; Sakuldaipeara, T.; Falkow, S. Identification of enterotoxigenic *Escherichia coli* by colony hybridization using three enterotoxin gene probes. J. Infect. Dis. 145:864–869, 1982.

Moulder, J. The relation of the psittacosis group (chlamydiae) to bacteria and viruses. Ann. Rev. Microbiol. 20:107–130, 1966.

Moulder, J.W. A primer for Chlamydiae. In: Chlamydial infections. Mårdh, P.-A.; Holmes, K.K.; Oriel, J.D.; Piot, P.; Schachter, J. eds. Amsterdam: Elsevier Biomedical Press, 1982, pp. 3–14.

Moulder, J.W.; Levy, N.J.; Schulman, L.P. Persistent infection of mouse fibroblasts (L cells) with *Chlamydia psittaci:* evidence for a cryptic form. Infect. Immun. 30:874–883, 1980.

Moulder, J.W.; Hatch, T.T.; Kuo, C.C.; Schachter, J.; Storz, J. Genus *Chlamydia.* In: Bergey's Manual of Systematic Bacteriology, Vol. 1. Krieg, N.R. ed. Baltimore: Williams & Wilkins, 1984, pp. 729–739.

Mourad, A.S.; Ramadan, M.; Rizk, M.A.; El-Addar, A.M.; Moursi, G.A. The TRIC agent in the female genital tract. A cytologic and virologic study in a trachomatous hyperendemic area. J. Egypt. Public Health Assoc. 51:55–76, 1976.

Mourad, A.; Sweet, R.L.; Sugg, N. Relative resistance to erythromycin in *Chlamydia trachomatis.* Antimicrob. Agents Chemother. 18:696–698, 1980.

Mulcahy, F.M.; Bignell, C.J.; Rajhumar, R.; Wangh, M.A.; Hetherington, J.W.; Ewing, R.; Whelan, P. Prevalence of chlamydial infection in acute epididymo-orchitis. Genitourin. Med. 63:16–18, 1987.

Mumtaz, G.; Mellars, B.J.; Ridgway, G.L.; Oriel, J.D. Enzyme immunoassay for the detection of *Chlamydia trachomatis* antigen in urethral and endocervical swabs. J. Clin. Pathol. 38:740–742, 1985.

Munday, P.E.; Johnson, A.P.; Thomas, B.J.; Taylor-Robinson, D. *Chlamydia trachomatis* proctitis. N. Engl. J. Med. 305:1158, 1981.

Murray, E.S. Review of clinical, epidemiological and immunological studies of guinea-pig inclusion conjunctivitis infection in guinea pigs. In: Nongonococcal Urethritis and Related Infections. Hobson, D.; Holmes, K.K. eds. Washington, D.C.: American Society for Microbiology, 1977, pp. 199–204.

Murray, E.S.; Fraser, C.E.O.; Peters, J.H.; McComb, D.E.; Nichols, R.L. The owl monkey as an experimental primate model for conjunctival trachoma infection. In: Trachoma and Related Disorders Caused by Chlamydial Agents. Nichols, R.L. ed. Amsterdam: Excerpta Medica, 1971, pp. 386–395.

Murray, E.S.; Charbonnet, L.T.; MacDonald, A.B. Immunity to chlamydial infections of the eye. I. The role of circulatory and secretory antibodies in resistance to reinfection with guinea pig inclusion conjunctivitis. J. Immunol. 110:1518–1525, 1973.

Müller-Schoop, J.W.; Wang, S.-P.; Munziger, J.; Schläpfer, H.U.; Knoblauch, M.;

Amman, R.W. *Chlamydia trachomatis* as possible cause of peritonitis and peri-hepatitis in young women. Br. Med. J. I:1022–1024, 1978.

Myhre, E.B.; Mårdh, P.-A. Unusual manifestations of *Chlamydia trachomatis* infections. In: *Chlamydia trachomatis* in Genital and Related Infections. Mårdh, P.-A.; Møller, B.R.; Paavonen, J. eds. Scand. J. Infect. Dis. Suppl. 32:122–126, 1982a.

Myhre, E.B.; Mårdh, P.-A. Antibody response in psittacosis. In: Chlamydial Infections. Mårdh, P.-A.; Holmes, K.K.; Oriel, J.D.; Piot, P.; Schachter, J. eds. Amsterdam: Elsevier Biomedical Press, 1982b, pp. 345–348.

Nabli, B. The effect of rifampicin on the growth of TRIC agents in embryonated eggs. In: Trachoma and Related Disorders caused by Chlamydial Agents. Nichols, R.L. ed. Amsterdam: Excerpta Medica, 1971, pp. 34–39.

Nagel, T.C.; Tagatz, G.E.; Campbell, B.F. Transmission of *Chlamydia trachomatis* by artificial insemination. Fertil. Steril. 46:959–960, 1986.

Nagington, J. Psittacosis/ornithosis in Cambridgeshire 1975–1983. J. Hyg. (Camb.) 92:9–19, 1984.

Naib, Z.M. Cytology of TRIC agent infection of the eye of newborn infants and their mothers' genital tracts. Acta Cytol. 14:390–395, 1970.

Nano, F.E.; Caldwell, H.D. Expression of the chlamydial genus-specific lipopolysac-charide epitope in *Escherichia coli*. Science 228:742–744, 1985.

Nayyar, K.C.; O'Neill, J.J.; Habbing, M.H.; Waugh, M.A. Isolation of *Chlamydia trachomatis* from women attending a clinic for sexually transmitted diseases. Br. J. Vener. Dis. 52:396–398, 1976.

Neinstein, L.S.; Inderlied, C. Low prevalence of *Chlamydia trachomatis* in the oropharynx of adolescents. Ped. Infect. Dis. 5:660–662, 1986.

Newhall, V.W.J.; Batteiger, B.; Jones, R.B. Analysis of human serological response to proteins of *Chlamydia trachomatis*. Infect. Immun. 38:1181–1189, 1982.

Newhall, V.W.J.; Terho, P.; Wilde III C.E.; Batteriger, B.E.; Jones, B.R. Serovar determination of *Chlamydia trachomatis* isolates using type-specific monoclonal antibodies. J. Clin. Microbiol. 23:333–338, 1986.

Nichols, B.A.; Setzer, P.Y.; Pang, F.; Dawson, C.R. New view of the surface projec-tions of *Chlamydia trachomatis*. J. Bacteriol. 164:344–349, 1985.

Nichols, R.L.; Bobb, A.A.; Haddad, N.A.; McComb, D.E. Immunofluorescent studies of the microbiologic epidemiology of trachoma in Saudi Arabia. Am. J. Ophthalmol. 63:1372–1408, 1967.

Nichols, R.L.; Snyder, J.C. Naturally acquired or artificially induced immunity to tra-choma. Vaccines against viral, rickettsial and bacterial diseases of man. PAHO/WHO Scientific publications 226:299–303, 1971.

Nichols, R.L.; Murray, E.S.; Nilsson, P.E. Use of enteric vaccines in protection against chlamydial infections of the genital tract and the eye of guinea pigs. J. Infect. Dis. 138:742–746, 1978.

Nielsen, P.B.; Christensen, J.D.; Frentz, G. A comparison of oxitetracycline and tri-methoprim in the treatment of *Chlamydia trachomatis* urethritis. Infection 12:274–275, 1984.

Nilsson, I.K.; Collen, S.; Mårdh, P.-A. Relationship between psychological and laboratory findings in patients with symptoms of non-acute prostatitis. In: Genital Infections and their complications. Danielsson, D.; Juhlin, L.; Mårdh, P.-A. eds. Stockholm: Almqvist & Wiksell International, 1975, pp. 133–144.

Nilsson, T.; Fischer, A.B. Acute epididymitis. Curr. Ther. Res. 26:732–737, 1979.

Nugent, R.P.; Berlin, L.; Rhoads, G.G.; Spence, M.; Quinn, T.; Polk, B.F. Risk factors for cervicitis and *Chlamydia trachomatis* in an inner city pregnant population. In: Chlamydial Infections. Oriel, D.; Ridgway, G.; Schachter, J.; Taylor-Robinson, D.; Ward, M. eds. Cambridge: Cambridge University Press, 1986, pp. 185–188.

Numazaki, K.; Chiba, S.; Moroboshi, T.; Kudoh, T.; Yamanaka, T.; Nakao, T. Comparison of enzyme linked immunosorbent assay and enzyme linked fluorescence immunoassay for detection of antibodies against *Chlamydia trachomatis*. J. Clin. Pathol. 38:345–350, 1985.

Nurminen, M.; Leinonen, M.; Saikku, P.; Mäkelä, P.H. The genus-specific antigen of *Chlamydia:* resemblance to the lipopolysaccharide of enteric bacteria. Science 220:1279–1281, 1983.

Nurminen, M.; Rietschel, E.T.; Brade, H. Chemical characterization of *Chlamydia trachomatis* lipopolysaccharide. Infect. Immun. 48:573–575, 1985.

Omori, T.; Ishii, S.; Harada, K.; Ishikawa, O.; Muruose, N.; Katada, M.; Araumi, W. Study of an infectious pneumonia in goats caused by virus. I. Isolation of the causative agent and characteristics. Exp. Rep. Gov. Exp. Sta. Anim. Hyg. (Tokyo) 27:101–119, 1953.

Omori, T.; Morimoto, T.; Harada, K.; Inaba, Y.; Ishii, S.; Matsumoto, M. Miyagawanella psittacosis-lymphogranuloma group of viruses. I. Excretion of goat pneumonia virus in feces. Jap. J. Exp. Med. 27:131–143, 1957.

O'Neill, M.B.; Moore, D.B. Periappendicitis: Clinical reality or pathologic curiosity. Am. J. Surg. 134:356–357, 1977.

Oriel, J.D. Chemotherapy. In: Chlamydial Infections. Oriel, D.; Ridgway, G.; Schachter, J.; Taylor-Robinson, D.; Ward, M. eds. Cambridge: Cambridge University Press, 1986, pp. 513–523.

Oriel, J.D.; Reeve, P.; Powis, P.; Miller, A.; Nicol, C.S. Chlamydial infection. Isolation of *Chlamydia trachomatis* from patients with non-specific genital infection. Br. J. Vener. Dis. 48:429–436, 1972.

Oriel, J.D.; Powis, P.A.; Reeve, P.; Miller, A.; Nicol, C.S. Chlamydial infections of the cervix. Br. J. Vener. Dis. 50:11–14, 1974.

Oriel, J.D.; Reeve, P.; Thomas, B.J.; Nicol, C.S. Infection with *Chlamydia* group A in men with urethritis due to *Neisseria gonorrhoeae*. J. Infect. Dis. 131:376–382, 1975.

Oriel, J.D.; Ridgway, G.L.; Reeve, P.; Beckingham, D.C.; Owen, J. The lack of effect of ampicillin plus probenecid given for genital infections with *Neisseria gonorrhoeae* on associated infections with *Chlamydia trachomatis*. J. Infect. Dis. 133:568–571, 1976.

Oriel, J.D.; Ridgway, G.L.; Tchamouroff, S. Comparison of erythromycin stearate and oxytetracycline in the treatment of nongonococcal urethritis: their efficacy against *Chlamydia trachomatis*. Scott. Med. J. 22:375–379, 1977.

Oriel, J.D.; Johnson, A.L.; Barlow, D.; Thomas, B.J.; Nayyar, K.; Reeve, P. Infection of the uterine cervix with *Chlamydia trachomatis*. J. Infect. Dis. 137:443–451, 1978.

Osser, S.; Persson, K. Epidemiologic and serodiagnostic aspects of chlamydial salpingitis. Obstet. Gynecol. 59:206–209, 1982.

Osser, S.; Persson, K. Postabortal pelvic infection associated with *Chlamydia trachomatis* and the influence of humoral immunity. Am. J. Obstet. Gynecol. 150:699–703, 1984.

Ostler, H.B.; Schachter, J.; Dawson, C.R. Acute follicular conjunctivitis of epizootic-origin feline pneumonitis. Arch. Ophthalmol. 82:587–591, 1969.

Oyelese, A.O.; Brunham, R.C.; Dowell, J.; Williams, T. Enhanced susceptibility of trypsinized HeLa cells to *Chlamydia trachomatis* infection. Eur. J. Clin. Microbiol. 6:594–595, 1987.

Paavonen, J. *Chlamydia trachomatis*-induced urethritis in female partners of men with nongonococcal urethritis. Sex. Transm. Dis. 6:69–71, 1979.

Paavonen, J.; Purola, E. Cytologic findings in cervical chlamydial infection. Med. Biol. 58:174–178, 1980.

Paavonen, J.; Valtonen, V. *Chlamydia trachomatis* as a possible cause of peritonitis and perihepatitis in a young woman. Br. J. Vener. Dis. 56:341–343, 1980.

Paavonen, J.; Vesterinen, E. *Chlamydia trachomatis* in cervicitis and urethritis in women. Scand. J. Infect. Dis. 32(Suppl):45–54, 1982.

Paavonen, J.; Mäkelä, P.H. Use of serologic methods in the diagnosis of pelvic inflammatory disease. In: Infections in Reproductive Health. Keith, L.G.; Berger, G.S.; Edelman, D.A. eds. Boston: MTP Press Ltd., 1984, pp. 209–236.

Paavonen, J.; Kousa, M.; Saikku, P.; Vesterinen, E.; Jansson, E.; Lassus, A. Examination of men with nongonococcal urethritis and their sexual partners for *Chlamydia trachomatis* and *Ureaplasma urealyticum*. Sex. Transm. Dis. 5:93–96, 1978a.

Paavonen, J.; Saikku, P.; Vesterinen, E.; Meyer, B.; Vartiainen, E.; Saksela, E. Genital chlamydial infections in patients attending a gynecologic outpatient clinic. Br. J. Vener. Dis. 54:257–261, 1978b.

Paavonen, J.; Vesterinen, E.; Meyer, B.; Saikku, P.; Suni, J.; Purola, E.; Saksela, E. Genital *Chlamydia trachomatis* infections in patients with cervical atypia. Obstet. Gynecol. 54:289–291, 1979.

Paavonen, J.; Kousa, M.; Saikku. P.; Kanerva, L.; Vartiainen, E.; Lassus, A. Treatment of nongonococcal urethritis with trimethoprim-sulfadiazine and placebo. A double-blind partner-controlled study. Br. J. Vener. Dis. 56:101–104, 1980.

Paavonen, J.; Saikku, P.; von Knorring, J.; Aho, K.; Wang, S.P. Association of infection with *Chlamydia trachomatis* with Fitz-Hugh–Curtis syndrome. J. Infect. Dis. 144:178, 1981.

Paavonen, J.; Vesterinen, E.; Mårdh, P.-A. Infertility as a sequelae of chlamydial pelvic inflammatory disease. In: *Chlamydia trachomatis* in Genital and Related Infections. Mårdh, P.-A.; Møller, B.R.; Paavonen, J. eds. Scand. J. Infect. Dis. Suppl. 32:73–76, 1982a.

Paavonen, J.; Vesterinen, E.; Meyer, B.; Saksela, E. Colposcopic and histologic findings in cervical chlamydial infection. Obstet. Gynecol. 59:712–715, 1982b.

Paavonen, J.; Aine, R.; Teisala, K.; Heinonen, P.K.; Punnonen, R.; Lehtinen, M.; Miettinen, A.; Grönroos, P. Chlamydial endometritis. J. Clin. Pathol. 38:726–732, 1985a.

Paavonen, J.; Aine, R.; Teisala, K.; Heinonen, P.K.; Punnonen, R. Comparison of endometrial biopsy and peritoneal fluid cytology with laparoscopy in the diagnosis of acute pelvic inflammatory disease. Am. J. Obstet. Gynecol. 151:645–650, 1985b.

Paavonen, J.; Kiviat, N.; Brunham, R.C.; Stevens, C.E.; Kuo, C.C.; Stamm, W.E.; Miettinen, A.; Soules, M.; Eschenbach, D.A.; Holmes, K.K. Prevalence and manifestations of endometritis among women with cervicitis. Am. J. Obstet. Gynecol. 152:280–286, 1985c.

Paavonen, J.; Critchlow, C.; DeRouen, T.; Kiviat, N.; Stevens, C.; Brunham, R.C.; Kuo, C.C.; Stamm, W.E.; Hyde, K.; Corey, L.; Eschenbach, D.A.; Holmes, K.K. Etiology of cervical inflammation. Am. J. Obstet. Gynecol. 154:556–567, 1986.

Paavonen, J.; Teisala, K.; Heinonen, P.K.; Aine, R.; Laine, S.; Lehtinen, M.; Miettinen, A.; Punnonen, R.; Grönroos, P. Microbiological and histopathological findings in acute pelvic inflammatory disease. Br. J. Obstet. Gynecol. 94:454–460, 1987.

Paavonen, J.; Kiviat, N.; Wølner-Hanssen, P.; Stevens, C.E.; Koutsky, L.; Critchlow, C.W.; DeRouen, T.; Holmes, K.K. Colposcopic manifestations of cervical and vaginal infections. Obstet. Gynecol. Surv. 43:373–381; 1988a.

Paavonen, J.; Roberts, P.L.; Stevens, C.E.; Wølner-Hanssen, P.; Brunham, R.C.; Hillier, S.; Stamm, W.E.; Kuo, C.-C.; Holmes, K.K.; Eschenbach, D.A. Treatment of mucopurulent cervicitis with doxycycline or amoxicillin. Am. J. Obstet. Gynecol. 1988b (in press).

Paavonen, T.; Andersson, L.C.; Adlercreutz, H. Sex hormone regulation of in vitro immune response. Estradiol enhances human B cell maturation via inhibition of suppressor T cells in pokeweed mitogen-stimulated cultures. J. Exp. Med. 154:1935–1945, 1981.

Page, L.A. Order II. Chlamydiales. In: Bergey's manual of determinative bacteriology, 8th Ed. Buchanan, R.E.; Gibbons, N.E. eds. Baltimore: Williams and Wilkins, 1974, pp. 914–918.

Palva, A. Nucleic acid spot hybridization for detection of Chlamydia trachomatis. FEMS Microbiol. Lett. 28:85–91, 1985.

Palva, A.; Jousimies-Somer, H.; Saikku, P.; Väänänen, P.; Söderlund, H.; Ranki, M. Detection of Chlamydia trachomatis by nucleic acid sandwich hybridization. FEMS Microbiol. Lett. 23:83–89, 1984.

Palva, A.; Korpela, K.; Lassus, A.; Ranki, M. Detection of Chlamydia trachomatis from genitourinary specimens by improved nucleic acid sandwich hybridization. FEMS Microbiol. Lett. 40:211–217, 1987.

Pao, C.C.; Lin, S.S.; Yang, T.E.; Soong, Y.K.; Lee, P.S.; Lin, J.Y. Deoxyribonucleic acid hybridization analysis for the detection of urogenital Chlamydia trachomatis infections in women. Am. J. Obstet. Gynecol. 156:195–199, 1987.

Paperny, D.M.; Hicks, R.; Rudoy, R. Chlamydial pelvic inflammatory disease in adolescents. J. Adolesc. Health Care 2:139–142, 1981.

Paran, H.; Heimer, D.; Sarov, I. Serological, clinical and radiological findings in adults with bronchopulmonary infections caused by Chlamydia trachomatis. Isr. J. Med. Sci. 22:823–827, 1986.

Pasco, W.J. Pet bird disease in southern California. Avian/Exotic Prac. 2:13–23, 1985.

Pasley, J.N.; Rank, R.G.; Hough, A.J., Jr.; Cohen, C.; Barron, A.L. Effects of varying doses of estradiol on chlamydial genital infection in ovariectomized guinea pigs. Sex. Transm. Dis. 12:8–13, 1985a.

Pasley, J.N.; Rank, R.G.; Hough, A.J., Jr.; Cohen, C.; Barron, A.L. Absence of progesterone effects on chlamydial genital infection in female guinea pigs. Sex. Transm. Dis. 12:155–158, 1985b.

Patamasucon, P.; Rettig, P.J.; Faust, K.L.; Kusmiecz, H.T.; Nelson, J.D. Oral v. topical erythromycin therapies for chlamydial conjunctivitis. Am. J. Dis. Child. 136:817–821, 1982.

Pattin, S.; Durosoir, J.L.; Doury, A.T.P. Le test de transformation lymphoblastique avec l'antigéne Bedsonien (TTL Bedsonien) dans les syndromes de Fiessiger-Leroy-Reiter anciens et récents et dans les spondylarthrites ankylosantes (in French). Rev. Rhum. Mal. Osteo-Articulaires 43:407–410, 1976.

Pattman, R.S. The significance of finding curved rods in the vaginal secretions of patients attending a genito-urinary medical clinic. In: Bacterial Vaginosis. Mårdh, P.-A.; Taylor-Robinson, D. eds. Stockholm: Almqvist & Wiksell International, 1984, pp. 143–146.

Patton, D.L. Immunopathology and histopathology of experimental chlamydial salpingitis. Rev. Infect. Dis. 7:746–753, 1985.

Patton, D.L.; Brunham, R.C.; Halbert, S.A.; Wang, S.-P.; Holmes, K.K. *Chlamydia trachomatis* salpingitis in the pig-tailed macaque. In: Chlamydial Infections. Mårdh, P.-A.; Holmes, K.K.; Oriel, J.D.; Piot, P.; Schachter, J. eds. Amsterdam: Elsevier Biomedical Press, 1982, pp. 399–402.

Patton, D.L.; Halbert, S.A.; Kuo, C.C.; Wang, S.P.; Holmes, K.K. Host response to primary *Chlamydia trachomatis* infection of the fallopian tube in pig-tailed monkeys. Fertil. Steril. 40:829–840, 1983.

Patton, D.L.; Kuo, C.-C.; Wang, S.-P.; Brenner, R.M.; Sternfeld, M.D.; Morse, S.A. Chlamydial salpingitis in subcutaneous fimbrial transplants in monkeys. In: Chlamydial Infections. Oriel, D.; Ridgway, G.; Schachter, J.; Taylor-Robinson, D.; Ward, M. eds. Cambridge: Cambridge University Press, 1986a, pp. 367–370.

Patton, D.L.; Moore, D.E.; Hicks, L.A.; Soules, M.R.; Spadoni, L.R. Tubal morphology in women with silent salpingitis. Pacific Coast Fertility Society Meeting, April 9–13, 1986b, San Diego, Abstracts.

Patton, D.L.; Kuo, C.C.; Wang, S.P.; Halbert, S.A. Distal tubal obstruction induced by repeated *Chlamydia trachomatis* salpingeal infections in pig-tailed macaques. J. Infect. Dis. 155:1292–1299, 1987a.

Patton, D.L.; Kuo, C.C.; Wang, S.P.; Brenner, R.M.; Strenfeld, M.D.; Morse, S.A.; Barnes, R.C. Chlamydial infection of subcutaneous fimbrial transplants in cynomolgus and rhesus monkeys. J. Infect. Dis. 155:229–235, 1987b.

Patton, D.L.; Cosgrove, P.A.; Kuo, C.-C.; Wang, S.-P. Subcutaneous autotransplant model for studying oculogenital infections with *Chlamydia trachomatis*. Proceedings of Eur. Soc. for Chlamydia Research, 1st Meeting, Bologna, Italy, May 30–June 1, 1988, p. 139.

Patton, S.F. Diagnostic Cytopathology of the Uterine Cervix. New York: S. Karger AG, 1978.

Peeling, R.; Maclean, I.W.; Brunham, R.C. In vitro neutralization of *Chlamydia tra-*

chomatis with monoclonal antibody to an epitope on the major outer membrane protein. Infect. Immun. 46:484–488, 1984.

Pépin, M.; Bailly, L.; Sourin, A.; Rodolakis, A. An enzyme-linked immunosorbent assay (ELISA) for the detection of chlamydial antibodies in caprine sera. Ann. Res. Vet. 16:393–398, 1985.

Perera, S.A.B.; Jones, C.; Srinkantha, V.; Ranawickrama, W.; Bhattacharyya, M.N. Leucocyte esterase test as rapid screen for non-gonococcal urethritis. Genitourin. Med. 63:380–383, 1987.

Perez-Martinez, J.A.; Storz, J. Antigenic diversity of *Chlamydia psittaci* of mammalian origin determined by microimmunofluorescence. Infect. Immun. 50:905–910, 1985.

Perez-Martinez, J.A.; Schmeer, N.; Storz, J. Bovine chlamydial abortion: serodiagnosis by modified complement fixation and indirect inclusion fluorescence tests and enzyme-linked immunosorbent assay. Am. J. Vet. Res. 47:1501–1506, 1986.

Perine, P.L.; Osoba, A.O. Lymphogranuloma venereum. In: Sexually Transmitted Diseases. Holmes, K.K.; Mårdh, P.A.; Sparling, F.; Wiesner, P. eds. New York: McGraw-Hill, 1984, pp. 281–291.

Persson, K. Chlamydial Infections. Aspects on Epidemiology and Immunity. Academic dissertation. University of Lund, 1986.

Persson, K.; Bröms M. *Chlamydia trachomatis* in lower respiratory tract infection in children, and the detection of spurious chlamydial IgM antibodies in the acute mononucleosis. Eur. J. Clin. Microbiol. 5:581–583, 1986.

Persson, K.; Rönnerstam, R.; Scanberg, L.; Pohla, M.A. Neonatal chlamydial eye infection: an epidemiological and clinical study. Br. J. Ophthalmol. 67:700–704, 1983.

Persson, K.; Rönnerstam, R.; Svanberg, L.; Polberger, S. Neonatal chlamydial conjunctivitis. Serologic investigation of mothers and infants. Arch. Dis. Child. 61:565–568, 1986.

Peterson, E.M.; de la Maza, L. Characterization of Chlamydia DNA by restriction endonuclease cleavage. Infect. Immun. 41:604–608, 1983.

Pether, J.V.S.; Noah, N.D.; Lau, Y.K.; Taylor, J.A.; Bowie, J.C. An outbreak of psittacosis in a boys' boarding school. J. Hyg. 92:337–343, 1984.

Phillips, R.S.; Hanff, P.A.; Kauffman, R.S.; Aronson, M.D. Use of a direct fluorescent antibody test for detecting *Chlamydia trachomatis* cervical infection in women seeking routine gynecologic care. J. Infect. Dis. 156:575–581, 1987.

Pittaway, D.E.; Winfield, A.C.; Maxson, W.; Daniell, J.; Herbert, C.; Wentz, A.C. Prevention of acute pelvic inflammatory disease after hysterosalpingography: Efficacy of doxycycline prophylaxis. Am. J. Obstet. Gynecol. 147:623–626, 1983.

Piura, B.; Sarov, I.; Kleinmann, D.; Chaimm, W.; Insier, V. Serum IgG and IgA antibodies specific for *Chlamydia trachomatis* in salpingitis patients as determined by the immunoperoxidase assay. Eur. J. Epidemiol. 1:110–116, 1985.

Poletti, F.; Medici, M.C.; Alinovi, A.; Menozzi, M.G.; Sacchini, P.; Stagni, G.; Toni, M.; Benolidi, D. Isolation of *Chlamydia trachomatis* from the prostatic cells in patients affected by nonacute abacterial prostatitis. J. Urol. 134:691–693, 1985.

Potter, M.E.; Kaufmann, A.F. Psittacosis in humans in United States 1975–77. J. Infect. Dis. 140:131–134, 1979.

Potter, M.E.; Kaufman, A.K.; Plikaytis, B.D. Psittacosis in the United States. MMWR. 32:27ss–31ss, 1983.

Poynard, T.; Mazeron, M.C.; Vacherot, B. Perihepatitie a *Chlamydia trachomatis* étude de cinq cas et revue de la litterature (in French). Gastroenterol. Clin. Biol. 6:321–325, 1982.

Pugh, S.F.; Slack, R.C.B.; Caul, E.O.; Paul, I.D.; Appleton, P.N.; Gatley, S. Enzyme aplified immunoassay: a novel technique applied to direct detection of *Chlamydia trachomatis* in clinical specimens. J. Clin. Pathol. 38:1139–1141, 1985.

Punnonen, R.; Terho, P.; Nikkanen, V.; Meurman, O. Chlamydial serology in infertile women by immunofluorescence. Fertil. Steril. 31:656–659, 1979.

Puolakkainen, M. Human chlamydial infections: aspects on serology. Academic dissertation. University of Helsinki, 1987.

Puolakkainen, M.; Saikku, P.; Leinonen, M.; Nurminen, M.; Väänänen, P.; Mäkelä, P.H. Chlamydial pneumonitis and its serodiagnosis in infants. J. Infect. Dis. 149:598–604, 1984.

Puolakkainen, M.; Saikku, P.; Leinonen, M.; Nurminen, M.; Väänänen, P.; Mäkelä, P.H. Comparative sensitivity of different serological tests for detecting chlamydial antibodies in perihepatitis. J. Clin. Pathol. 38:929–932, 1985.

Puolakkainen, M.; Vesterinen, E.; Purola, E.; Saikku, P.; Paavonen, J. Persistence of chlamydial antibodies after pelvic inflammatory disease. J. Clin. Microbiol. 23:924–928, 1986.

Puolakkainen, M.; Kousa, M.; Saikku, P. Clinical conditions associated with positive complement fixation serology for Chlamydiae. Epidem. Inf. 98:101–108, 1987a.

Puolakkainen, M.; Palva, A.; Julkunen, I.; Ranki, M.; Saikku, P. Comparison of culture, enzyme immunoassay and nucleic acid sandwich hybridization in diagnosis of genital *Chlamydia trachomatis* infections. Fifth International Symposium on Rapid Methods and Automation in Microbiology and Immunology, Florence, 4–6 November, 1987b, p. 322.

Puolakkainen, M.; Saikku, P. *Chlamydia trachomatis* infections in Finland. In: Proceedings of Society of Chlamydia Research, 1st Meeting, Bologna, Italy, May 30–June 1, 1988, p. 139.

Puolakkainen, M.; Ukkonen, P.; Saikku, P. Import of psittacine birds and chlamydial infections in Finland. Lancet ii:287–288, 1988.

Purola, E.; Paavonen, J. Routine cytology as a diagnostic aid in chlamydial cervicitis. Scand. J. Infect. Dis. 32 (Suppl):55–58, 1982.

Qvigstad, E.; Skaug, K.; Jerve, F.; Fylling, P.; Ulstrup, J.C. Pelvic inflammatory disease associated with *Chlamydia trachomatis* infection after therapeutic abortion. A prospective study. Br. J. Vener. Dis. 59:189–192, 1983.

Qvigstad, E.; Onsrud, M.; Skaug, T. T cell proliferative responses to *Chlamydia trachomatis* antigen in vitro in patients with a history of gynaecological infection. Br. J. Vener. Dis. 60:132, 1984.

Quinn, T.C.; Goodell, S.E.; Mkrtichian, E.; Schuffler, M.D.; Wang, S.P.; Stamm, W.E.; Holmes, K.K. *Chlamydia trachomatis* proctitis. N. Engl. J. Med. 305:195–200, 1981a.

Quinn, T.C.; Corey, L.; Chaffee, R.G.; Schuffler, M.D.; Brancato, F.P.; Holmes, K.K. The etiology of anorectal infections in homosexual men. Am. J. Med. 71:395–406, 1981b.

Quinn, T.C.; Warfield, P.; Kappus, E.; Barbacci, M.; Spence, M. Screening for *Chlamydia trachomatis* infection in an inner-city population: a comparison of diagnostic methods. J. Infect. Dis. 152:419–423, 1985.

Quinn, T.C.; Gupta, P.K.; Burkamn, R.T.; Kappus, E.W.; Barbacci, M.; Spence, M.R. Detection of *Chlamydia trachomatis* cervical infection: a comparison of Papanicolaou and immunofluorescent staining with cell culture. Am. J. Obstet. Gynecol. 157:394–399, 1987.

Radkowski, M.A.; Kranzler, J.K.; Beem, M.O.; Tipple, M.A. Chlamydial pneumonia in infants: radiography in 125 cases. Am. J. Roentg. 137:703–706, 1981.

Ragnaud, J.M.; Dupon, M.; Echinard, E.; Lacut, J.Y.; Aubertin, J. Les manifestations hépatiques de la psittacose (in French). Gastroenterol. Clin. Biol. 10:234–237, 1986.

Rake, G.; Eaton, M.D.; Shaffer, M.F. Similarities and possible relationships among viruses psittacosis, meningopneumonitis and lymphogranuloma venereum. Proc. Soc. Exp. Biol. Med. 48:528–531, 1941.

Rank, R.G.; Barron, A.L. Effect of antithymocyte serum on the course of chlamydial genital infection in female guinea-pigs. Infect. Immun. 41:876–879, 1983a.

Rank, R.G.; Barron, A.L. Humoral immune response in acquired immunity to chlamydial genital infection of the female guinea-pigs. Infect. Immun. 39:463–465, 1983b.

Rank, R.G.; White, H.J.; Barron, A.L. Humoral immunity in the resolution of genital infection in female guinea-pigs infected with the agent of guinea-pig inclusion conjunctivitis. Infect. Immun. 26:573–579, 1979.

Rank, R.G.; White, H.J.; Hough, A.J. Jr.; Pasley, J.N.; Barron, A.L. Effect of estradiol on chlamydial genital infection of female guinea pigs. Infect. Immun. 38:699–705, 1982.

Rank, R.G.; Hough, A.J., Jr.; Jacobs, R.F.; Cohen, C.; Barron, A.L. Chlamydial pneumonitis induced in newborn guinea pigs. Infect. Immun. 48:153–158, 1985.

Rapoza, P.A.; Quinn, T.C.; Kiessling, L.A.; Green, W.R.; Taylor, H.R. Assessment of neonatal conjunctivitis with a direct immunofluorescent monoclonal antibody stain for *Chlamydia*. J. Am. Med. Assoc. 255:3369–3373, 1986.

Räsänen, L., Lehtinen, M.; Lehto, M.; Paavonen, J.; Leinikki, P. Polyclonal response of human lymphocytes to *Chlamydia trachomatis*. Infect. Immun. 54:28–31, 1986.

Rees, E.; Treatment of pelvic inflammatory disease. Am. J. Obstet. Gynecol. 138:1042–1047, 1980.

Rees, E.; Tait, I.A.; Hobson, D.; Johnson, F.W.A. *Chlamydia* in relation to cervical infection and pelvic inflammatory disease. In: Nongonococcal Urethritis and Related Infections. Hobson, D.; Holmes, K.K. Washington, D.C.: American Society for Microbiology, 1977a, pp. 67–76.

Rees, E.; Tait, I.A.; Hobson, D.; Johnson, F.W.A. Perinatal chlamydial infection. In: Nongonococcal Urethritis and Related Infections. Hobson, D.; Holmes, K.K. eds. Washington, D.C.; American Society for Microbiology, 1977b, pp. 140–147.

Reeve, P.; Taverne, J. Some properties of the complement-fixing antigens of the agents of trachoma and inclusion blennorrhea and the relationship of the antigens to the developmental cycle. J. Gen. Microbiol. 27:501–508, 1962.

Reeve, P.; Owen, J.; Oriel, J.D. Laboratory procedures for the isolation of *Chlamydia trachomatis* from the human genital tract. J. Clin. Pathol. 28:910–914, 1975.

Regan, J.A.; Chao, S.; James, L.S. Premature rupture of membranes, preterm delivery, and group B streptococcal colonization of mothers. Am. J. Obstet. Gynecol. 141:184–186, 1981.

Regan, R.L.; Dathan, J.R.E.; Treharne, J.D. Infective endocarditis with glomerulonephritis associated with cat chlamydia (*Chlamydia psittaci*) infection. Br. Heart J. 42:349–352, 1978.

Reichert, J.A.; Valle, R.F. Fitz-Hugh–Curtis syndrome: a laparoscopic approach. J. Am. Med. Assoc. 236:266–268, 1976.

Rettig, P.J. Infections due to *Chlamydia trachomatis* from infancy to adolescence. Pediatr. Infect. Dis. 5:449–457, 1986a.

Rettig, P.J.; Rollerson, W.J.; Macks, M.I. In vitro activity of six fluoroquinolones against *Chlamydia trachomatis*. In Chlamydial Infections. Oriel, J.D.; Ridgway, G.; Schachter, J.; Taylor-Robinson, D.; Ward, M. eds. Cambridge: Cambridge University Press, 1986b, pp. 528–531.

Richmond, S.J. Chlamydial group antigen in McCoy cells infected with *Chlamydia trachomatis* and *Chlamydia psittaci*. FEMS Microbiol. Lett. 8:47–50, 1980.

Richmond, S.J.; Hilton, A.L.; Clarke, S.K.R. Chlamydial infection. Role of *Chlamydia* subgroup A in non-gonococcal and post-gonococcal urethritis. Br. J. Vener. Dis. 48:437–444, 1972.

Richmond, S.J.; Caul, E.O. Fluorescent antibody studies in chlamydial infections. J. Clin. Microbiol. 1:345–352, 1975.

Richmond, S.J.; Milne, J.D.; Hilton, A.L.; Caul, E.O. Antibodies to *Chlamydia trachomatis* in cervicovaginal secretions. Relation to serum antibodies and current infection. Sex. Transm. Dis. 7:11–15, 1980.

Richmond, S.J.; Mearns, G.; Storey, C. Sensitive immune dot-blot test for diagnosis of *Chlamydia trachomatis* infection. In: Proceedings of the Eur. Soc. for Chlamydia Research, 1st Meeting, Bologna, Italy, May 30–June 1, 1988, p. 253.

Ridgway, G.L.; Owen, J.M.; Oriel, J.D. A method for testing the antibiotic susceptibility of *Chlamydia trachomatis* in a cell culture system. J. Antimicrob. Chemother. 2:71–76, 1976.

Ripa, K.T.; Mårdh, P.-A. Cultivation of *Chlamydia trachomatis* in cycloheximide-treated McCoy cells. J. Clin. Microbiol. 6:328–331, 1977.

Ripa, K.T.; Mårdh, P.A.; Thelin, I. *Chlamydia trachomatis* urethritis in men attending a venereal disease clinic: A culture and therapeutic study. Acta Dermatovener. (Stockholm) 58:175–179, 1978a.

Ripa, K.T.; Svensson, L.; Mårdh, P.-A.; Weström, L. *Chlamydia trachomatis* cervicitis in gynecologic outpatients. Obstet. Gynecol. 52:698–702, 1978b.

Ripa, K.T.; Møller, B.R.; Mårdh, P.-A.; Freundt, E.A.; Melsen, F. Experimental acute salpingitis in grivet monkeys provoked by *Chlamydia trachomatis*. Acta Pathol. Microbiol. Scand. B87:65–70, 1979.

Robbins, J.B. Vaccines for prevention of encapsulated bacterial diseases: current status, problems and prospects for future. Immunochemistry 15:839–854, 1978.

Roberts, W.; Grist, N.E.; Giroud, P. Human abortion associated with infection by ovine abortion agent. Br. Med. J. 222:37, 1967.

Robertson, J.N.; Ward, M.E.; Conway, D.; Caul, E.O. Chlamydial and gonococcal antibodies in sera of infertile women with tubal obstruction. J. Clin. Pathol. 40:377–383, 1987.

Rodaniche, E.C.; Kirsner, J.B.; Palmer, W.L. The relationship between lymphogranuloma venereum and regional eneteritis: an etiologic study of 4 cases with negative results. Gastroenterology 1:687–689, 1943.

Rompalo, A.M.; Price, C.B.; Roberts, P.L.; Stamm, W.E. Potential value of rectal screening cultures for *Chlamydia trachomatis* in homosexual men. J. Infect. Dis. 153:888–892, 1986.

Rönnerstam, R.; Persson, K.; Hansson, H.; Renmarker, K. Prevalence of chlamydial eye infection in patients attending an eye clinic, a VD clinic, and in healthy persons. Br. J. Ophthalmol. 69:385–388, 1985.

Roongpisuthipong, A.; Grimes, D.A.; Hagdu, A. Is the Papanicolaou smear useful for diagnosing sexually transmitted diseases? Obstet Gynecol 69:820–824, 1987.

Rosenfeld, D.L.; Seidman, S.M.; Bronson, R.A.; Scholl, G.M. Unsuspected chronic inflammatory disease in the infertile female. Fertil. Steril. 39:44–48, 1983.

Rothermel, C.D.; Byrne, G.I.; Havell, E.A. Effect of interferon on the growth of *Chlamydia trachomatis* in mouse fibroblasts (L cells). Infect. Immunol. 39:362–370, 1983.

Rothermel, C.D.; Rubin, B.Y.; Murray, H.W. Interferon is the factor in lymphokine that activates human macrophages to inhibit intracellular *Chlamydia psittaci* replication. J. Immunol. 131:2542–2544, 1983.

Rotterdam, H. Chronic endometritis. A clinicopathological study. Pathol. Ann. 13:209–231, 1978.

Rowe, D.S.; Aicardi, E.Z.; Dawson, C.R.; Schachter, J. Purulent ocular discharge in neonates. Pediatrics 63:628–632, 1979.

Rowland, G.F.; Forsey, T.; Moss, T.R.; Steptoe, D.C.; Hewitt, J.; Darougar, S. Failure of in vitro fertilization and embryo replacement following infection with *Chlamydia trachomatis*. J. In Vitro Fertil. Emb. Transf. 2:151–155, 1985.

Sacks, D.L.; Rota, T.R.; MacDonald, A.B. Separation and partial characterization of a type-specific antigen from *Chlamydia trachomatis*. J. Immunol. 121:204–208, 1978.

Sacks, D.L.; MacDonald, A.B. Isolation of a type-specific antigen from *Chlamydia trachomatis* by sodium dodecyl sulfate-polyacrylamide gel electrophoresis. J. Immunol. 122:136–139, 1979.

Saiki, R.K.; Scharf, S.; Falcona, F.; Mullis, K.B.; Horn, G.T.; Erlich, H.A.; Arnheim, N. Enzymatic amplification of beta-globin genomic sequences and restriction site analysis for diagnosis of sickle cell anemia. Science 230:1350–1354, 1985.

Saikku, P. *Chlamydia* TWAR and its epidemiology. In: Proceedings of the Eur. Soc. for Chlamydia Research, 1st Meeting, Bologna, Italy, May 30–June 1, 1988, pp. 7–10.

Saikku, P.; Paavonen, J. Single-antigen immunofluorescence test for chlamydial antibodies. J. Clin. Microbiol. 8:119–122, 1978.

Saikku, P.; Wang, S.P. *Chlamydia trachomatis* immunotypes in Finland. Acta Pathol. Microbiol. Immunol. Scand. B95:131–134, 1987.

Saikku, P.; Paavonen, J.; Väänänen, P.; Vaheri, A. Solid-phase enzyme immunoassay for chlamydial antibodies. J. Clin. Microbiol. 17:22–27, 1983.

Saikku, P.; Wang, S.-P.; Kleemola, M.; Brander, E.; Rusanen, E.; Grayston, J.T. An epidemic of mild pneumonia due to an unusual *Chlamydia psittaci* strain. J. Infect. Dis. 151:832–839, 1985.

Saikku, P.; Puolakkainen, M.; Leinonen, M.; Nurminen, M.; Nissinen, A. Cross-reactivity between Chlamydiazyme and *Acinetobacter* strains. N. Engl. J. Med. 314:922–923, 1986a.

Saikku, P.; Visakorpi, R.; Kleemola, M.; Wang, S.-P.; Grayston, J.T. *Chlamydia psittaci* TWAR-strains as a frequent cause of military epidemics in Finland. In: Chlamydial Infections. Oriel, J.D.; Ridgway, G.; Schachter, J.; Taylor-Robinson, D.; Ward, M. eds. Cambridge: Cambridge University Press, 1986b, pp. 333–336.

Saikku, P.; Wang, S.P.; Kleemola, M.; Ekman, M.R.; Grayston, J.T. Rapid diagnosis in military TWAR chlamydia pneumonia epidemics with the microimmunofluorescence test. Fifth International Symposium on Rapid Methods and Automation in Microbiology and Immunology. Florence. 4–6 November, 1987, p. 432.

Saikku, P.; Leinonen, M.; Mattila, K.; Ekman, M.-R.; Nieminen, M.S.; Mäkelä, P.H.; Huttunen, J.; Valtonen, V. Serological evidence of an assocation of a novel chlamydia, TWAR, with chronic coronary heart disease and myocardial infarction. Lancet ii:983–986, 1988.

Salari, S.H.; Ward, M.E. Polypeptide composition of *Chlamydia trachomatis*. J. Gen. Microbiol. 123:197–207, 1981.

Saltz, G.R.; Linneman, C.C.; Brookman, R.R.; Rauh, J.L. *Chlamydia trachomatis* cervical infections in female adolescents. J. Pediatr. 98:981–985, 1981.

Sanders, L.L.; Harrison, H.; Washington, A.E. Treatment of sexually transmitted chlamydial infections. J. Am. Med. Assoc. 255:1750–1756, 1986.

Sandström, I. Etiology and diagnosis of neonatal conjunctivitis. Academic dissertation. University of Stockholm, 1987.

Sandström, K.I.; Bell, T.A.; Chandler, J.W.; Wang, S.-P.; Kuo, C.-C.; Foy, H.M.; Grayston, J.T.; Cooney, M.; Smith, A.; Holmes, K.K. Diagnosis of neonatal purulent conjunctivitis caused by *Chlamydia trachomatis* and other organisms. In: Chlamydial Infections. Mårdh, P.-A.; Holmes, K.K., Oriel, J.D.; Piot, P.; Schachter, J. eds. Amsterdam: Elsevier Biomedical Press, 1982, pp. 217–220.

San Joaquin, V.H.; Rettig, P.J.; Newton, J.Y.; Marks, M.I. Prevalence of chlamydial antibodies in children. Am. J. Dis. Child. 136:425–427, 1982.

San Joaquin, V.H.; Rettig, P.R. Role of *Chlamydia trachomatis* in upper-respiratory-tract infections in children. J. Infect. Dis. 154:193, 1987.

Sarner, M.; Wilson, R.J. Erythema nodosum and psittacosis: Report of five cases. Br. Med. J. 2:1469–1470, 1965.

Sarov, I.; Becker, Y. Trachoma agent DNA. J. Mol. Biol. 42:581–589, 1969.

Schaad, U.B.; Rossi, E. Infantile chlamydial pneumonia: a review based on 115 cases. Eur. J. Pediatr. 138:105–109, 1982.

Schachter, J. Chlamydial infections. N. Engl. J. Med. 298:428–435, 490–495, 540–549, 1978.

Schachter, J. Confirmatory serodiagnosis of lymphogranuloma venereum proctitis may yield false-positive results due to other chlamydial infections of the rectum. Sex. Transm. Dis. 8:26–28, 1981.

Schachter, J. Biology of *Chlamydia trachomatis*. In Sexually Transmitted Diseases.

Holmes, K.K.; Mårdh, P.-A.; Sparling, F.; Wiesner, P. eds. New York: McGraw-Hill, 1984, pp. 243–257.

Schachter, J. Immunodiagnosis of sexually transmitted diseases. Yale J. Biol. Med. 58:443–452, 1985.

Schachter, J Chlamydiae. In: Manual of Clinical Immunology, 3rd Ed. Rose, N.R.; Friedman, H.; Fahey, J.L. eds. Washington, D.C.: American Society for Microbiology, 1986a, pp. 587–592.

Schachter, J. Human *Chlamydia psittaci* infection. In: Chlamydial Infections. Oriel, D.; Ridgway, G.; Schachter, J.; Taylor-Robinson, D.; Ward, M. eds. Cambridge: Cambridge University Press, 1986b, pp. 311–320.

Schachter, J. *Chlamydia psittaci:* reemergence of a forgotten pathogen. N. Engl. J. Med. 315:189–191, 1986c.

Schachter, J. Human *Chlamydia psittaci* infection. In: Chlamydial Infections. Oriel, D.; Ridgway, G.; Schachter, J.; Taylor-Robinson, D.; Ward, M., eds. Cambridge: Cambridge University Press, 1986d, pp. 311–320.

Schachter, J.; Meyer, K.F. Lymphogranuloma venereum. II. Characterization of some recently isolated strains. J. Bacteriol. 99:636–638, 1969.

Schachter, J.; Dawson, C.R. Lymphogranuloma venereum. J. Am. Med. Assoc. 236:915–916, 1976.

Schachter, J.; Dawson, C.R. Comparative efficiency of various diagnostic methods for chlamydial infection. In: Nongonococcal Urethritis and Related Infections. Hobson, D.; Holmes, K.K. eds. Washington, D.C.: American Society for Microbiology, 1977, pp. 337–341.

Schachter, J.; Dawson, C.R. Human Chlamydial Infections. Littleton, MA: PSG, 1978.

Schachter, J.; Caldwell, H. Chlamydiae. Ann. Rev. Microbiol. 34:285–309, 1980.

Schachter, J.; Dawson, C.R. Chlamydial infections, a worldwide problem. Epidemiology and implications for trachoma therapy. Sex. Transm. Dis. 8:167–174, 1981.

Schachter, J.; Grossman, M. Chlamydial infections. Annu. Rev. Med. 32:45–61, 1981.

Schachter, J.; Osoba, A.O. Lymphogranuloma venereum. Br. Med. Bull. 39:151–154, 1983.

Schachter, J.; Martin, D.H. Failure of multiple passages to increase chlamydial recovery. J. Clin. Microbiol. 25:1851–1853, 1987.

Schachter, J.; Barnes, M.G.; Jones, J.T.; Engleman, E.P.; Meyer, K.F. Isolation of Bedsoniae from joints of patients with Reiter's syndrome. Proc. Soc. Exp. Biol. Med. 122:283–285, 1966.

Schachter, J.; Smith, D.E.; Dawson, C.R. Lymphogranuloma venereum. I. Comparison of the Frei test, complement fixation test, and isolation of the agent. J. Infect. Dis. 120:372–375, 1969.

Schachter, J.; Hill, E.C.; King, E.B.; Coleman, V.R.; Jones, P.; Meyer, K.F. Chlamydial infection in women with cervical neoplasia. Am. J. Obstet. Gynecol. 123:753–757, 1975a.

Schachter, J.; Hanna, L.; Hill, E.C.; Massad, G.; Sheppard, C.W.; Conte, J.E., Jr.; Cohen, S.N.; Meyer, K.F. Are chlamydial infections the most prevalent venereal disease? J. Am. Med. Assoc. 231:1252–1255, 1975b.

Schachter, J.; Lum, I.; Gooding, C.A.; Ostler, B. Pneumonitis following inclusion blennorrhoea. J. Pediatr. 87:779–780, 1975c.

Schachter, J.; Sugg, N.; Sung, M. Psittacosis: The reservoir persists. J. Infect. Dis. 137:44–49, 1978.

Schachter, J.; Cles, L.; Ray, R.; Hines, P.A. Failure of serology in diagnosing chlamydial infections of the female genital tract. J. Clin. Microbiol. 10:647–649, 1979a.

Schachter, J.; Holt, J.; Goodner, E.; Grossman, M.; Sweet, R.; Mills, J. Prospective study of chlamydial infection in neonates. Lancet ii:377–380, 1979b.

Schachter, J.; Grossman, M.; Holt, J.; Sweet, R.; Spector, S. Infection with *Chlamydia trachomatis:* Involvement of multiple anatomic sites in neonates. J. Infect. Dis. 139:232–234, 1979c.

Schachter, J.; Hill, E.C.; King, E.B.; Heilbron, D.C.; Ray, R.M.; Margolis, A.J.; Greenwood, S.A. *Chlamydia trachomatis* and cervical neoplasia. J. Am. Med. Assoc. 248:2134–2138, 1982a.

Schachter, J.; Grossman, M.; Azimi, P.M. Serology of *Chlamydia trachomatis* in infants. J. Infect. Dis. 146:530–535, 1982b.

Schachter, J.; Banks, J.; Sung, M.; Sweet, R. Hydrosalpinx as a consequence of chlamydial salpingitis in the guinea pig. In: Chlamydial Infections. Mårdh, P.-A.; Holmes, K.K.; Oriel, J.D.; Piot, P.; Schachter, J. eds. Amsterdam: Elsevier Biomedical Press, 1982c, pp. 371–374.

Schachter, J.; Cles, L.D.; Ray, R.M.; Hesse, F.E. Is there immunity to chlamydial infections of the human genital tract? Sex. Transm. Dis. 10:123–125, 1983.

Schachter, J.; Sweet, R.L.; Grossmann, M.; Landers, D.; Robbie, M.; Bishop, E. Experience with the routine use of erythromycin for chlamydial infections in pregnancy. N. Engl. J. Med. 314:276–279, 1986a.

Schachter, J.; Grossman, M.; Sweet, R.L.; Holt, J.; Bishop, E. Prospective study of perinatal transmission of *Chlamydia trachomatis.* J. Am. Med. Assoc. 27:3374–3377, 1986b.

Schaefer, C.; Harrison, H.R.; Boyce, W.T.; Lewis, M. Illnesses in infants born to women with *Chlamydia trachomatis* infection. Am. J. Dis. Child. 139:127–133, 1985.

Schildt, B.E.; Eisemann, B. Peritoneal absorption of Cr51-tagged erythrocytes. Its influence by pneumoperitoneum and Fowler's position. Acta Clin. Scand. 119:397–410, 1960.

Schiøtz, H.; Csángo, P.A. A prospective study of *Chlamydia trachomatis* in first trimester abortion. Am. Clin. Res. 17:60–63, 1985.

Schmeer, N.; Perez-Martinez, J.A.; Schnorr, K.; Storz, J.; Krauss, H. Analysis of the IgG response of cattle to natural and experimental chlamydial infections. Proceedings of the IVth International Symposium of Veterinary Laboratory Diagnosticians, Amsterdam, 1986a, pp. 472–475.

Schmeer, N.; Muller, H.P.; Krauss, H. Differences in IgG 1 and IgG 2 responses of goats to chlamydial abortions and to clinically inapparent infections detected by the western blot technique. J. Vet. Med. B. 33:751–757, 1986b.

Schröder, R. Beiträge zur normalen und pathologischen Anatomie des Endometriums (in German). Arch. Geburtsh. Gynäkol. 83:668, 1921.

Schultz, R.M.; Kleinschmidt, W.J. Functional identity between murine interferon and macrophage activating factor. Nature 305:239–240, 1983.

Schultz, R.M.; Kleinschmidt, W.J. Functional identity between murine interferon and macrophage activating factor. Nature 305:239–240, 1983.

Scott, B.D.; Fortenberry, J.D. Postgonococcal conjunctivitis due to *Chlamydia trachomatis*. Sex. Trans. Dis. 13:172–173, 1986.

Sellors, J.W.; Mahony, J.B.; Chernesky, M.A.; Rath, D.J. Tubal factor infertility: An association with prior chlamydial infection in asymptomatic salpingitis. Fertil. Steril. 49:451, 1988.

Sezer, F.N. The cytology of trachoma. Am. J. Ophthalmol. 34:1709–1713, 1951.

Semchyschyn, S. Fitz-Hugh and Curtis syndrome. J. Reprod. Med. 22:45–48, 1979.

Senanayake, P.; Kramer, D.G. Contraception and the etiology of pelvic inflammatory disease: new perspectives. Am. J. Obstet. Gynecol. 138:852–860, 1980.

Shafer, M.A.; Irwin, C.E.; Sweet, R.L. Acute salpingitis in the adolescent female. J. Pediatr. 100:339, 1982.

Shafer, M.A.; Beck, A.; Blain, B.; Dole, P.; Irwin, C.E., Jr.; Sweet, R.; Schachter, J. *Chlamydia trachomatis:* important relationships to race, contraception, lower genital tract infection, and Papanicolaou smear. J. Pediatr. 104:141–146, 1984.

Shafer, M.A.; Chew, K.L.; Kromhout, L.K.; Beck, A.; Sweet, R.C.; Schachter, J.; King, E.B. Chlamydial endocervical infections and cytologic findings in sexually active female adolescents. Am. J. Obstet. Gynecol. 151:765–771, 1985.

Shafer, M.A.; Weiss, A.; Moscicki, B.; Schachter, J. Performance of the urinary leucocyte esterase dipstick as a screening device to predict *C. trachomatis* and *N. gonorrhoeae* urethritis in asymptomatic adolescent males. Fifth International Symposium on Rapid Methods and Automation in Microbiology and Immunology, Florence, 4–6 November, 1987, p. 463.

Shatkin, A. *Chlamydia trachomatis* infections in USSR. In: Proceedings of the Eur. Soc. for Chlamydia Research, 1st Meeting, Bologna, Italy, May 30–June 1, 1988, p. 34.

Sheldon, W.H.; Wall, M.; Slade, J.R.; Heyman, A. Lymphogranuloma venereum of supraclavicular lymph nodes with mediastinal lymphadenopathy and pericarditis. Am. J. Med. 5:320, 1948.

Shemer, Y.; Sarov, I. Inhibition of growth of *Chlamydia trachomatis* by human gamma interferon. Infect. Immun. 48:592–596, 1985.

Shewen, P.E. Chlamydial infections in animals: a review. Cond. Vet. 21:2–11, 1980.

Shiao, L.; Wang, S.P.; Grayston, J.T. Sensitivity and resistance of TRIC agents to penicillin, tetracycline and sulpha drugs. Am. J. Ophthalmol. 63:532–542, 1967.

Shurin, P.A.; Alpert, S.; Rosner, B.; Driscoll, S.G.; Lee, Y.H.; McCormack, W.M.; Santamarina, B.A.G.; Kass, E.H. Chorioamnionitis and colonization of the newborn infant with genital mycoplasmas. N. Engl. J. Med. 293:5–8, 1975.

Siboulet, A.; Galestin, P. Arguments in favour of a virus aetiology of non-gonococcal urethritis illustrated by 3 cases of Reiter's syndrome. Br. J. Vener. Dis. 38:209–211, 1962.

Simmons, P.D.; Vosmik, F. Cervical cytology in nonspecific genital infection: an aid to diagnosis. Br. J. Vener. Dis. 50:313–314, 1974.

Singh, M.; Sugathan, P.S.; Bhujivala, R.A. Human colostrum for prophylaxis against sticky eyes and conjunctivitis in the newborn. J. Trop. Pediatr. 28:35–37, 1982.

Slaney, L.; Plummer, F.; Ronald, R.R.; Degagne, P.; Hoban, D.; Brunham, R.C. In vitro activity of azithromycin (AZM) against *Neisseria gonorrhoeae* (gc), *Haemophilus ducreyi* (Hd) *Chlamydia trachomatis* and *Chlamydia psittaci*. In Abstracts of the 1987 ICAAC, Abstract No. 728, p. 1224.

Smith, D.E.; James, P.G.; Schachter, J.; Engleman, E.P.; Meyer, K.F. Experimental bedsonial arthritis. Arthr. Rheum. 16:21–29, 1973.

Smith, E.B.; Custer, R.P. The histopathology of lymphogranuloma venereum. J. Urol. 63:546, 1950.

Smith, J.W.; Rogers, R.E.; Katz, B.P.; Brickler, J.F.; Lineback, P.L.; van der Pol, B.; Jones, B.R. Diagnosis of chlamydial infection in women attending antenatal and gynecology clinics. J. Clin. Microbiol. 25:868–872, 1987.

Socialstyrelsens Allmänna Råd och Anvisningar angående *Chlamydia trachomatis* infektioner (in Swedish). Stockholm 1987.

Söderlund, G.; Kihlström, E. Effect of methylamine and monodansylcadaverine on the susceptibility of McCoy cells to *Chlamydia trachomatis* infection. Infect. Immun. 40:543–541, 1983.

Soldati, M.; Intini, C.; Isetta, A.M.; Ghione, M.; Larghini, F. Further studies on experimental infection of the mouse with trachoma agents. Ophthalmology. Proceedings of the XXI International Congress, Mexico, 8–14, March 1970. Excerpta Medica International Congress Series No. 222.

Soldati, M.; Verini, M.A.; Isetta, A.M.; Ghione, M. Immunization researches in the field of trachoma. Some laboratory and clinical contributions. In: Trachoma and Related Disorders Caused by Chlamydial Agents. Nichols, R.L. ed. Amsterdam: Excerpta Medica, 1971, pp. 407–417.

Sompolinsky, B.; Richmond, S.J. Growth of *Chlamydia trachomatis* in McCoy cells treated with cytochalasin B. Appl. Microbiol. 28:912–914, 1974.

Sowa, S.; Sowa, J.; Collier, L.H.; Blyth, W. Trachoma and allied infections in a Gambian village. Special Report Series, Medical Research Council, No. 308, HMSO, London, 1965.

Spence, M.R.; Barbacci, M.; Kappus, E.; Quinn, T. A correlative study of Papanicolaou smear fluorescent antibody, and culture for the diagnosis of *Chlamydia trachomatis*. Obstet. Gynecol. 68:691–195, 1986.

Spiegel, C.A.; Amsel, R.; Eschenbach, D.A.; Schoenknecht, F.; Holmes, K.K. Anaerobic bacteria in nonspecific vaginitis. N. Engl. J. Med. 303:601–607, 1980.

Staargardt, K. Über Epithelzellveränderungen beim Trachom und andern Conjunctivalerkrankungen (in German). Arch. Ophthalmol. 69:525–542, 1909.

Stajano, C. La reaccion frenica en ginecologica (in Spanish). Semana Med. Buenos Aires, 27:243–248, 1920.

Stålhandske, P.; Pettersson, U. Identification of DNA viruses by membrane filter hybridization. J. Clin. Microbiol. 15:744–747, 1982.

Stamm, W.E. Diagnosis of *Neisseria gonorrhoeae* and *Chlamydia trachomatis* infections using antigen detection methods. Diagnostic Microbiol. Infect. Dis. 4(Suppl):935–1005, 1986.

Stamm, W.E.; Cole, B. Asymptomatic *Chlamydia trachomatis* urethritis in men. Sex. Trans. Dis. 13:163–165, 1986.

Stamm, W.E.; Holmes, K.K. Measures to control *Chlamydia trachomatis* infections: an assessment of new national policy guidelines. J. Am. Med. Assoc. 256:1176–1178, 1986.

Stamm, W.E.; Suchland, R. Antimicrobial activity of U-70138F (paldimycin) roxithromycin (RU 965), and ofloxacin (ORF 18489) against *Chlamydia trachomatis* in cell culture. Antimicrob. Agents Chemother. 30:806–807, 1986.

Stamm, W.E.; Wagner, K.F.; Amsel, R.; Alexander, E.R.; Turck, M.; Counts, G.W.; Holmes, K.K. Causes of the acute urethral syndrome in women. N. Engl. J. Med. 303:409–415, 1980.

Stamm, W.E.; Quinn, T.C.; Mkrtichian, E.E.; Wang, S.-P.; Schuffler, M.D.; Holmes, K.K. *Chlamydia trachomatis* proctitis. In: Chlamydial Infections. Mårdh, P.-A.; Holmes, K.K.; Oriel, J.D.; Piot, P.; Schachter, J. eds. Amsterdam: Elsevier Biomedical Press, 1982, pp. 111–114.

Stamm, W.E.; Tam, M.; Koester, M.; Cles, L. Detection of *Chlamydia trachomatis* inclusions in McCoy cell cultures with fluorescein-conjugated monoclonal antibodies. J. Clin. Microbiol. 17:666–668, 1983.

Stamm, W.E.; Holmes, K.K. *Chlamydia trachomatis* infections of the adult. In: Sexually Transmitted Diseases. Holmes, K.K.; Mårdh, P.-A.; Sparling, P.F.; Wiesner, P.J. eds. New York: McGraw-Hill, 1984, pp. 258–269.

Stamm, W.E.; Harrison, H.R.; Alexander, E.R.; Cles, L.D.; Spence, M.R.; Quinn, T.C. Diagnosis of *Chlamydia trachomatis* infections by direct immunofluorescence staining of genital secretions, a multicenter trial. Ann. Intern. Med. 101:638–641, 1984a.

Stamm, W.E.; Koutsky, L.A.; Benedetti, J.K.; Jourden, J.L.; Brunham, R.C.; Holmes, K.K. *Chlamydia trachomatis* urethral infections in men. Prevalence, risk factors, and clinical manifestations. Ann. Intern. Med. 100:47–51, 1984b.

Stamm, W.E.; Quinan, M.E.; Johnson, C.; Starcher, T.; Holmes, K.K.; McCormack, W.M. Effect of treatment regimens for *Neisseria gonorrhoeae* on simultaneous infection with *Chlamydia trachomatis*. N. Engl. J. Med. 310:545–549, 1984c.

Stamm, W.E.; Running, K.; McKevitt, M.; Counts, G.W.; Turck, M.; Holmes, K.K. Treatment of the acute urethral syndrome. N. Engl. J. Med. 304:956–958, 1986.

Stary, A.; Kopp, W.; Gebhart, W.; Söltz-Szöts, J. Culture versus direct specimen test: comparative study of infections with *Chlamydia trachomatis* in Viennese prostitutes. Genitourin. Med. 61:258–260, 1985.

Staub, H. Virusabort in einem Ziegenbestand (in German). Dtsch. Tierärztl. Wschr. 66:98–99, 1959.

Stellmacher, H.; Kielstein, P.; Horsch, F.; Martin, J. Zur Bedeutung der Chlamydieninfektion des Schweines unter besonder Berucksichtigung der Pneumonien (in German). Monatsh. Veterinaermed. 38:601–606, 1983.

Stenberg, K.; Mårdh, P.-A. Persistent neonatal chlamydial infection in a six-year-old child. Lancet ii:1978–1979, 1986.

Stenberg, K.; Mårdh, P.-A. Comparison of the value of different methods for the diagnosis of chlamydial conjunctivitis. In Abstracts of 3rd Eur. Conf. of Clin. Microbiol., The Hague, May 10–14, 1987, p. 41.

Stephens, R.S.; Kuo, C.C. *Chlamydia trachomatis* species-specific epitope detected on mouse pneumonitis biovar outer membrane protein. Infect. Immun. 45:790–791, 1984.

Stephens, R.S.; Tam, M.R.; Kuo, C.-C.; Nowinski, R.C. Monoclonal antibodies to *Chlamydia trachomatis*: antibody specificities and antigen characterization. J. Immunol. 128:1083–1089, 1982a.

Stephens, R.S.; Chen, W.J.; Kuo, C.-C. Effects of corticosteroids and cyclophosphamide on a mouse model of *Chlamydia trachomatis* pneumonitis. Infect. Immun. 35:680–684, 1982b.

Stephens, R.S.; Kuo, C.C.; Tam, M.R. Sensitivity of immunofluorescence with monoclonal antibodies for detection of *Chlamydia trachomatis* inclusions in cell culture. J. Clin. Microbiol. 16:4–7, 1982c.

Stephens, R.S.; Kuo, C.C.; Newport, G.; Agabian, M. Molecular cloning and expression of *Chlamydia trachomatis* major outer membrane protein antigens in *Escherichia coli*. Infect. Immun. 47:713–718, 1985.

Stephens, R.S.; Inouye, C.J.; Wagar, E.A. A species-specific major outer membrane protein domain. In: Chlamydial Infections. Oriel, D.; Ridgway, G.; Schachter, J.; Taylor-Robinson, D.; Ward, M. eds. Cambridge: Cambridge University Press, 1986, pp. 110–113.

Storz, J. Psittacosis agents as a cause of polyarthritis in cattle and sheep. Vet. Med. Rev. 2(3):125–139, 1961.

Storz, J. Chlamydia and Chlamydia-Induced Diseases. Springfield, IL: Charles Thomas, 1971.

Storz, J.; Krauss, H. Chlamydial infections. In: Handbuch der bakteriellen Infektionen bei Tieren. Band V, 1. Auflage. Blobel, H.; Schliesser, Th. eds. Jena: Gustav Fisher Verlag, 1985, pp. 447–531.

Strauss, J. Microbiologic and epidemiologic aspects of duck ornithosis in Czechoslovakia. Am. J. Ophthalmol. 63:1246–1259, 1967.

Stumpf, P.G.; March, C.M. Febrile morbidity following hysterosalpingography: identification of risk factors and recommendations for prophylaxis. Fertil. Steril. 33:487–492, 1980.

Sueltenfuess, E.A.; Pollard, M. Cytochemical assay of interferon produced by duck hepatitis virus. Science 139:595–598, 1963.

Sulaiman, M.Z.C.; Foster, J.; Pugh, S.F. Prevalence of *Chlamydia trachomatis* in homosexual men. Genitourin. Med. 63:179–181, 1987.

Sundal, E.; Stalder, G.A. Perihepatitis gonorrhoica (Fitz-Hugh-Curtis syndrome). Schweitz. Med. Wschr. 110:540–543, 1980.

Svensson, L.; Mårdh, P.-A. Treatment of acute salpingitis, with special reference to *Chlamydia trachomatis*. In: *Chlamydia trachomatis* in Genital and Related Infections. Mårdh, P.-A.; Møller, B.R.; Paavonen, J. eds. Scand. J. Infect. Dis. Suppl. 32:182–190, 1982.

Svensson, L.; Weström, L.; Ripa, K.T.; Mårdh, P.-A. Differences in some clinical and laboratory parameters in acute salpingitis related to culture and serologic findings. Am. J. Obstet. Gynecol. 138:1017–1021, 1980.

Svensson, L.; Weström, L.; Mårdh, P.-A. *Chlamydia trachomatis* in women attending a gynecological out-patient clinic with lower genital tract infection. Br. J. Vener. Dis. 57:259–262, 1981a.

Svensson, L.; Weström, L.; Mårdh, P.-A. Acute salpingitis with *Chlamydia trachomatis* infection from the Fallopian tubes, clinical, cultural and serological findings. Sex. Transm. Dis. 8:51–55, 1981b.

Svensson, L.; Mårdh, P.-A.; Weström, L. Infertility after acute salpingitis with special reference to *Chlamydia trachomatis*. Fertil. Steril. 40:322–329, 1983.

Svensson, L.; Mårdh, P.-A.; Weström, L. Contraceptives and salpingitis. J. Am. Med. Assoc. 251:2553–2555, 1984.

Svensson, L.; Mårdh, P.-A.; Ahlgren, M.; Nordenskjöld, F. Ectopic pregnancy and antibodies to *Chlamydia trachomatis*. Fertil. Steril. 44:313–317, 1985.

Swanson, J.; Eschenbach, D.A.; Alexander, E.R.; Holmes, K.K. Light and electron microscopic study of *Chlamydia trachomatis* infection of the cervix. J. Infect. Dis. 131:678–687, 1975.

Sweet, R.L. Pelvic inflammatory disease: Etiology, diagnosis, and treatment. Sex. Trans. Dis. 8(Suppl):308–315, 1981.

Sweet, R.L. Chlamydial salpingitis and infertility. Fertil. Steril. 38:530–532, 1982.

Sweet, R.L.; Draper, D.L.; Schachter, J.; Microbiology and pathogenesis of acute salpingitis as determined by laparoscopy: What is the appropriate site to sample. Am. J. Obstet. Gynecol. 138:985–989, 1980.

Sweet, R.L.; Schachter, J.; Robbie, M.O. Failure of beta-lactam antibiotics to eradicate *Chlamydia trachomatis* in the endometrium despite apparent clinical cure of acute salpingitis. J. Am. Med. Assoc. 250:2641–2645, 1983.

Sweet, R.L.; Landers, D.V.; Walker, C.; Schachter, J. *Chlamydia trachomatis* infection and pregnancy outcome. Am. J. Obstet. Gynecol. 156:824–833, 1987.

Swenson, C.E.; Schachter, J. Infertility as a consequence of chlamydial infection of the upper genital tract in female mice. Sex. Transm. Dis. 11:64–67, 1984.

Swenson, C.E.; Donegan, E.; Schachter, J. *Chlamydia trachomatis*-induced salpingitis in mice. J. Infect. Dis. 148:1101–1107, 1983.

Swenson, C.E.; Sung, M.L.; Schachter, J. The effect of tetracycline treatment on chlamydial salpingitis and subsequent fertility in the mouse. Sex. Trans. Dis. 13:40–44, 1986.

Szybalski, W. Use of cesium sulfate for equilibrium density gradient centrifugation. Meth. Enzymol. 12B:330–360, 1968.

Tack, K.J.; Petterson, P.K.; Rasp, F.L.; O'Leary, M.; Hanto, D.; Simmons, R.L.; Sabath, L.D. Isolation of *Chlamydia trachomatis* from the lower respiratory tract of adults. Lancet i:117–120, 1980.

Tait, I.A.; Rees, E.; Holson, D.; Byng, R.E., Tweedie, M.C.K. Chlamydial infection of the cervix in contacts of men with nongonococcal urethritis. Br. J. Vener. Dis. 56:37–45, 1980.

Tam, M.R.; Stamm, W.E.; Handsfield, H.H.; Stephens, R.; Kuo, C.-C.; Holmes, K.K.; Ditzenberger, K.; Krieger, M.; Nowinski, R.C. Culture-independent diagnosis of *Chlamydia trachomatis* using monoclonal antibodies. N. Engl. J. Med. 310:1146–1150, 1984.

T'ang, F.F.; Chang, H.L.; Huang, Y.T.; Wang, K.C. Studies on the etiology of trachoma with special reference to isolation of the virus in chick embryo. Chin. Med. J. 75:429–447, 1957.

Taylor, H.R.; Prendergast, R. Attempted oral immunization with chlamydial lipopolysaccharide ml-unit vaccine. Invest. Ophthalmol. Vis. Sci. 28:1722–1726, 1987.

Taylor, H.R.; Prendergast, R.A.; Dawson, C.R.; Schachter, J.; Silverstein, A.M. An animal model for cicatrizing trachoma. Invest. Ophthalmol. Vis. Sci. 21:422–433, 1981.

Taylor, H.R.; Johnson, S.L.; Prendergast, R.A.; Schachter, J.; Dawson, C.R.; Silverstein, A.M. An animal model of trachoma: II, The importance of repeated infection. Invest. Ophthalmol. Vis. Sci. 23:507–515, 1982a.

Taylor, H.R.; Prendergast, R.A.; Dawson, C.R.; Schachter, J.; Silverstein, A.M. Animal model of trachoma: III. The necessity of repeated exposure to live *Chlamydia*. In:

Chlamydial infections. Mårdh, P.-A.; Holmes, K.K.; Oriel, J.D.; Piot, P.; Schachter, J. eds. Amsterdam: Elsevier Biomedical Press, 1982b, pp. 387–390.

Taylor, H.R.; Schachter, J.; Caldwell, H.D. The stimulus for conjunctival inflammation in trachoma. In: Human Chlamydial Infections. Oriel, D.; Ridgway, G.; Schachter, J.; Taylor-Robinson, D.; Ward, M. eds. Cambridge: Cambridge University Press, 1986, pp. 167–170.

Taylor, H.R.; Johnson, J.; Schachter, J.; Caldwell, H.; Prendergast, R. Pathogenesis of trachoma: the stimulus for inflammation. J. Immunol. 138:3023–3027, 1987a.

Taylor, H.R.; West, S.K.; Katala, S.; Foster, A. Trachoma: evaluation of a new grading scheme in the United Republic of Tanzania. Bull. WHO 65(4):485–488, 1987b.

Taylor-Robinson, D. The role of animal models in chlamydial research. In: Human Chlamydial Infections. Oriel, D.; Ridgway, G.; Schachter, J.; Taylor-Robinson, D.; Ward, M. eds. Cambridge: Cambridge University Press, 1986, pp. 355–366.

Taylor-Robinson, D.; Evans, R.T.; Confalik, E.D.; Prentice, M.J.; Munday, P.E.; Csonka, G.W.; Oates, J.K. *Ureaplasma urealyticum* and *Mycoplasma hominis* in chlamydial and in non-chlamydial non-gonococcal urethritis. Br. J. Vener. Dis. 55:30–35, 1979.

Taylor-Robinson, D.; McCormack, W.M. The genital mycoplasmas. N. Engl. J. Med. 302:1063–1067, 1980.

Taylor-Robinson, D.; Purcell, R.H.; London, W.T.; Sly, D.L.; Thomas, B.J.; Evans, R.T. Microbiological, serological, and histopathological features of experimental *Chlamydia trachomatis* urethritis in chimpanzees. Br. J. Vener. Dis. 57:36–40, 1981.

Taylor-Robinson, D.; Tuffrey, M.; Falder, P. Some aspects of animal models for *Chlamydia trachomatis* genital infections. In: Chlamydial Infections. Mårdh, P.-A.; Holmes, K.K.; Oriel, J.D.; Piot, P.; Schachter, J. eds. Amsterdam: Elsevier Biomedical Press, 1982, pp. 375–378.

Taylor-Robinson, D.; Furr, P.M.; Hanna, N.F. Microbiological and serological study of non-gonococcal urethritis with special reference to *Mycoplasma genitalium*. Genitourin. Med. 61:319–324, 1985.

Taylor-Robinson, D.; Thomas, B.J.; Osborne, M.F. Evaluation of enzyme immunoassay (Chlamydiazyme) for detecting *Chlamydia trachomatis* in genital tract specimens. J. Clin. Pathol. 40:194–196, 1987.

Teare, E.L.; Sexton, C.; Lim, F.; McManus, T.; Uttley, A.H.C.; Hodgson, J. Conventional tissue culture compared with rapid immunofluorescence for identifying *Chlamydia trachomatis* in specimens from patients attending a genitourinary clinic. Genitourin. Med. 61:379–382, 1985.

Teisala, K.; Heinonen, P.K.; Aine, R.; Punnonen, R.; Paavonen, J. Second laparoscopy after treatment of acute pelvic inflammatory disease. Obstet. Gynecol. 69:343–346, 1987.

Terho, P. *Chlamydia trachomatis* in non-specific urethritis. Br. J. Vener. Dis. 54:251–256, 1978.

Terho, P.; Matikainen, M.T. Detection of *Chlamydia trachomatis* antigen by radioimmunoassay. J. Immunoass. 2:239–262, 1981.

Terho, P.; Meurman, O. Chlamydial serum IgG, IgA and local IgA antibodies in patients with genital-tract infections measured by solid-phase radioimmunoassay. J. Med. Microbiol. 14:77–87, 1981.

Thelin, I.; Mårdh, P.-A. Contact-tracing in genital chlamydial infection. In: *Chlamydia trachomatis* in Genital and Related Infections. Mårdh, P.-A.; Møller, B.R.; Paavonen, J. eds. Scand. Infect. Dis. Suppl. 32:163–166, 1982.

Thelin, I.; Wennström, A.M.; Mårdh, P.-A. Contact-tracing in patients with genital chlamydial infection. Br. J. Vener. Dis. 56:259–262, 1980.

Thomas, B.J.; Reeve, P.; Oriel, J.D. Simplified serological test for antibodies to *Chlamydia trachomatis*. J. Clin. Microbiol. 4:6–10, 1976.

Thomas, B.J.; Evans, R.T.; Hutchinson, G.R.; Taylor-Robinson, D. Early detection of chlamydial inclusions combining the use of cycloheximide-treated McCoy cells and IF staining. J. Clin. Microbiol. 6:285–292, 1977.

Thomas, B.J.; Evans, R.T.; Hawkins, D.A.; Taylor-Robinson, D. Sensitivity of detecting *Chlamydia trachomatis* elementary bodies in smears by use of a fluorescein labelled monoclonal antibody: comparison with conventional chlamydial isolation. J. Clin. Pathol. 37:812–816, 1984.

Thomas, G.B.; Sbarra, A.J.; Feingold, M.; Cetralo, C.L.; Shakr, C.; Newton, E.; Selvarej, R.J. Antimicrobial activity of amniotic fluid against *Chlamydia trachomatis, Mycoplasma hominis,* and *Ureaplasma urealyticum.* Am. J. Obst. Gynecol. 158:16–22, 1988.

Thompson, S.E.; Hager, W.D.; Wong, K.H., Lopez, B., Ramsey, C., Allen, S.D.; Stargel, M.D.; Thornsberry, C.; Benigno, B.B.; Thompson, J.D.; Shulman, J.A. The microbiology and therapy of acute pelvic inflammatory disease in hospitalized patients. Am. J. Obst. Gynecol. 136:179–186, 1980.

Thompson, S.E.; Lopez, B.; Wong, K.H.; Ramsey, C.; Thomas, J.; Reising, C.; Jenks, B.; Peacock, W.; Sanderson, M.; Goforth, S.; Zaidi, A.; Miller, R.; Klein, L. A prospective study of *Chlamydia* and *Mycoplasma* infections during pregnancy: relation to pregnancy outcome and maternal morbidity. In: Chlamydial infections. Mårdh, P.-A.; Holmes, K.K.; Oriel, J.D.; Piot, P.; Schachter, J. eds. Amsterdam: Elsevier Biomedical Press, 1982, pp. 155–158.

Thygeson, P. The present status of laboratory research in trachoma. Bull. WHO 19:129–152, 1958.

Thygeson, P.; Mengert, W.F. The virus of inclusion conjunctivitis: Further observations. Arch. Ophthalmol. 15:377–410, 1936.

Thygeson, P.; Stone, W.F., Jr. Epidemiology of inclusion conjunctivitis. Arch. Ophthalmol. 27:91–122, 1942.

Thylefors, B.; Dawson, C.R.; Jones, B.R.; West, S.K.; Taylor, H.R. A simple system for the assessment of trachoma and its complications. Bull. WHO 65(4):477–483, 1987.

Timms, P.; Eaves, F.W.; Girjes, A.A.; Lavino, M.F. Comparison of *C. psittaci* isolates by restriction endonuclease and DNA probe analysis. Infect. Immun. 56:287–290, 1988.

Tipple, M.A.; Beem, M.O.; Saxon, E.M. Clinical characteristics of the afebrile pneumonia associated with *Chlamydia trachomatis* infection in infants less than 6 months of age. Pediatrics 63:192–197, 1979.

Tjiam, K.H.; van Heijst, B.Y.M.; de Roo, J.C.; de Beer, A.; van Joost, T.H.; Michel, M.F.; Stolz, E. Survival of *Chlamydia trachomatis* in different transport media and at different temperatures: diagnostic implications. Br. J. Vener. Dis. 60:92–94, 1984.

Tjiam, K.H.; Zeilmaker, G.H.; Alberda, A.T.H.; van Heijst, B.Y.M.; de Roo, J.C.; Polak-Vogelzang, A.A.; van Joost, T.H.; Stolz, E.; Michel, M.F. Prevalence of antibodies to *Chlamydia trachomatis, Neisseria gonorrhoeae*, and *Mycoplasma hominis* in infertile women. Genitourin. Med. 61:175–178, 1985.

Tjiam, K.H.; van Heijst, B.Y.M.; van Zuuren, A.; Wagenwoort, J.H.T.; van Joost, T.; Stolz, E.; Michel, M.F. Evaluation of an enzyme immunoassay for the diagnosis of chlamydial infections in urogenital specimens. J. Clin. Microbiol. 23:752–754, 1986.

Todd, W.J.; Caldwell, H.D. The interaction of *Chlamydia trachomatis* with host cells: ultrastructural studies of the mechanism of release of a biovar II strain from HeLa 229 cells. J. Infect. Dis. 151:1037–1044, 1985.

Toomey, K.E.; Rafferty, M.P.; Stamm, W.E. Unrecognized high prevalence of *Chlamydia trachomatis* cervical infection in an isolated Alaskan Eskimo population. J. Am. Med. Assoc. 258:53–56, 1987.

Tozzo, P.J. Semen analysis of unilateral epididymitis. N.Y. State J. Med. 68:2769–2770, 1968.

Treharne, J.D.; Darougar, S.; Jones, R.B. Modification of the micro-IF test to provide a routine serodiagnostic test for chlamydial infection. J. Clin. Pathol. 30:510–517, 1977.

Treharne, J.D.; Darougar, S.; Simmons, P.D.; Thin, R.N. Rapid diagnosis of chlamydial infection of the cervix. Br. J. Vener. Dis. 54:403–408, 1978a.

Treharne, J.D.; Dwyer, R.St.C.; Darougar, S.; Jones, B.R.; Daghfous, T. Anti-chlamydial antibody in tears and sera, and serotypes of *Chlamydia trachomatis* isolated from school children in southern Tunisia. Br. J. Ophthalmol. 62:509–515, 1978b.

Treharne, J.D.; Ripa, K.T.; Mårdh, P.-A.; Svensson, L.; Weström, L.; Darougar, S. Antibodies to *Chlamydia trachomatis* in acute salpingitis. Br. J. Vener. Dis. 55:26–29, 1979.

Trimbos, J.B.; Arentz, N.P.W. The efficiency of the cytobrush versus the cotton swab in the collection of endocervical cells in cervical smears. Acta Cytologica 30:261–263, 1986.

Tuffrey, M.; Taylor-Robinson, D. Progesterone as a key factor in the development of a mouse model for genital tract infection with *Chlamydia trachomatis*. FEMS Microbiol. Lett. 12:111–115, 1981.

Tuffrey, M.; Falder, P.; Taylor-Robinson, D. Genital-tract infection and disease in nude and immunologically competent mice after inoculation of a human strain of *Chlamydia trachomatis*. Br. J. Exp. Pathol. 63:539–546, 1982.

Tuffrey, M.; Falder, P.; Thomas, B.; Taylor-Robinson, D. The distribution and effect of *Chlamydia trachomatis* in CBA mice inoculated genitally intra-articularly, or intra-venously. Med. Microbiol. Immunol. 173:539–546, 1984a.

Tuffrey, M.; Falder, P.; Taylor-Robinson, D. Reinfection of the mouse genital tract with

Chlamydia trachomatis: the relationship of antibody to immunity. Br. J. Exp. Pathol. 65:51–58, 1984b.

Tuffrey, M.; Falder, P.; Taylor-Robinson, D. A mouse model of chlamydial salpingitis and subsequent infertility. In: Chlamydial Infections. Oriel, D.; Ridgway, G.; Schachter, J.; Taylor-Robinson, D.; Ward, M. eds. Cambridge: Cambridge University Press, 1986a, pp. 380–383.

Tuffrey, M.; Falder, P.; Taylor-Robinson, D. Salpingitis in mice induced by human strains of *Chlamydia trachomatis.* Br. J. Exp. Pathol. 67:605–616, 1986b.

Uyeda, C.T.; Welborn, P.; Ellison-Birang, N.; Shunk, K.; Tsaouse, B. Rapid diagnosis of chlamydial infections with the MikroTrak direct test. J. Clin. Microbiol. 20:948–950, 1984.

Väänänen, P.; Lassus, A.; Saikku, P. Direct detection of *Chlamydia trachomatis* in clinical samples. Ann. Clin. Res. 17:64–65, 1985.

Vasudeva, K.; Thrasher, T.V.; Richart, R.M. Chronic endometritis: A clinical and electron microscopic study. Am. J. Obstet. Gynecol. 112:749–757, 1972.

Vaughan-Jackson, J.D.; Dunlop, E.M.C.; Darougar, S.; Treharne, J.D.; Taylor-Robinson, D. Urethritis due to *C. trachomatis.* Br. J. Vener. Dis. 53:180–183, 1977.

Vinje, O.; Fryjordet, A.; Brun, A.L.; Møller, P.; Mellbye, O.J.; Kåss, E. Laboratory findings in chronic prostatitis, with special reference to immunological and microbiological aspects. Scand. J. Urol. Nephrol. 17:191–197, 1983.

Viswalingam, N.D.; Wishart, M.S.; Woodland, R.M. Adult chlamydial ophthalmia (paratrachoma). Br. Med. Bull. 39:123–127, 1983.

Volkert, M.; Matthiesen, M. An ornithosis related antigen from a coccoid bacterium. Acta Pathol. Microbiol. Scand. 39:117–126, 1956.

Wachendörfer, J. Auftreten und Bekämpfung der psittakose/ornithose in der Bundesrepublik Deutchland (in German). Tierarztl. Prax. 12:455–467, 1984.

Wager, G.P. Puerperal infectious morbidity: relationship to route of delivery and to antepertum *Chlamydia trachomatis* infection. Am. J. Obstet. Gynecol. 138:1028–1033, 1980.

Waites, K.B.; Crouse, D.T.; Nelson, K.G.; Rudd, P.T.; Canupp, K.C.; Ramsey, C.; Cassell, G.H. Chronic *Ureaplasma urealyticum* and *Mycoplasma hominis* infections of central nervous system in preterm infants. Lancet i:17–21, 1988.

Wallin, J.; Thompson, S.E.; Zaidi, A.; Wong, K.H. Urethritis in women attending an STD clinic. Br. J. Vener. Dis. 57:50–54, 1981.

Wang, S.-P. A micro-immunofluorescence method. A study of antibody response to TRIC organisms in mice. In: Trachoma and Related Disorders caused by Chlamydial Agents. Nichols, R.L. ed. Amsterdam: Excerpta Medica, 1971, pp. 273–288.

Wang, S.-P.; Grayston, J.T. Classification of trachoma virus strains by protection of mice from toxic death. J. Immunol. 90:849–856, 1963.

Wang, S.-P.; Grayston, J.T. Pannus with experimental trachoma and inclusion conjunctivitis agent infection of Taiwan monkey. Am. J. Ophthalmol. 63:1133–1145, 1967.

Wang, S.-P.; Grayston, J.T. Immunologic relationship between genital TRIC, lymphogranuloma venereum, and related organisms in a new microtiter indirect immunofluorescence test. Am. J. Ophthalmol. 70:367–374, 1970.

Wang, S.-P.; Grayston, J.T. Local and systemic antibody response to trachoma eye infection in monkeys. In: Trachoma and Related Disorders caused by Chlamydial Agents. Nichols, R.L. ed. Amsterdam: Excerpta Medica, 1971, pp. 217–232.

Wang, S.-P.; Grayston, J.T. Human serology in *Chlamydia trachomatis* infections with micro-immunofluorescence. J. Infect. Dis. 130:388–379, 1974.

Wang, S.-P.; Grayston, J.T. Micro immunofluorescence antibody responses in *Chlamydia trachomatis* infections, a review. In: Chlamydial infections. Mårdh, P.-A.; Holmes, K.K.; Oriel, J.D.; Piot, P.; Schachter, J. eds. Amsterdam: Elsevier Biomedical Press, 1982, pp. 301–316.

Wang, S.-P.; Grayston, J.T. Micro-IF serology of *Chlamydia trachomatis*. In: Medical Virology. III. de la Maza, L.; Peterson, E. (eds.) Amsterdam: Elsevier Biomedical Press, 1984, pp. 87–116.

Wang, S.-P.; Grayston, J.T. Microimmunofluorescence serological studies with the TWAR organism. In: Chlamydial Infections. Oriel, D.; Ridgway, G.; Schachter, J.; Taylor-Robinson, D.; Ward, M. eds. Cambridge: Cambridge University Press, 1986, pp. 329–332.

Wang, S.-P.; Grayston, J.T.; Alexander, E.R. Trachoma vaccine studies in monkeys. Am. J. Ophthalmol. 63:1615–1630, 1967.

Wang, S.-P.; Grayston, J.T.; Alexander, E.R.; Holmes, K.K. Simplified microimmunofluorescence test with trachoma-lymphogranuloma venereum (*Chlamydia trachomatis*) antigens for use as a screening test for antibody. J. Clin. Microbiol. 1:250–255, 1975.

Wang, S.-P.; Grayston, J.T.; Kuo, C.-C.; Alexander, E.R.; Holmes, K.K. Serodiagnosis of *Chlamydia trachomatis* infection with the micro-immunofluorescence test. In: Nongonococcal Urethritis and Related Infections. Hobson, D.; Holmes, K.K. eds. Washington, D.C.: American Society for Microbiology, 1977, pp. 237–248.

Wang, S.-P.; Eschenbach, D.A.; Holmes, K.K.; Wager, G.; Grayston, J.T. *Chlamydia trachomatis* infection in Fitz-Hugh–Curtis syndrome. Am. J. Obstet. Gynecol. 138:1034–1038, 1980.

Wang, S.-P.; Kuo, C.-C.; Barnes, R.C.; Stephens, R.S.; Grayston, J.T. Immunotyping of *Chlamydia trachomatis* with monoclonal antibodies. J. Infect. Dis. 152:791–800, 1985.

Ward, M.E. Outstanding problems in chlamydial cell biology. In: Chlamydial Infections. Oriel, D.; Ridgway, G.; Schachter, J.; Taylor-Robinson, D.; Ward, M. eds. Cambridge: Cambridge University Press, 1986, pp. 3–14.

Ward, M.E.; Treharne, J.D.; Murray, A. Antigenic specificity of human antibody to Chlamydia in trachoma and lymphogranuloma venereum. J. Gen. Microbiol. 132:1599–1610, 1986.

Ward, M.E.; Conlan, W., Clarke, I.N. Prospects for chlamydial vaccine development. In: Proceedings of the Eur. Soc. for Chlamydia Research, 1st Meeting, Bologna, Italy, May 30–June 1, 1988, pp. 121–123.

Washington, A.E. Economic costs of pelvic inflammatory disease and ectopic pregnancy. Int. Meeting of Int. Soc. for STD research, Brighton, September 1–5, 1985.

Washington, A.E.; Cates, W.; Zaidi, A. Hospitalization for pelvic inflammatory disease. Epidemiology and trends in the United States, 1975–1981. J. Am. Med. Assoc. 251:2529–2533, 1984.

Washington, A.E.; Gove, S.; Schachter, J.; Sweet, R.L. Oral contraceptives, *Chlamydia trachomatis* and pelvic inflammatory disease. A word of caution about protection. J. Am. Med. Assoc. 253:2246–2250, 1985.

Washington, A.E.; Arno, P.S.; Brooks, M.A. Economic cost of pelvic inflammatory disease. J. Am. Med. Assoc. 255:1735–1738, 1986.

Washington, A.E.; Johnson, R.E.; Sanders, L.L., Jr. *Chlamydia trachomatis* infections in the United States. What are they costing us? J. Am. Med. Assoc. 257:2070–2072, 1987.

Wasserheit, J.N.; Bell, T.A.; Kiviat, N.B.; Wølner-Hansson, P.; Zabriskie, V.; Kirby, B.; Prince, E.C.; Holmes, K.K.; Stamm, W.E.; Eschenbach, D.A. Microbial causes of proven inflammatory disease and efficacy of clindamycin and tobramycin. Ann. Intern. Med. 104:187–193, 1986.

Watkins, J.F.; MacKenzie, A.M.R. Pulmonary infection of adult white mice with the Te55 strain of trachoma virus. J. Gen. Microbiol. 30:43–52, 1963.

Watkins, N.G.; Hallow, W.J.; Moss, A.B.; Caldwell, H.D. Ocular delayed hypersensitivity: a pathogenetic mechanism of chlamydial conjunctivitis in guinea pigs. Proc. Natl. Acad. Sci. USA 83:7480–7484, 1986.

Watkins, N.G.; Caldwell, H.D.; Hackstadt, T. Chlamydial hemagglutinin identified as lipopolysaccharide. J. Bact. 169:3826–3828, 1987.

Watts, D.H.; Eschenbach, D.A. The role of *Chlamydia trachomatis* in postpartum endometritis. In: Chlamydial Infections. Oriel, D.; Ridgway, G.; Schachter, J.; Taylor-Robinson, D.; Ward, M. eds. Cambridge: Cambridge University Press, 1986, pp. 245–248.

Webberley, J.M.; Matthews, R.S.; Andrews, J.M.; Wise, R. Commercially available fluorescein-conjugated monoclonal antibody for determining the in vitro activity of antimicrobial agents against *Chlamydia trachomatis*. Eur. J. Clin. Microbiol. 6.587 589, 1987.

Weisburg, W.G.; Hatch, T.T.; Woese, C.R. Eubacterial origin of chlamydiae. J. Bacteriol. 167:570–574, 1986.

Weiss, E.; Schramek, S.; Weilson, N.W.; Newman, L.W. Deoxyribonucleic acid heterogeneity between human and murine strains of *Chlamydia trachomatis*. Infect. Immun. 2:24–28, 1970.

Weiss, S.G.; Newcomb, R.W.; Beem, M.O. Pulmonary assessment of children after chlamydial pneumonia of infancy. J. Pediatr. 108:659–664, 1986.

Wenman, W.M.; Lovett, M.A. Expression in *E. coli* of *Chlamydia trachomatis* antigen recognized during human infection. Nature 269:68–70, 1982.

Wenman, W.M.; Meuser, R.U. *Chlamydia trachomatis* elementary bodies possess proteins which bind to eucaryotic cell membranes. J. Bacteriol. 165:602–607, 1986.

Wentworth, B.B. Use of gentamicin in the isolation of subgroup A *Chlamydia*. Antimicrob. Agents Chemother. 3:698–702, 1973.

Wentworth, B.B.; Alexander, E.R. Isolation of *Chlamydia trachomatis* by use of 5-iodo-2-deoxyuridine-treated cells. Appl. Microbiol. 27:912–916, 1974.

Westergaard, L.; Philipsen, T.; Scheibel, J. Significance of cervical *Chlamydia trachomatis* infection in postabortal pelvic inflammatory disease. Obstet. Gynecol. 60:322–325, 1982.

Weström, L. Effect of acute pelvic inflammatory disease on fertility. Am. J. Obstet. Gynecol. 121:707–713, 1975.

Weström, L. Incidence, prevalence, and trends of acute pelvic inflammatory disease and its consequences in industrialized countries. Am. J. Obstet. Gynecol. 138:880–892, 1980.

Weström, L.; Mårdh, P.A. Chlamydial salpingitis. Br. Med. Bull. 39:138–144, 1983a.

Weström, L.; Mårdh, P.A. Pelvic inflammatory disease: epidemiology, diagnosis, clinical manifestations and sequelae. In: International Perspectives on Neglected Sexually Transmitted Diseases: Impact on Venereology, Infertility, and Maternal and Infant Health. Holmes, K.K.; Mårdh, P.A. eds. Washington, D.C.: Hemisphere Publishing Co., 1983b, pp. 235–250.

Weström, L.; Mårdh, P.A.; Salpingitis. In: Sexually Transmitted Diseases. Holmes, K.K.; Mårdh, P.A.; Sparling, F.; Wiesner, P. eds. New York: McGraw-Hill, 1984a, pp. 615–633.

Weström, L.; Bengtsson, L.P.; Mårdh, P.-A. The risk of pelvic inflammatory disease in women using intrauterine contraceptive devices as compared to non-users. Lancet ii:221–224, 1976.

Weström, L.; Iosif, S.; Svensson, L.; Mårdh, P.A. Infertility after acute salpingitis: Results of treatment with different antibiotics. Curr. Ther. Res. 6(Suppl):752–759, 1979.

Weström, L.; Bengtsson, L.P.; Mårdh, P.-A. Incidence, trends and risks of ectopic pregnancy in a defined population of women. Br. Med. J. 282:15–18, 1981.

Weström, L.; Svensson, L.; Wølner-Hanssen, P.; Mårdh, P.A. Chlamydial and gonococcal infections in a defined population of women. Scand. J. Infect. Dis. 32(Suppl)157–162, 1982.

Weström, L.; Bekassy, Z.; Svensson, L.; Blomberg, J.; Mårdh, P.-A. Use of data bases for follow-up cervical cytology in women culture positive for sexually transmittableagents. Abstract. In: Abstracts of Int. Conjoint STD Meeting, Montreal, June 17–21, 1984b, p. 156.

Whittum-Hudson, J.A.; Prendergast, R.A.; Taylor, H.R. Changes in conjunctival lymphocyte populations induced by oral immunization with Chlamydia trachomatis. Curr. Eye Res. 5:973–979, 1986.

WHO Symposium. Guide to the laboratory diagnosis of trachoma. World Health Organization, Geneva, 1975.

Wiedner, W.; Schiefer, H.J.; Ebner, H.; Brunner, H. Nongonococcal urethritis: leucocyte counts in urethral secretions correlated to chlamydial and ureaplasmal infections. Eur. J. Sex. Trans. 3:207–211, 1986.

Wiedner, W.; Schiefer, H.J.; Garbe, C. Acute nongonococcal epididymitis: aetiological and therapeutic aspects. Drugs 34 (Suppl. 1):111–117, 1987.

Wilhelmus, K.R.; Robinson, N.M.; Tredici, L.L.; Jones, D.B. Conjunctival cytology of adult chlamydial conjunctivitis. Arch. Ophthalmol. 104:691–193, 1986.

Williams, D.M.; Schachter, J.; Drutz, D.J.; Sumaya, C.V. Pneumonia due to Chlamydia trachomatis in the immunocompromised (nude) mouse. J. Infect. Dis. 143:238–241, 1981.

Williams, D.M.; Schachter, J.; Grubbs, B. Studies of the immunity to the pneumonitis agent of mice (murine *Chlamydia trachomatis*). In: Chlamydial Infections. Mårdh, P.-A.; Holmes, K.K.; Oriel, J.D.; Piot, P.; Schachter, J. eds. Amsterdam: Elsevier Biomedical Press, 1982a: pp. 225–228.

Williams, D.M.; Schachter, J.; Grubbs, B.; Sumaya, C.V. The role of antibody in host defence against the agent of mouse pneumonitis. J. Infect. Dis. 145:200–205, 1982b.

Willigan, D.A.; Beamer, P.D. Isolation of a transmissible agent from pericarditis of swine. J. Am. Vet. Med. Assoc. 126:118–122, 1955.

Wills, J.M.; Gruffyd-Jones, T.J.; Richmond, S.J.; Gaskell, R.M.; Boume, F.J. Effect of vaccination on feline *Chlamydia psittaci* infection. Infect. Immun. 55:2653–2657, 1987.

Wills, P.J.; Johnson, L.; Thompson, R.G. Isolation of *Chlamydia* using McCoy cells and Buffalo green monkey cells. J. Clin. Pathol. 37:120–121, 1984.

Wilsmore, A.J.; Dawson, M.; Arthur, M.J.; Davies, D.C. The use of a delayed hypersensitivity test and long-acting oxytetracycline in a flock affected with ovine enzootic abortion. Br. Vet. J. 142:557, 1986.

Wilson, M.C.; Millou-Velasco, F.; Tielsch, J.M.; Taylor, H.R. Direct-smear fluorescent antibody cytology as a field diagnostic tool for trachoma. Arch. Ophthalmol. 104:688–690, 1986.

Winkler, B.; Reumann, W.; Mitaa, M.; Gallo, L.; Richart, R.; Crum, C.P. Endometritis: A histological and immunohistochemical analysis. Am. J. Surg. Pathol. 8:771–778, 1984.

Wong, S.Y.; Gray, E.S.; Buxton, D. Acute placentitis and spontaneous abortion caused by *Chlamydia psittaci* of sheep origin: a histological and ultrastructural study. J. Clin. Pathol. 38:707–711, 1985.

Wong, S.Y.; Buxton, D.; McKinlay, A.W.; Keeling, J.; Gray, E.S. Pathology of human acute placentitis caused by ovine *Chlamydia psittaci*. In: Chlamydial Infections. Oriel, D.; Ridgway, G.; Schachter, J.; Taylor-Robinson, D.; Ward, M. eds. Cambridge: Cambridge University Press, 1986, pp. 341–344.

Woodland, R.M.; Darougar, S. Feline keratoconjunctivitis: an animal model of persistent chlamydial conjunctivitis. In: Chlamydial Infections. Oriel, D.; Ridgway, G.; Schachter, J.; Taylor-Robinson, D.; Ward, M. eds. Cambridge: Cambridge University Press, 1986, pp. 412–415.

Woodland, R.M.; El-Sheikh, H.; Darougar, S.; Squires, S. Sensitivity of immunoperoxidase and immunofluorescent staining for detecting chlamydia in conjunctival scrapings and in cell culture. J. Clin. Pathol. 31:1073–1077, 1978.

Woodland, R.M.; Johnson, A.P.; Tuffrey, M. Animal models of chlamydial infection. Br. Med. Bull. 39:175–180, 1983.

Woodland, R.M.; Kirton, R.P.; Darougar, S. Sensitivity of mitomycin-C treated McCoy cells for isolation of *Chlamydia trachomatis* from genital specimens. Eur. J. Clin. Microbiol. 6:653–656, 1987.

Woolfi, H.J.M.G.; Watt, L. Chlamydial infection of the urogenital tract in promiscuous and non-promiscuous women. Br. J. Vener. Dis. 53:93–95, 1977.

Woolridge, R.L.; Grayston, J.T.; Perrin, E.B.; Yang, C.Y.; Cheng, K.H.; Chang, I.H. Natural history of trachoma in Taiwan school children. Am. J. Ophthalmol. 63:1313–1320, 1967.

Worm, A.M.; Petersen, C.S. Transmission of chlamydial infections to sexual partners. Genitourin. Med. 63:19–21, 1987.

Worm, A.M.; Avnstorp, C.; Petersen, C.S. Erythromycin for four or seven days against *Chlamydia trachomatis*. Genitourin. Med. 61:283, 1985.

Wreghitt, T.G.; Taylor, C.E.D. Incidence of respiratory tract chlamydial infections and importation of psittacine birds. Lancet i:582, 1988.

Wyrick, P.B.; Brownridge, E.A. Growth of *Chlamydia psittaci* in macrophages. Infect. Immun. 19:1054–1060, 1978.

Wyrick, P.B.; Brownridge, E.A.; Ivins, B.E. Interaction of *Chlamydia psittaci* with mouse peritoneal macrophages. Infect. Immun. 19:1061–1067, 1978.

Wølner-Hanssen, P. Manifestations and pathogenesis of chlamydial pelvic inflammatory disease. Academic dissertation, University of Lund, Sweden, 1985.

Wølner-Hanssen, P. Oral contraceptive use modifies the manifestations of pelvic inflammatory disease. Br. J. Obstet. Gynecol. 93:619–624, 1986.

Wølner-Hanssen, P.; Mårdh, P.A. In vitro tests of the adherence of *Chlamydia trachomatis* to human spermatozoa. Fertil. Steril. 42:102–107, 1984.

Wølner-Hanssen, P.; Weström, L.; Mårdh, P.-A. Perihepatitis and chlamydial salpingitis. Lancet i:901–904, 1980.

Wølner-Hanssen, P.; Svensson, L.; Weström, L.; Mårdh, P.-A. Isolation of *Chlamydia trachomatis* from the liver capsule in Fitz-Hugh–Curtis syndrome. N. Engl. J. Med. 306:113, 1982a.

Wølner-Hanssen, P.; Mårdh, P.-A.; Møller, B.R.; Weström, L. Endometrial infection in women with chlamydial salpingitis. Sex. Transm. Dis. 9:84–88, 1982b.

Wølner-Hanssen, P.; Weström, L.; Mårdh, P.-A. Chlamydial perihepatitis. In: *Chlamydia trachomatis* in Genital and Related Infections. Mårdh, P.-A.; Møller, B.R.; Paavonen, J. eds. Scand. J. Infect. Dis. Suppl. 32:77–82, 1982c.

Wølner-Hanssen, P.; Weström, L.; Mårdh, P.-A. Influence of amniotic fluid on the formation of chlamydial inclusions in McCoy cell cultures. In: Chlamydial Infections. Mårdh, P.-A.; Holmes, K.K.; Piot, P.; Oriel, D.; Schachter J. eds. Amsterdam: Elsevier Biomedical Press, 1982d, pp. 283–286.

Wølner-Hanssen, P.; Mårdh, P.-A.; Svensson, L.; Weström, L. Laparoscopy in women with chlamydial infection and pelvic pain: a comparison of patients with and without salpingitis. Obstet. Gynecol. 61:299–303, 1983.

Wølner-Hanssen, P.; Svensson, L.; Mårdh, P.A.; Weström, L. Laparoscopic findings and contraceptive usage in women with signs and symptoms suggestive of acute salpingitis. Obstet. Gynecol. 66:233–238, 1985.

Wølner-Hanssen, P.; Patton, D.L.; Stamm, W.E.; Holmes, K.K. Severe salpingitis in pig-tailed macaques after repeated cervical infections followed by a single tubal inoculation with *Chlamydia trachomatis*. In: Chlamydial Infections. Oriel, D.; Ridgway, G.; Schachter, J.; Taylor-Robinson, D.; Ward, M. eds. Cambridge: Cambridge University Press, 1986a, pp. 371–347.

Wølner-Hanssen, P.; Eschenbach, D.A.; Paavonen, J.; Holmes, K.K. Treatment of pelvic inflammatory disease: Use of doxycycline with an appropriate beta-lactam while we wait for better data. J. Am. Med. Assoc. 256:3262–3264, 1986b.

Wølner-Hanssen, P.; Paavonen, J.; Stevens, C.E.; Koutsky, L.; Eschenbach, D.A.;

Kiviat, N.; Critchlow, C.; DeRouen, T.; Holmes, K.K. Pelvic inflammatory disease and contraception. Multivariable analysis of cases and controls infected with *C. trachomatis, N. gonorrhoeae,* or neither organisms. Int. Soc. STD Res., 7th Int. Meeting, August 2–5, 1987, Atlanta, Georgia, Abstract 182.

Wølner-Hanssen, P.; Paavonen, J.; Kiviat, N.; Landers, D.; Sweet, R.L.; Eschenbach, D.A.; Holmes, K.K. Ambulatory treatment of suspected pelvic inflammatory disease with Augmentin with or without doxycycline. Am. J. Obstet. Gynecol. 158:577–579, 1988a.

Wølner-Hanssen, P.; Krieger, J.N.; Stevens, C.E.; Koutsky, L.; Critchlow, C.; DeRouen, T.; Holmes, K.K. Vaginal trichomoniasis: a cross-sectional study of clinical manifestations, adjusting for effects of coinfection in randomly selected STD clinic women. JAMA 1988b (in press).

Wølner-Hanssen, P.; Paavonen, J.; Kiviat, N.; Young M.; Eschenbach, D.A.; Holmes, K.K. Out patient treatment of pelvic inflammatory disease with cefoxitin and doxycycline. Obstet. Gynecol. 71:595–600, 1988b.

Yli-Kerttula, U.I.; Kataja, J.M.; Vilppula, A.H. Salpingitis and cervicitis in uro-arthritis. Clin. Rheumatol. 3:169–172, 1984.

Yoder, B.L.; Stamm, W.E.; Koester, C.M.; Alexander, E.R. Microtest procedure for isolation of *Chlamydia trachomatis.* J. Clin. Bact. 13:1036–1039, 1986.

Yong, E.C.; Chinn, J.S.; Caldwell, H.D.; Kuo, C.-C. Reticulate bodies as a single antigen in *Chlamydia trachomatis* serology with micro-IF. J. Clin. Microbiol. 10:351–356, 1979.

Yong, E.C.; Klebanoff, S.J.; Kuo, C.-C. Toxic effect of human polymorphonuclear leucocytes on *Chlamydia trachomatis.* Infect. Immun. 37:422–426, 1982.

Yong, E.C.; Chi, E.Y.; Chen, W.J.; Kuo, C.-C. Degradation of *Chlamydia trachomatis* in human polymorphonuclear leucocytes: an ultrastructural study of peroxidase-positive phagolysosomes. Infect. Immun. 53:427–431, 1986.

Yong, A.P.; Grayson, M.L. Psittacosis–a review of 135 cases. Med. J. Aust. 148:228–233, 1988.

Zdrodowska-Stefanov, B. *Chlamydia trachomatis* infections in Poland. In: Proceedings of the Eur. Soc. for Chlamydia Research, 1st Meeting, Bologna, Italy, May 30–June 1, 1988, p. 28.

Zouari, A.; Dehan, M.; Magny, J.F.; Saby, M.A.; Ropert, J.C.; Gabilan, J.C. Apnées révélatrices d'une infection à *Chlamydia trachomatis* chez un prématuré (in French). Arch. Fr. Pediatr. 43:187–189, 1986.

Index